LIT: The Simple Protocol for Dental Photography in the Age of Social Media

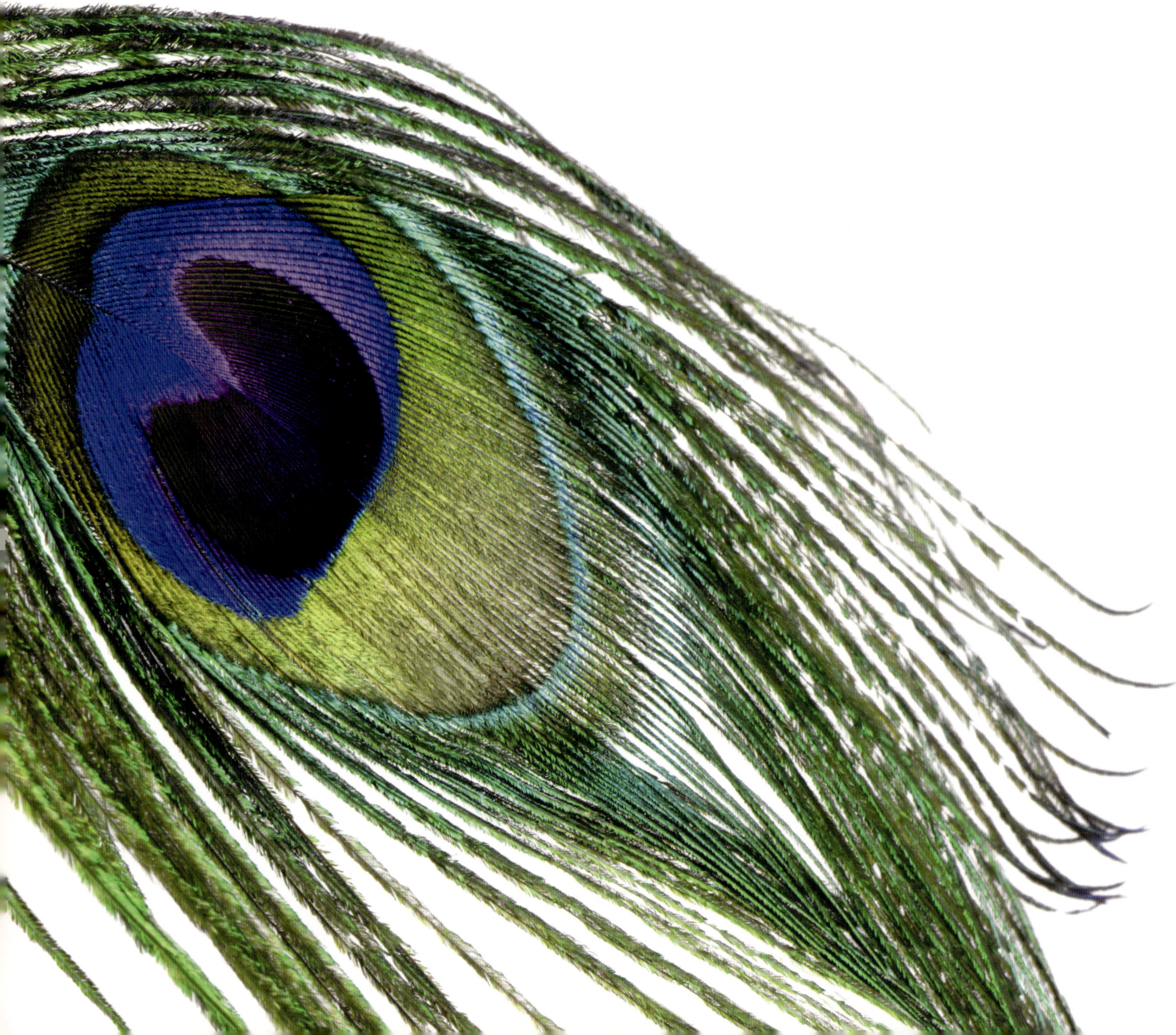

LIT

The Simple Protocol for Dental Photography in the Age of Social Media

MIGUEL A. ORTIZ, DMD

Prosthodontist, Private Practice
Boston, Massachusetts

Founder of www.DentLit.com

QUINTESSENCE PUBLISHING

Berlin, Barcelona, Chicago, Istanbul, London, Mexico City, Milan,
Moscow, Paris, Prague, São Paulo, Seoul, Tokyo, Warsaw

Library of Congress Cataloging-in-Publication Data

Names: Ortiz, Miguel A. (Miguel Angel), 1982 July 3- author.
Title: Lit : the simple protocol for dental photography in the age of social media / Miguel A. Ortiz.
Description: Batavia, IL : Quintessence Publishing Co, Inc., [2019] |
Includes bibliographical references.
Identifiers: LCCN 2019010145 | ISBN 9780867158021 (hardcover)
Subjects: LCSH: Dental photography. | Photography--Economic aspects. |
Dentistry--Practice. | MESH: Photography, Dental--methods | Marketing | Social Media
Classification: LCC TR708 .O78 2019 | NLM TR 708 | DDC 779/.9617--dc23
LC record available at https://lccn.loc.gov/2019010145

QUINTESSENCE PUBLISHING USA

Quintessence Publishing Co, Inc
411 N Raddant Road
Batavia, IL 60510
www.quintpub.com

5 4 3 2 1

Editor: Bryn Grisham
Designer: Sue Zubek

Printed in China

I love you, Colleen.

Contents

1 Fundamentals of Photography 1

2 Dental Photography Equipment 61

3 Portrait Photography 79

4 Intraoral Photography 105

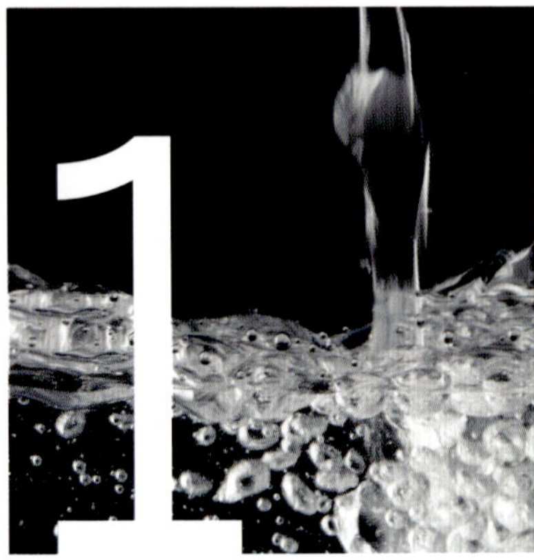

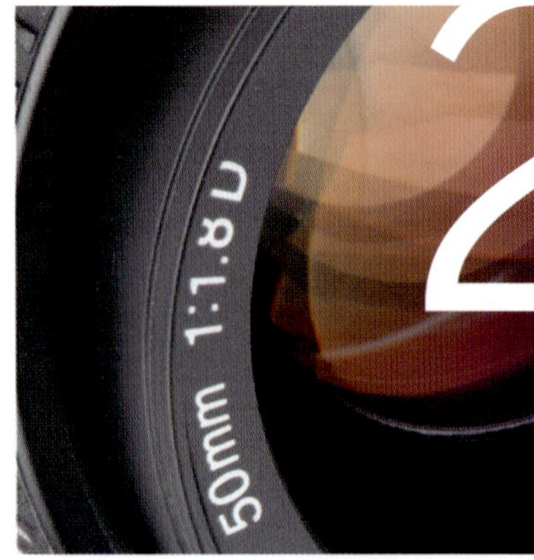

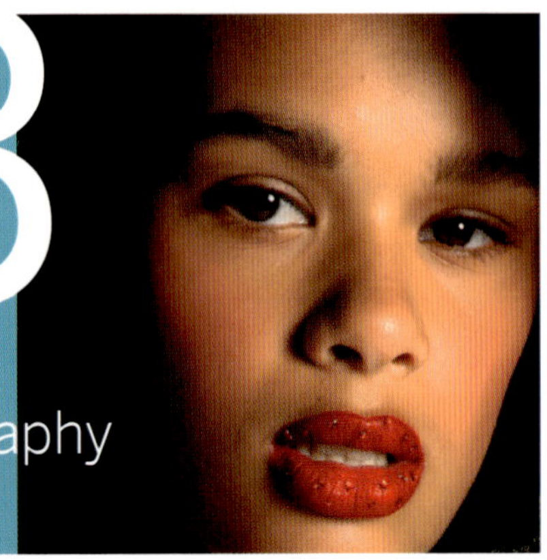

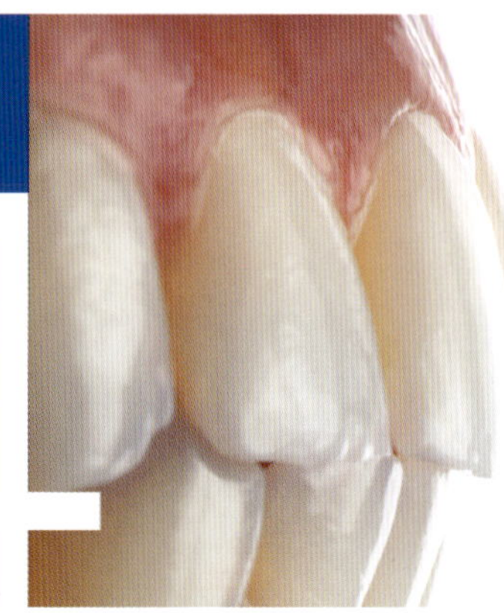

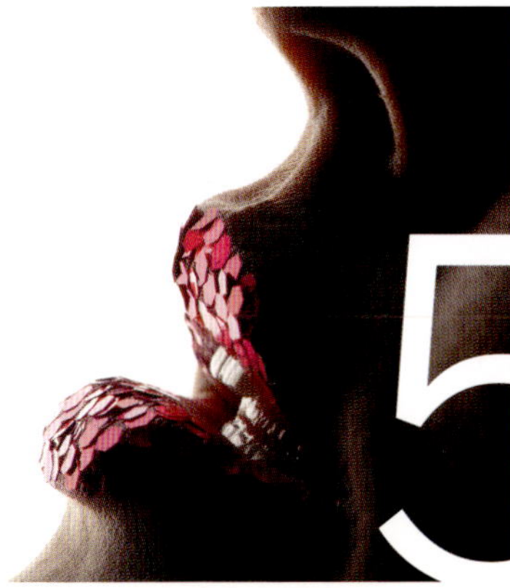

5 Artistic Dental Photography 139

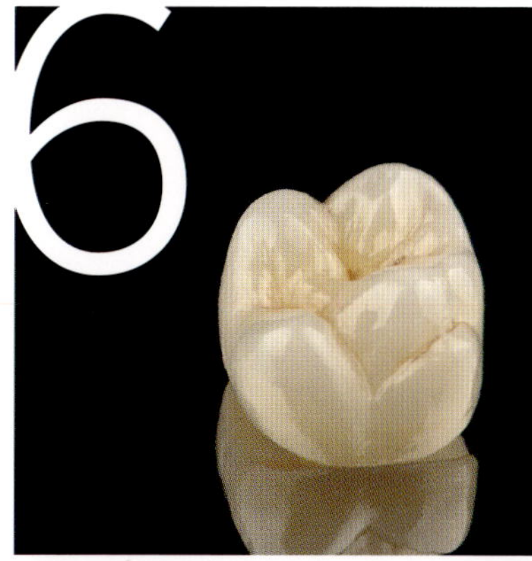

6 Dental Photography and Communication with the Dental Laboratory 167

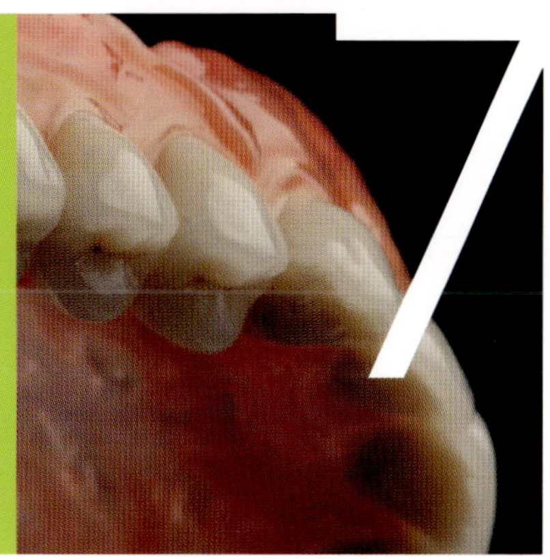

7 Dental Laboratory Photography 185

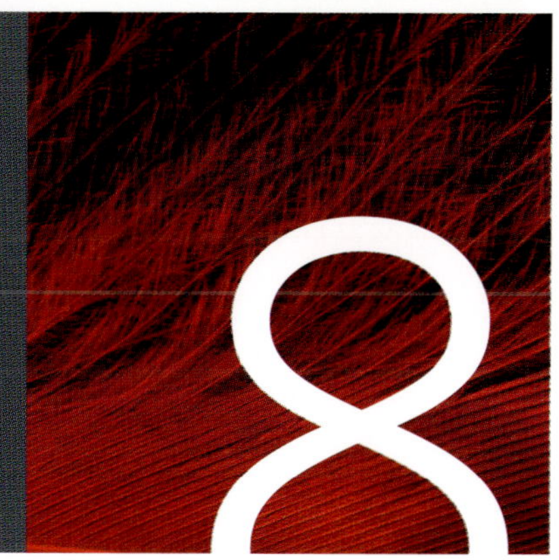

8 Marketing and Social Media 213

Foreword

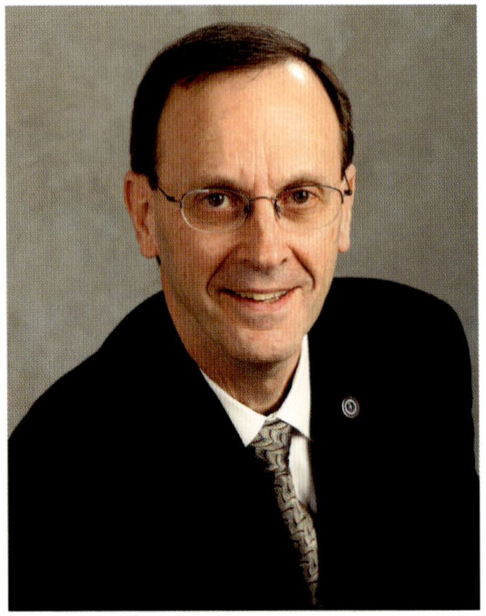

Lee M. Jameson, DDS, MS
Interim Head
Department of Restorative Dentistry
College of Dentistry
University of Illinois Chicago

Professor and Dean Emeritus
Northwestern University Dental School
Evanston, Illinois

Past President of the American
Prosthodontic Society and the
American College of Prosthodontics

With the publication of this book, Dr Miguel A. Ortiz has made a significant contribution to the growing discourse on artistic dental photography. This outstanding book is a fusion of museum-quality photography, down-to-earth instruction taken from his experience in private practice, and savvy tips for social media marketing. Through his creative photographic lens Dr Ortiz tells a story of patient prosthodontic care that goes beyond the traditional mechanics of photographic documentation. He simplifies complex concepts so that private practitioners can understand how to effectively incorporate photographic documentation into modern dental care. The ideas that are presented here will enable you to artistically communicate your transformational patient stories.

Dr Ortiz's personal writing style makes readers feel as if he is talking directly to them. The content echoes his popular dental photography courses by outlining the essentials of photography as well as the equipment that dentists need. He then devotes significant text to the most underestimated aspect of dental photography—lighting. The interaction between light sources, diffusers, working distances, and angulations—and their effect on exposure, shadows, depth of field, texture, and chromaticity—receives considerable emphasis, along with shade evaluation and intraoral and portrait photography. The final chapter of Dr Ortiz's book is an essential primer on how to get the best results from social media to link your practice with your target patient population and how to use Instagram's dynamic platform to interact with other professionals.

This magnificent book takes you on a journey of visual beauty that will enhance professional communication, documentation, and marketing for any practitioner who sets high standards and wants to optimize their dental practice.

Preface

***LIT* is a book in search of the perfect smile.** You might think that as a dental photographer I'm obsessed with every smile. But you'd be wrong. The smile that led to this work is the one I'll never get to photograph—your smile.

It took me over a year to create and deliver the best 1-day hands-on dental photography course in the world. But it took a decade of trial and error to acquire the knowledge and experience to make it even possible (lots of money too, as my photography budget can attest). My mission was to save my colleagues all that time and money and then gift wrap it into a sleek 1-day package.

Let me set the stage for you: any city in the world, 35 dental professionals, models, a makeup artist, lights, an interactive presentation, and me. We are all there, learning the fundamentals of photography, camera settings, accessories, intraoral protocols, lighting principles, laboratory photography, etc. Then the time comes when everyone splits into small groups with a model who is ready to smile for them. The students (you) try to remember and apply everything I just taught. They try to get that great shot, the one you've seen so many times on social media from people you believed to be especially talented—the Gods of Dental Photography. That. Perfect. Shot.

And there it is: The Smile. Not the one in the photos, not the one on the models, but the smile on my students' faces. My colleagues. Your smile. You get it—the shot—and look around to tell others. "Look! I got it!" Then it spreads, moving through the room like a wave. Everyone gets it. Along with the smile comes the realization that this isn't so hard after all, if you only know the fundamentals, the lighting, and a few little tricks. It was always right there. You've had the tools all along. You just didn't know how to use them properly.

Let me tell you, when it comes to dental photography, I'm an atheist. There are no gods. It's just practice and understanding. This is usually when the questioning starts.

"But Miguel, that's it? I place the light here and position myself there and I'm done?"

"I don't need a fancy camera? Or 10 lenses, or a bulky lighting setup?"

"What do you mean I don't need the ring flash anymore?"

"Are you telling me I can take this picture in my tiny office?"

Yes! Yes! Yes! That is exactly what I am saying. It's simple. It really is.

LIT was born because I got addicted to my colleagues' smiles. I have simplified and demystified the art of dental photography. I start with the fundamentals. I do not attempt to teach you only how to take pictures of pretty lips and glossy teeth. I teach you how to be a photographer, to take ALL pictures. Any picture.

Imagine you are learning to drive a car for the first time and your instructor only teaches you how to drive around your own block. Well I wouldn't want to be there when you get to the highway for the first time. Or experience that first rain. I will teach you to drive under any conditions. Where, when, and how far you go is up to you.

First, the fundamentals of photography are displayed here using simple visual scenarios and analogies. Then, we will move into portrait photography. Why portrait? Because it is the best way to practice the fundamentals you've just learned. Portrait is about understanding your camera, the light, and the space around you. It's the perfect start when you learn to shoot in manual mode. Believe me, you don't want to practice that while someone is holding retractors in their mouth. Once you've mastered portrait photography—and trust me it's pretty straightforward—then we'll talk about the equipment you need: cameras, lenses, lighting, accessories, etc.

At this point you're now equipped with the knowledge to walk into dental photography heaven. "What's that?" you might ask. A full intraoral protocol that can be done in a small office, in 10 minutes, without you or your patient having to move. No moving the chair, no moving the light, no moving yourself. Yes, you read that right. *LIT* brings you "The Simple Protocol."

Historically, dental photography books have stopped right here. But I didn't. It's the 21st century after all, and who doesn't want to perfect the artsy dental photography that you now see all over social media—Facebook, Instagram, and whatever fancy new app comes along next. In this book, you'll learn all the tricks and techniques to take those amazing artistic shots yourself, because guess what? It's not that hard to do. It really isn't.

As a dental technician myself, I have also dedicated a full chapter to my fellow technicians who want to showcase their work too. This book is for you as well. I give you all you need in order to photograph your craft, your art, and your passion in the laboratory.

Lastly, I close with something that has never been discussed at this level: how to use and understand the online marketplace and social media for your private practice. No, I am not talking about that silly weekly post that some company places for you on your clinic's Facebook page—the one that reminds your patients of the importance of flossing daily. Neither am I talking about how to get your page to rank higher on Google. Everyone is playing that game, and there's very little winning involved. I'm talking about a deeper understanding of how online marketing and social media really works: Google, Facebook, Instagram, AB testing, landing pages, building audiences, retargeting, the Pixel, etc—strategies that most of you have never even heard of are filling up the schedule in clinics near you.

I give you *LIT*. The first simplified but complete dental photography book. It will change the way you take photos, and you will use these skills forever. I know you'll love it, and that makes me smile too.

1

Fundamentals of Photography

The Big 5

The Big 5 refers to the five main concepts that are most important in dental photography. These 5 concepts will empower you to have complete control over your photographic results. Learn the Big 5 and you will be the boss of Manual Mode. Drop Auto Mode forever. You paint your own picture, not the camera.

EXPOSURE

APERTURE

SHUTTER SPEED

DEPTH OF FIELD

WHITE BALANCE

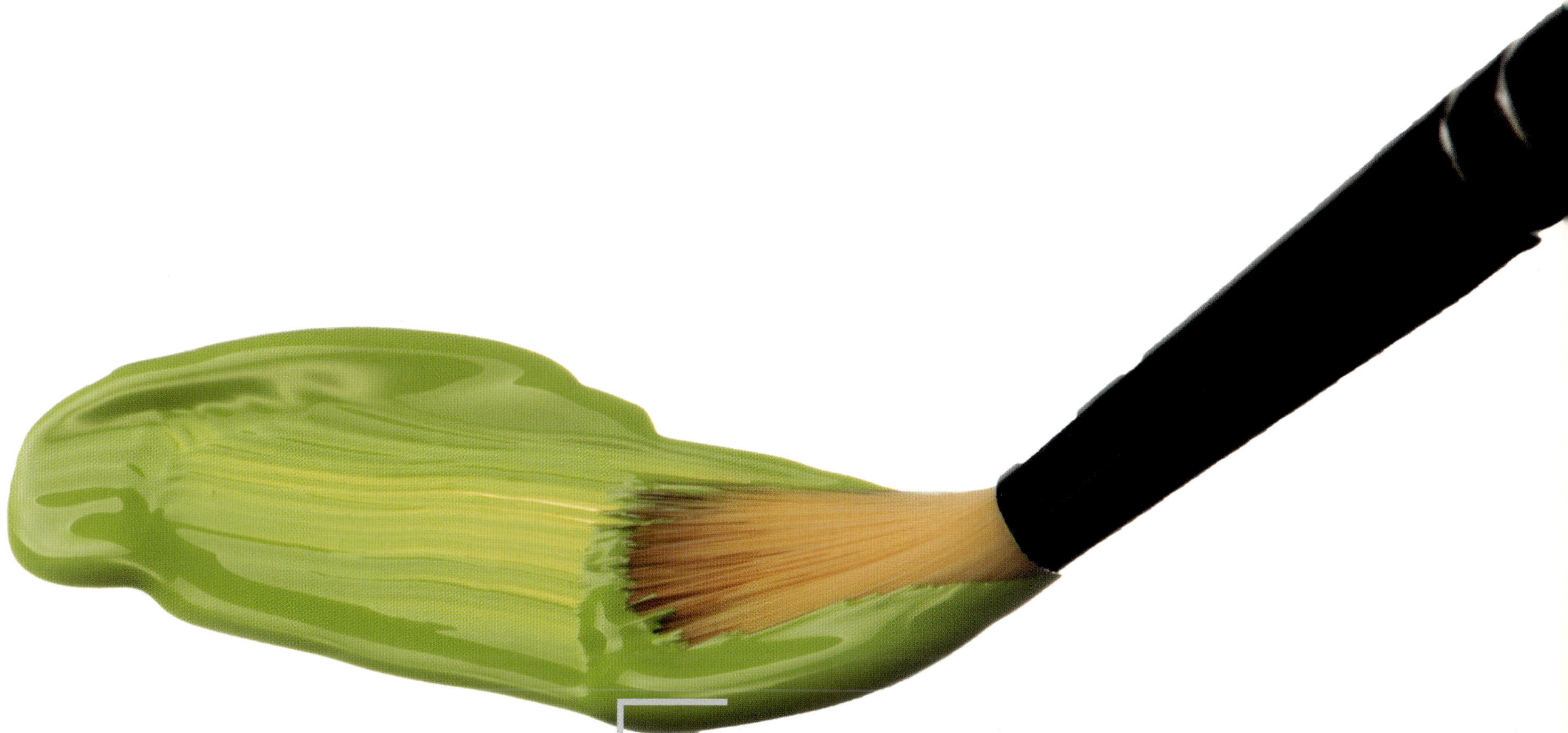

1/5: Exposure

EXPOSURE

The total amount of **light** that will reach the digital sensor inside your camera.

Water in a bucket

The most important concept in dental photography is *exposure*, because every other concept in photography is based on the understanding of exposure. Luckily, it is not an extremely complicated idea, so let's tackle it.

Exposure could be compared to the notion of water in a bucket. Imagine you have a bucket and you want to use a garden hose to fill it up with water. Your bucket is the digital sensor, the water is the light, and your hose is your lens. In this analogy, exposure is the AMOUNT of water that you put into the bucket.

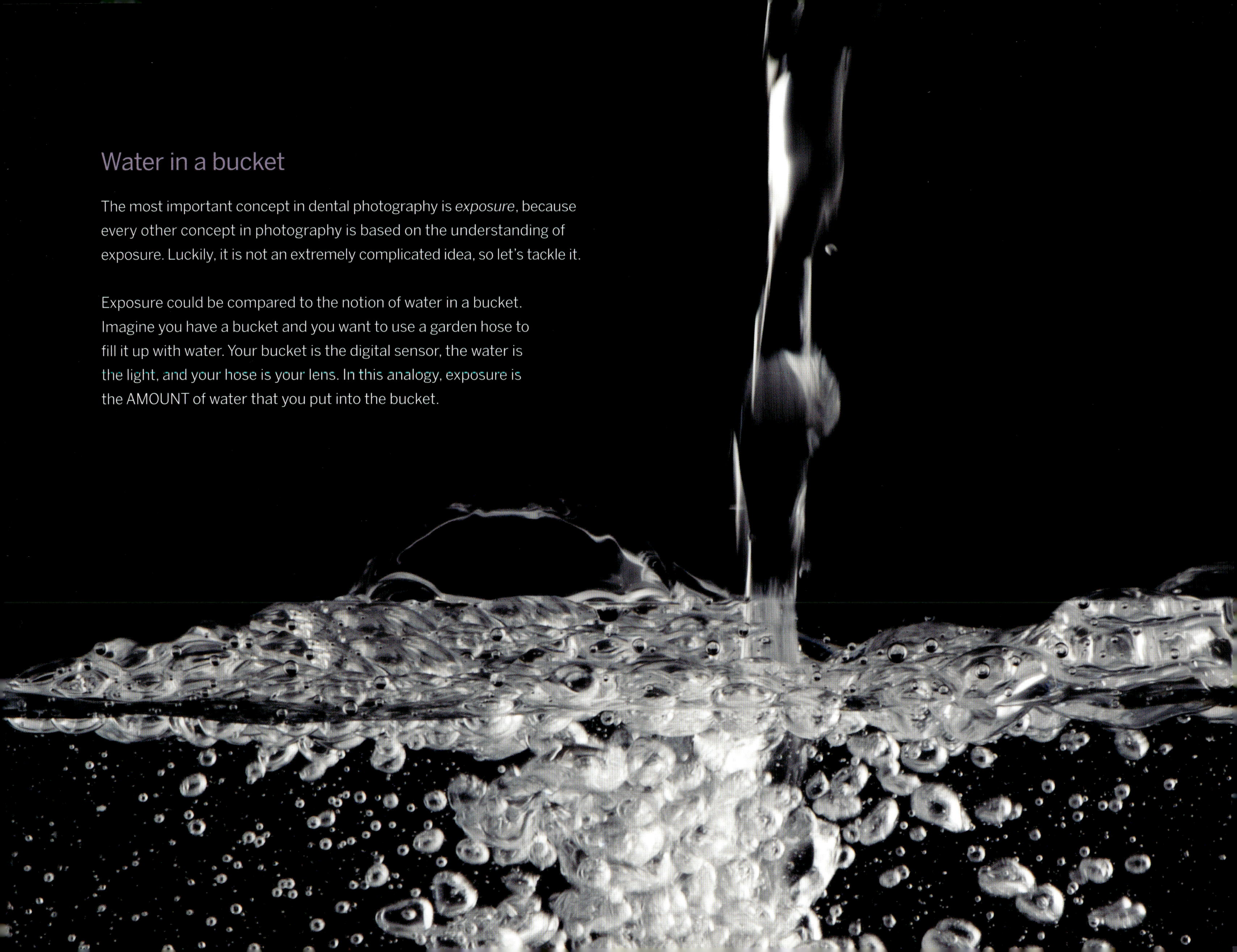

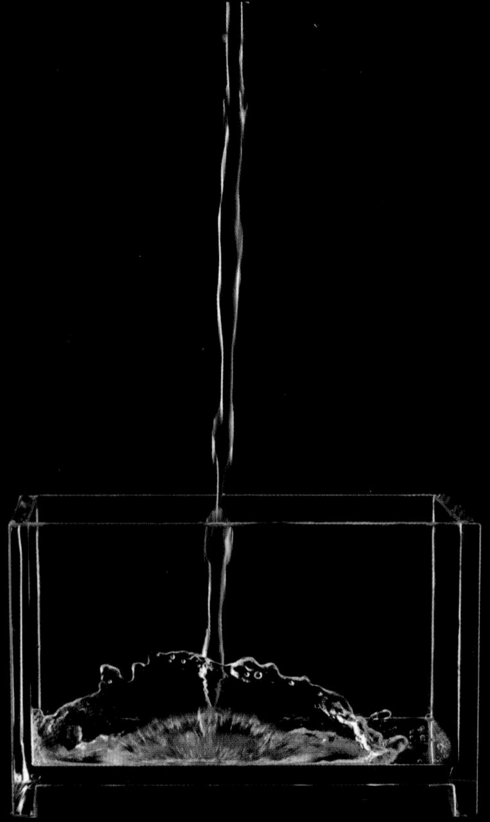

Underexposed

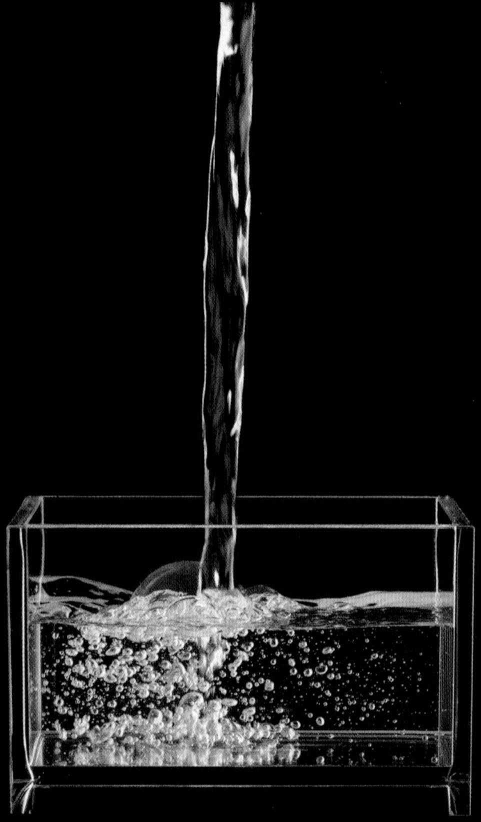

Correctly exposed

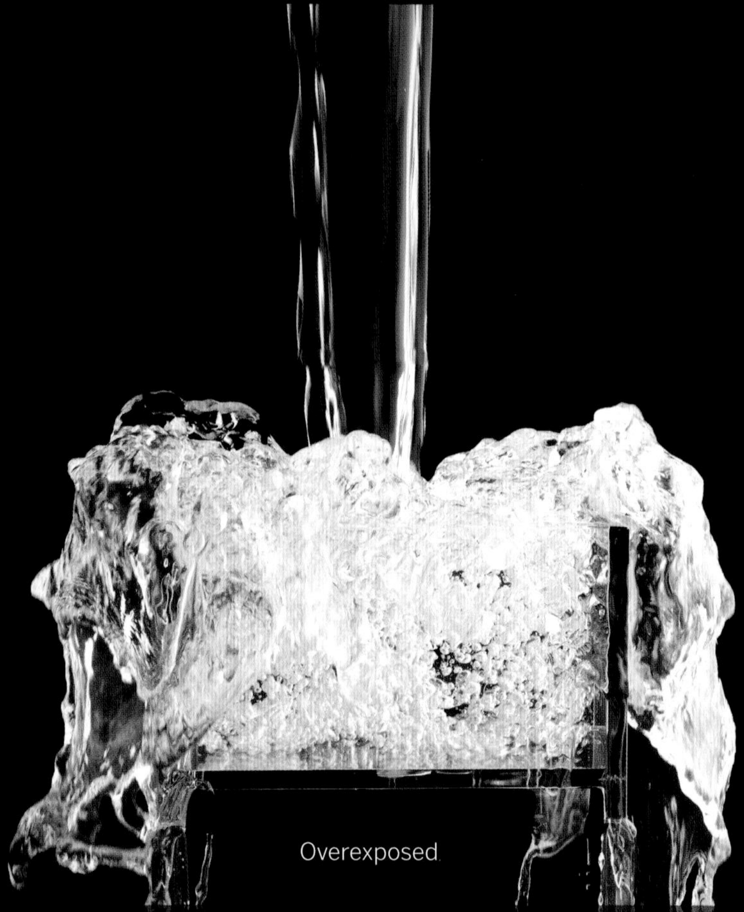

Overexposed

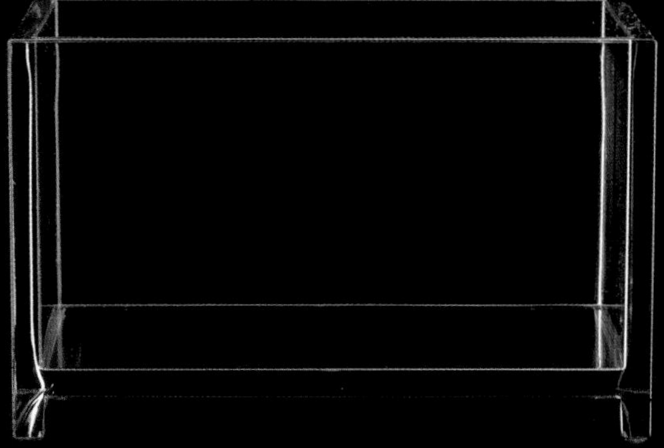

Large bucket = Full-frame sensor

Small bucket = Cropped sensor

We can have large or small buckets (sensor sizes), minimally filled buckets (underexposure), buckets filled to the desired mark (correct exposure), or a bucket so full that it's spilling water out (overexposure). We can have pure water (temperature-calibrated light) or colored water (noncalibrated light). Your hose (lens) could be of different diameters (aperture). We might use a wide-diameter hose or a very narrow-diameter hose, allowing us to deliver more or less water (light) to the bucket (sensor). Alternatively, the water pressure (light intensity) could be high or low, delivering more or less water (photons) in a given amount of time (exposure time). Lastly, opening and closing the water nozzle quickly (fast shutter speed)—allowing water to flow only at discrete intervals of time—is also an option. Or you can leave it open (long exposure), resulting in an endless amount of water being delivered to the bucket.

We will learn later that not all buckets (camera sensors) are the same size, and yes, size matters.

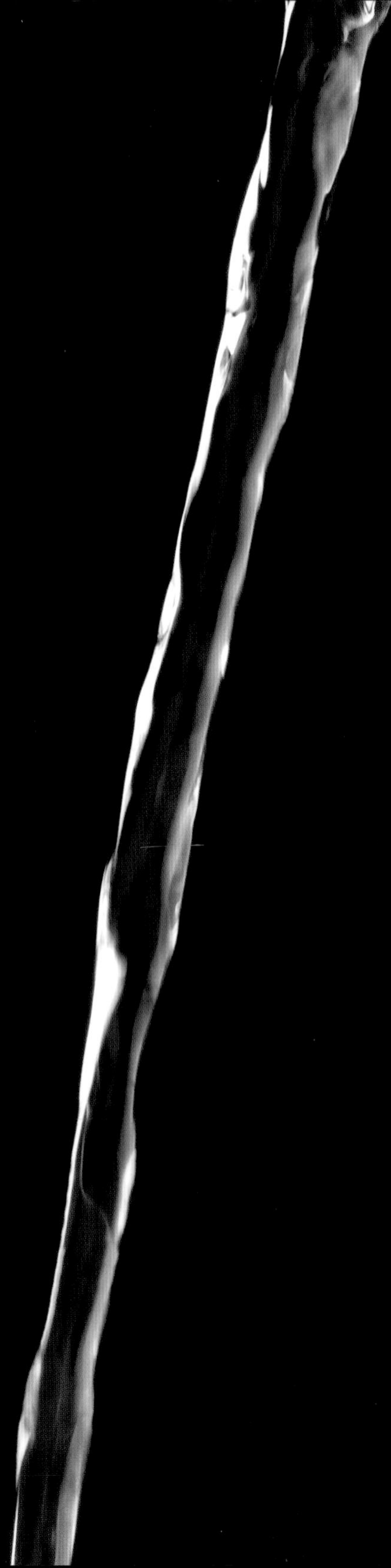

As you can see, the concept of filling up a bucket can be broken up into several components, all of which can be manipulated. One thing we know for sure is that, when it comes to filling up a bucket, you have full control over how you do it. You can control what kind of liquid you fill it with and how much and how fast that liquid pours into the bucket. When it comes to getting light to your camera sensor, you have the same control.

At the end of this book, you will be in full command of your camera settings and you will fill that sensor with light exactly how you want it.

water in a bucket

Once again, EXPOSURE is the AMOUNT of light that reaches the digital sensor in your camera. Without light there is no photography. Now that you fully understand what exposure is, we can begin learning how to fill that bucket.

The Big 5: 1 down, 4 to go....

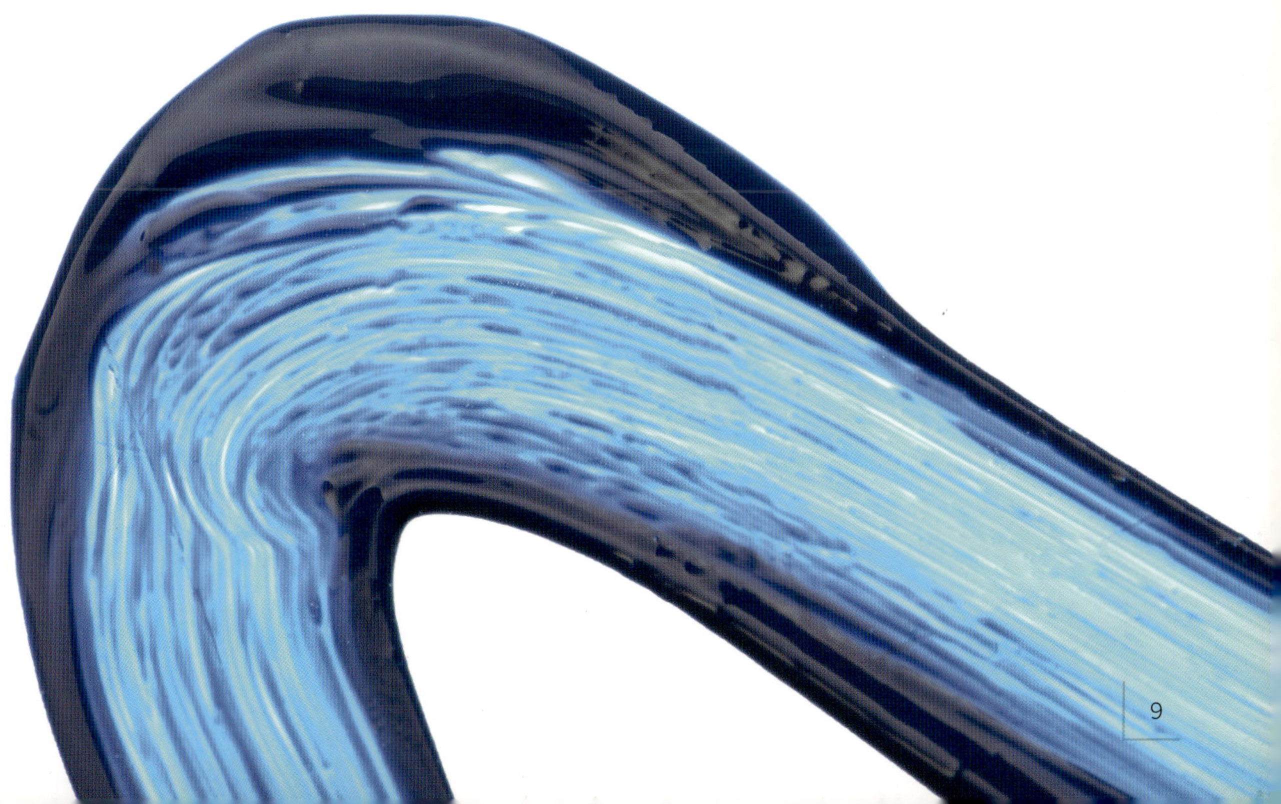

2/5: Aperture

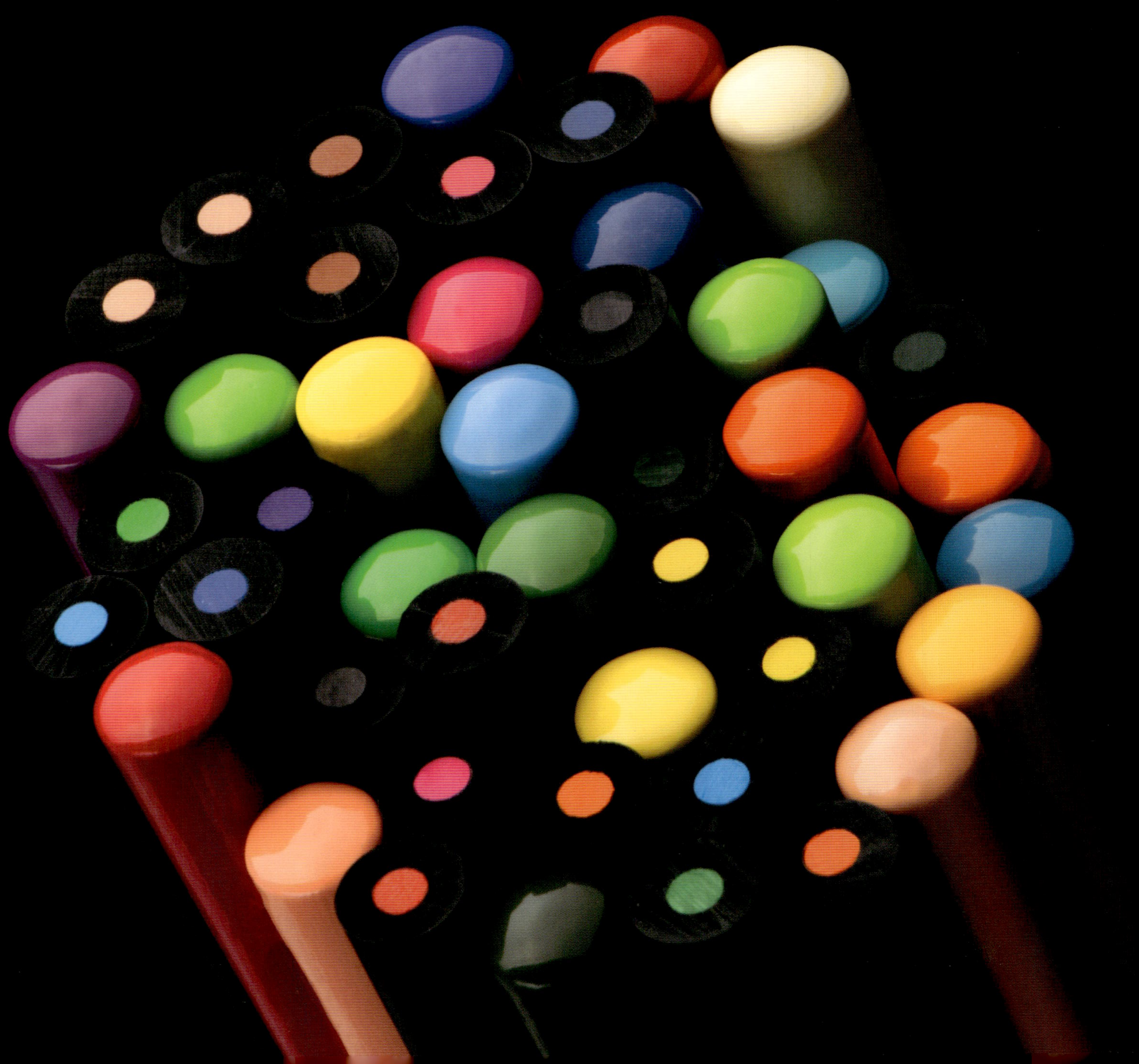

APERTURE

An adjustable opening inside your lens that allows you to **control how much** light reaches the sensor.

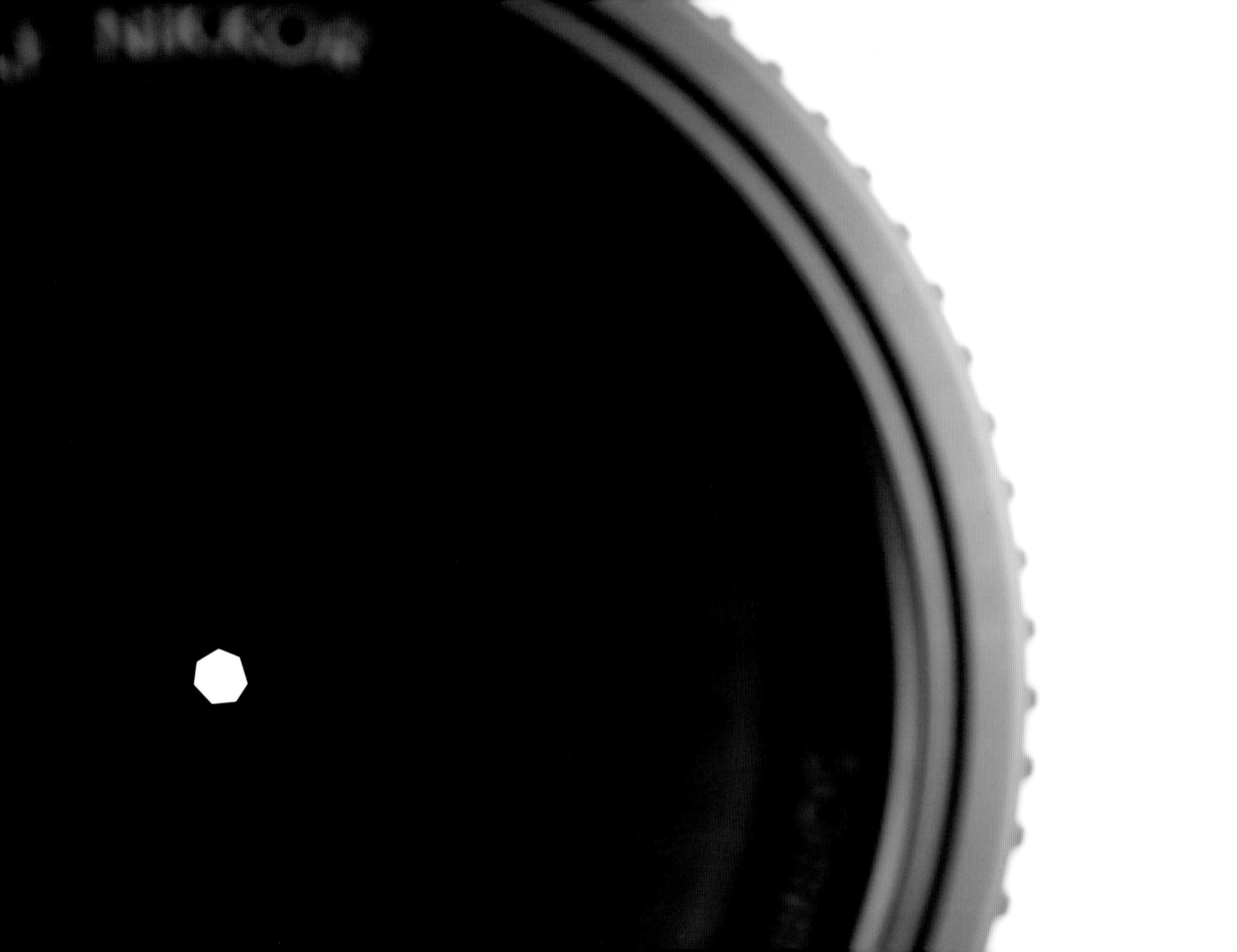

Aperture is the area of a spherical opening inside the camera lens that is designed to be adjustable. It can go from a very small round hole to an opening almost as large as the lens itself. This mechanical device inside your lens is used to control how much light can come through and reach the sensor. It is a way of controlling exposure, among other things.

Early photographers in the 19th century quickly realized that they could not control the amount of light reaching the photographic plates. Back then, overflowing the bucket meant a lot of money lost on photographic plates. So they created the diaphragm. They did not need to look too far for inspiration on the design. It was right in front of their eyes, right in front of your eye. Think of your eyes—your pupils. Your pupils work in the exact same manner as the mechanism in the lens that is used to modify the aperture. That mechanism is called the *diaphragm*, by the way. Your pupils open and close to allow more or less light to reach the sensors in your eyes. Remember those cones and rods from anatomy class?

At night, when you are in your room and the lights are off, your brain tells your pupils to open up wide in order to allow more light to come in. It does that to help you avoid stepping on that Lego that was left on the floor by your 4-year-old child. I sure know how painful that is. On the other hand, as you are lying in bed contemplating that first patient of the upcoming morning, with your pupils wide open, your spouse walks in and turns on the lights. As you reach to cover your eyes, your pupils immediately contract to accommodate for the sudden burst of light, allowing less light to reach the retinal sensor, so you don't have to scream at your partner for the unnecessary torture that just occurred.

This is exactly the same in photography. The diaphragm in the lens is like the pupil. It can be opened wide or closed down to a small orifice in order to control how much light we allow to reach the sensor.

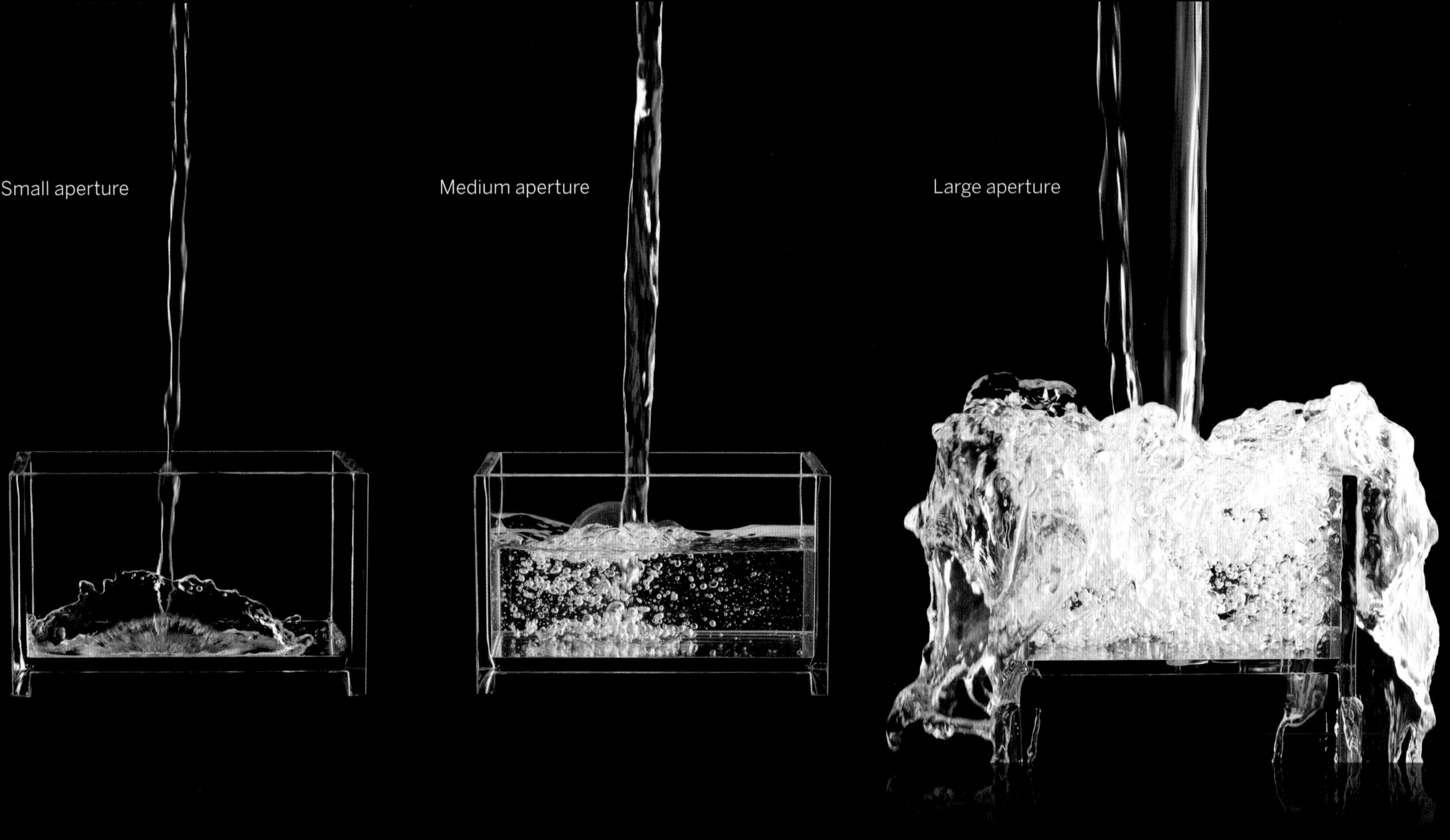

APERTURE = SIZE OF THE HOSE

F-stop

The way we modify the aperture in our DSLR (digital single-lens reflex) cameras is by changing the f-stop (also called the *f-number*). This number is one of two main values that are readily available for modification in all DSLR cameras. Most cameras will dedicate the most accessible and obvious controls to change the aperture with the f-stop and the shutter speed. We will talk about shutter speed in the upcoming section.

F-stop (aperture) is noted in a discrete geometric scale. f/1, f/1.4, f/2, f/2.8, f/4, f/5.6, f/8, f/11, f/16, f/22, f/32, f/45, f/64, f/90, f/128, etc. A value of 1 depicts a fully open diaphragm. From f/1 to f/1.4, the area of the circular opening **decreases by half**. Same as from f/1.4 to f/2 and from f/2 to f/2.8, etc.

Because the area of the aperture decreases by half every time we move up one stop on the scale, half the amount of light can get through that aperture to the sensor. It is because of this that the first conundrum arises. Pay attention next.

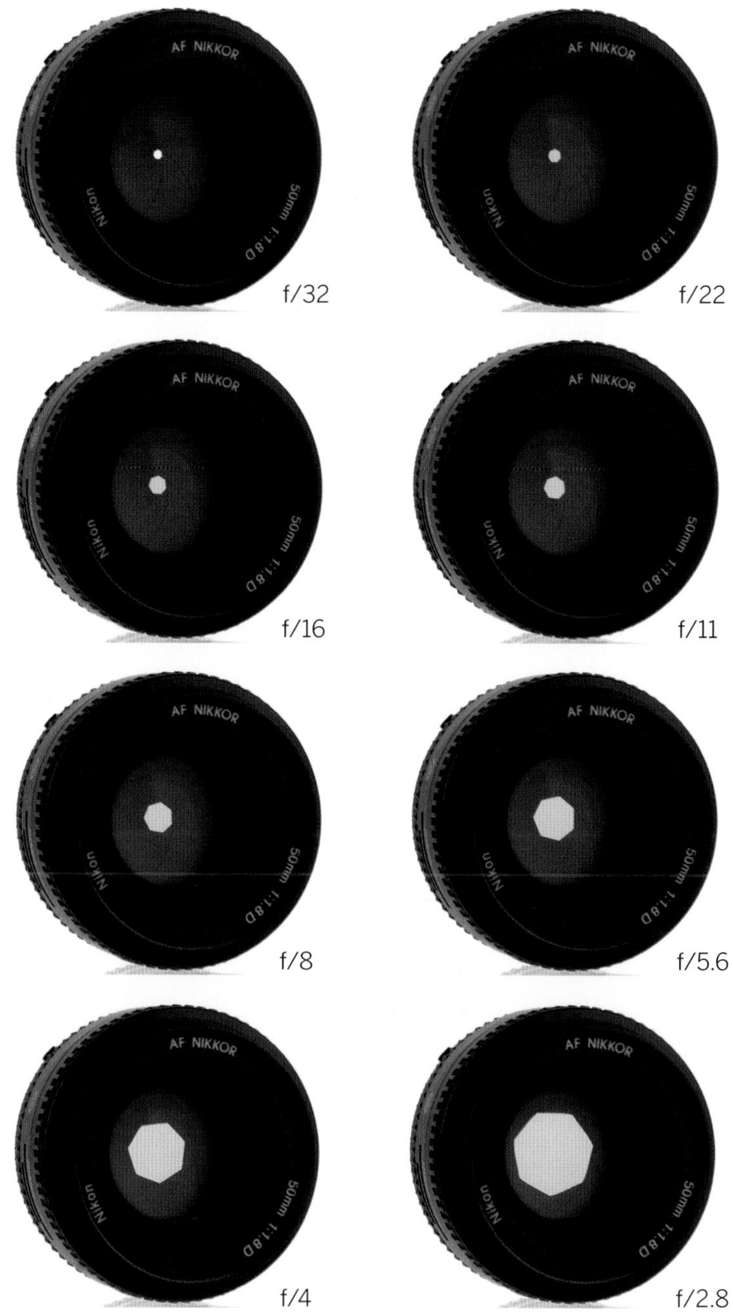

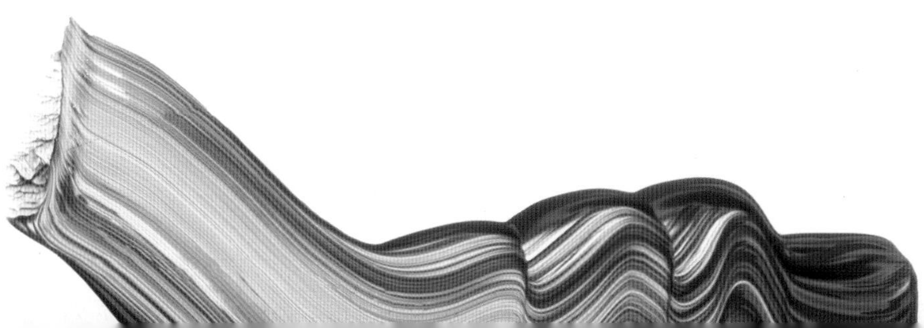

Here is where most beginners will make their first mistake. A picture will be taken that is underexposed (too dark). The photographer will remember that you can increase the exposure by modifying the aperture, and then will increase the aperture value. But remember that increasing the aperture value (f-stop) decreases the circular area in the diaphragm, which lets less light reach the sensor. If you want more light, the f-stop has to be reduced. If you take a photo at f/16 and it is underexposed, then you need to use maybe f/11 or f/9.

THE HIGHER THE F-STOP VALUE, THE SMALLER THE APERTURE. LESS LIGHT WILL REACH THE SENSOR, RESULTING IN LOWER EXPOSURE.

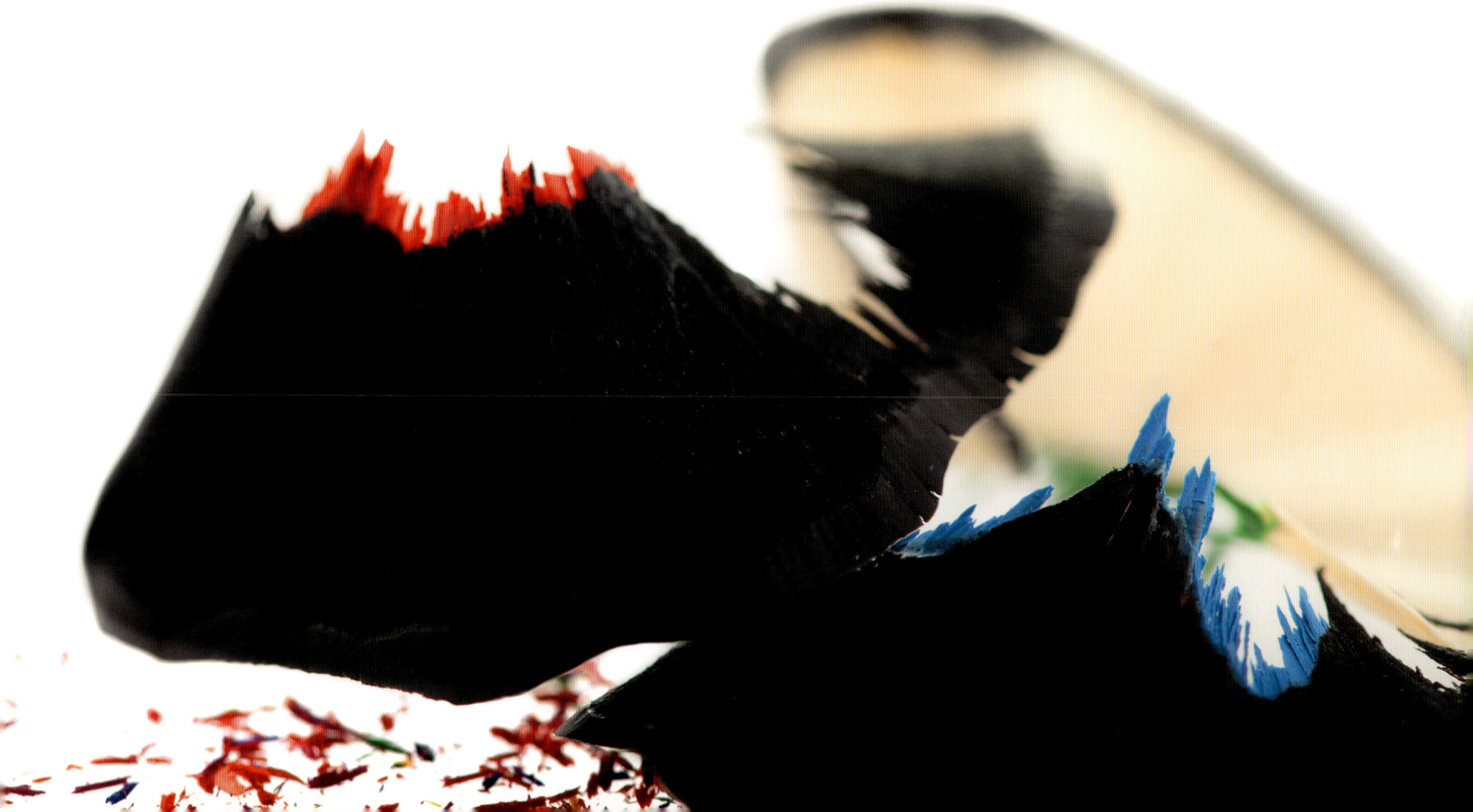

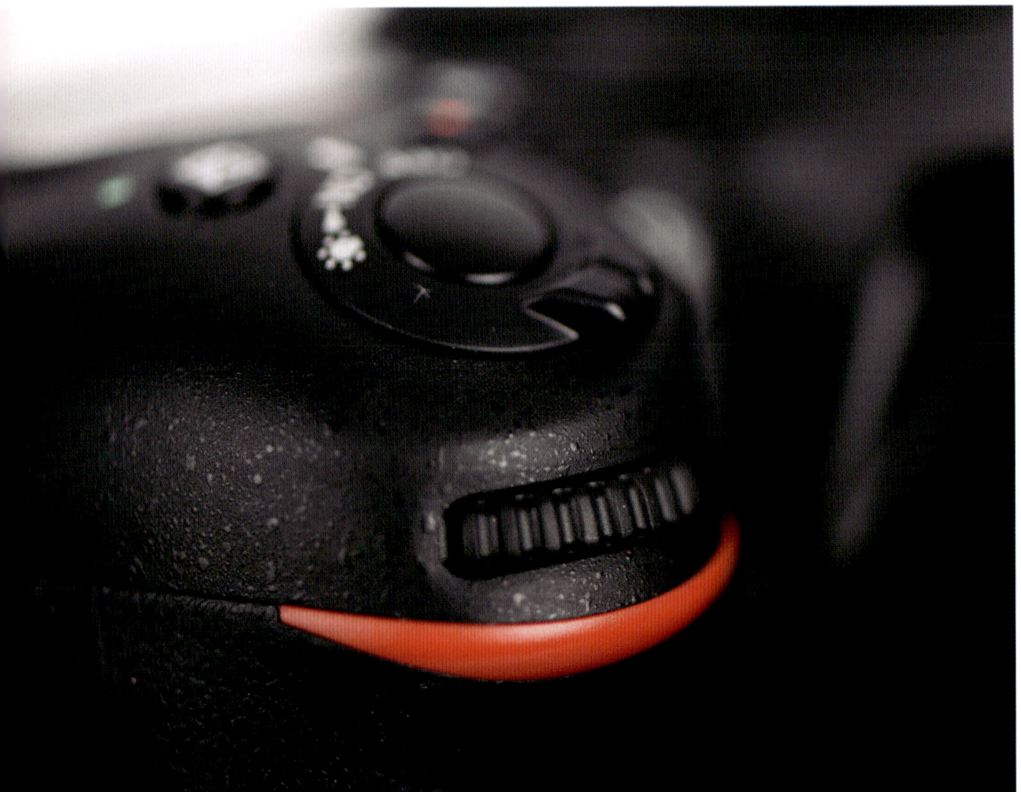

Dials

All men are created equal said our friend Thomas, but all cameras are not. However, I can say with confidence that if your camera has a dial—a small wheel-like mechanism on the top right area—it is highly likely that that dial is used to modify the f-stop, the shutter speed, or both. Some Nikon cameras come with two dials, one for each function of f-stop and shutter speed. Most Canon cameras have only one dial. That dial most likely changes the shutter speed if turned. However, there is a function button with black and white + and – signs that, when held down, switches the function of the dial to control f-stop instead of shutter speed.

Believe it or not, it is not a speed at all.

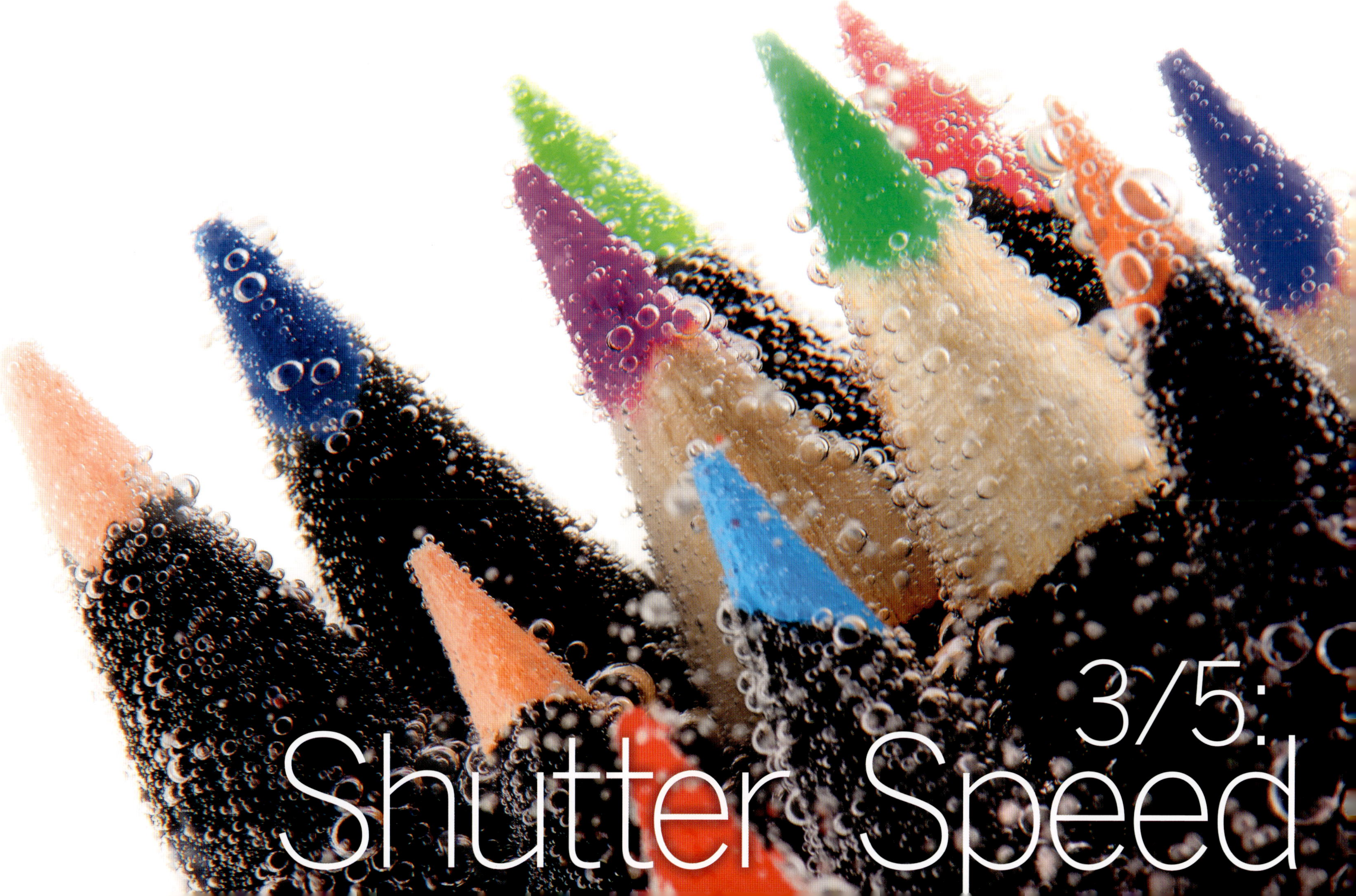

3/5: Shutter Speed

SHUTTER SPEED

The **time** that you allow the sensor to be exposed to the incoming light.

Shutter speed is not a velocity as the name implies. It is more of a time interval. It is the time that we allow the sensor to be exposed to the incoming light.

How do we do this? We use a shutter, which is a curtain in front of the sensor that opens and closes when we push the... The what? What do we push? It is easy to remember: We push the shutter release button.

So now you know: The button we push to take the photo is called the *shutter release* because it releases the shutter (curtain in front of the sensor) and allows the light to reach it.

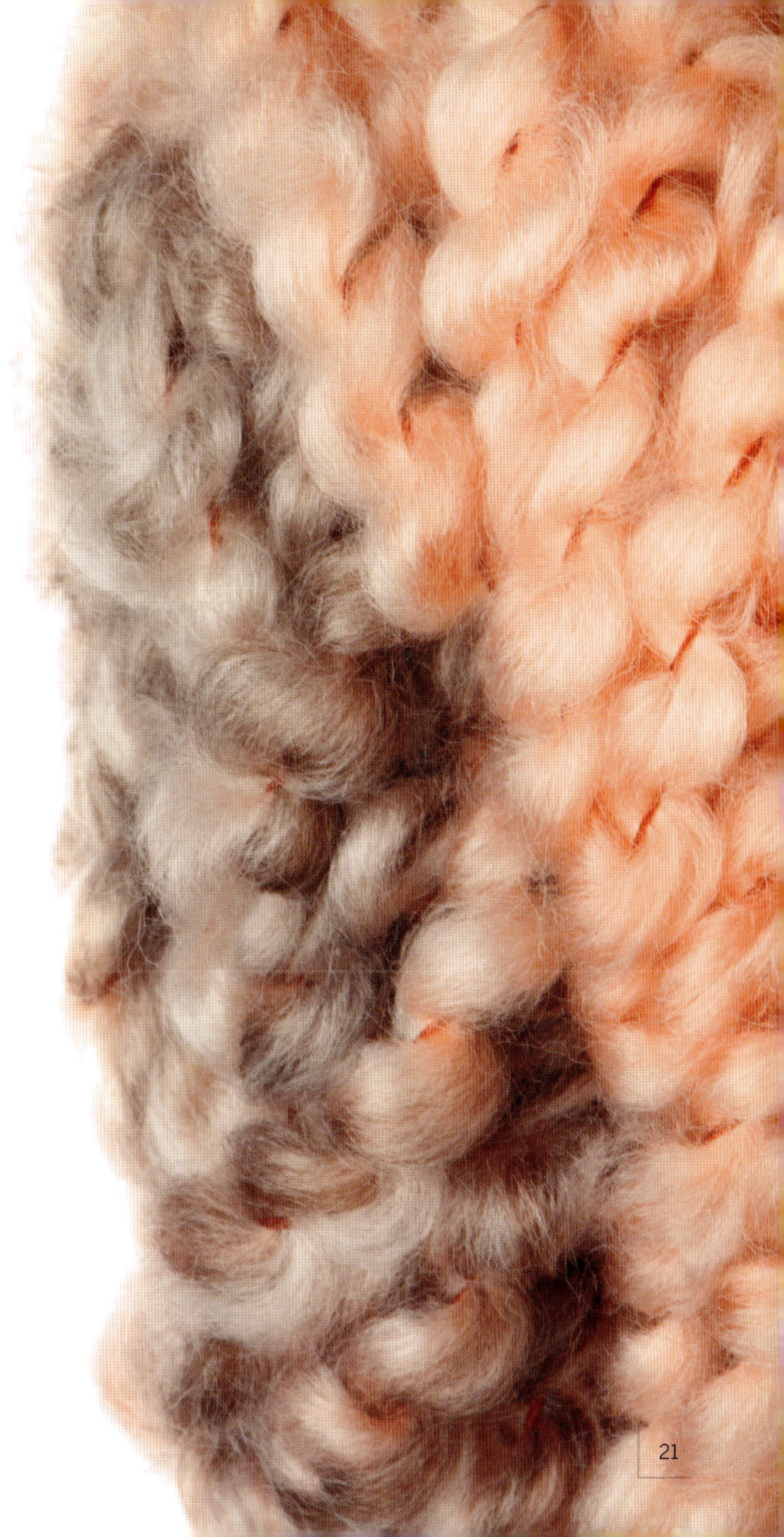

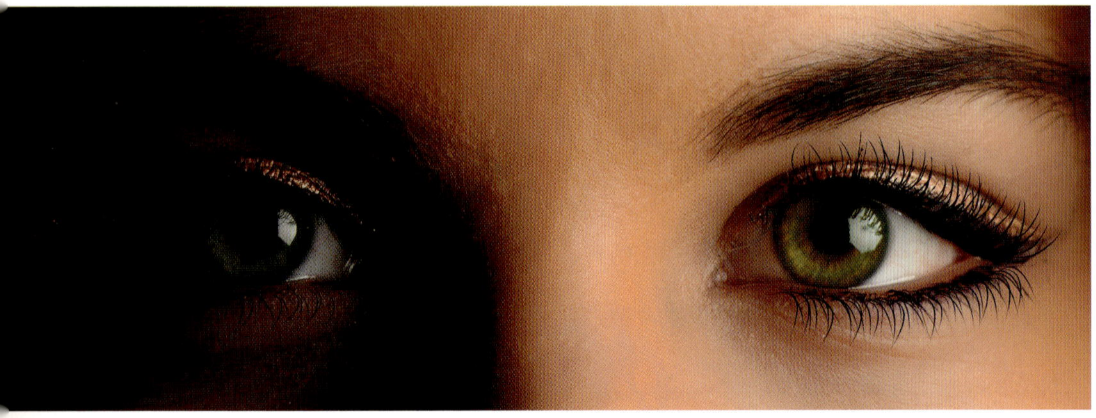

Imagine you are a camera. Your eye is the lens. But there is one big difference. The camera always has its eye (shutter) closed. Light does not reach the sensor. When you push the shutter release button, the shutter opens and closes very fast to allow light in to reach the sensor. That small amount of time that the shutter is open is called the *shutter speed*.

Shutter speed is measured in fractions of a second.
For example: 1/100 s, 1/125 s, 1/160 s, etc.

Shutter speed is a fraction.
Blink and you'll miss it.

If you have a Canon camera, chances are you have one dial and one button that allows that dial to be used for two different functions. Natively, the dial is used to modify shutter speed. Pressing the function button will allow you to change the f-stop (aperture) using the same dial. The picture on the right shows the "Av +/−" button on the Canon camera that switches the function of the dial wheel from shutter speed to f-stop.

On a Nikon camera, sometimes you have two dials, one for each function. This is a generalization, especially with manufacturers using the touchscreen to modify these parameters more and more.

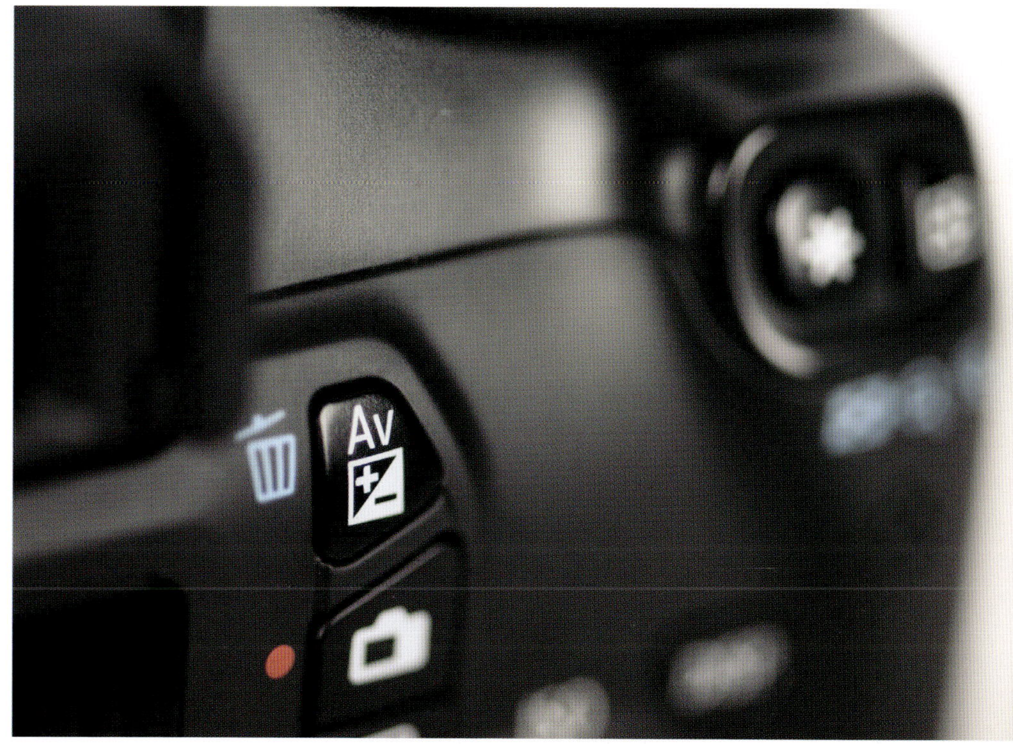

What is shutter speed used for?

What is the main "role" of shutter speed? To allow more or less time for light to reach the sensor. So, if you take a photo at a shutter speed of $1/100$ s (that is one 100th of a second), and that photo is overexposed (too much light), how should we modify the shutter speed to correct the exposure? If you said increase the shutter speed you were right. Increasing the shutter speed, however, means increasing the denominator in the fraction, for example from 100 to 160; $1/160$ s is less time for that curtain to be open than $1/100$ s. Remember, it is a fraction.

Shutter speed and motion

Fast or slow shutter speeds allow you to capture or eliminate motion, respectively. If you have a blurry photo, chances are that you have introduced motion into the picture. While the shutter was open, either you or your subject moved. It is for this reason that if we want to minimize blur or motion on a photo, we need to have a fast shutter speed. Fast shutter speeds in dentistry are those of $1/125$ s or above. The curtain opens and closes so fast that there is no time to capture motion, unless of course you are purposely shaking your camera. On the other hand, if you want to capture motion, such as water flowing or car lights moving on a highway at night, you want to reduce the shutter speed. You want that shutter open for longer. But remember, the longer it is open, the more blur you will introduce and the greater the chance your photo will be overexposed.

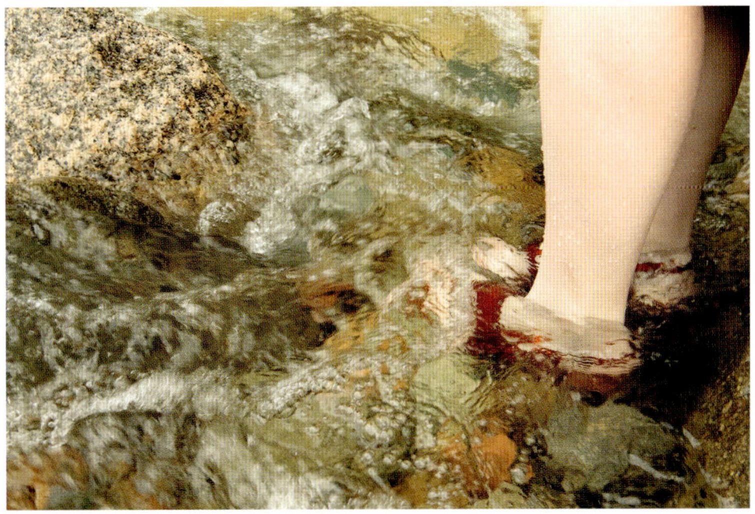

Shutter speed 1/200 s, f/5.6

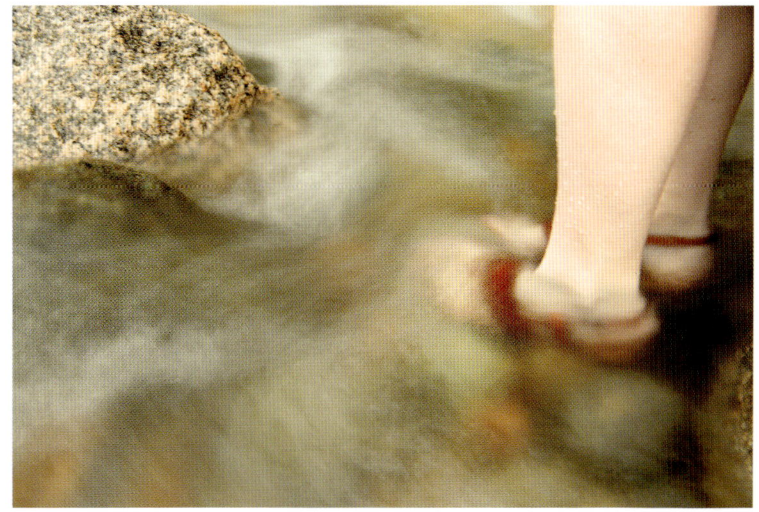

Shutter speed 1 s, f/32

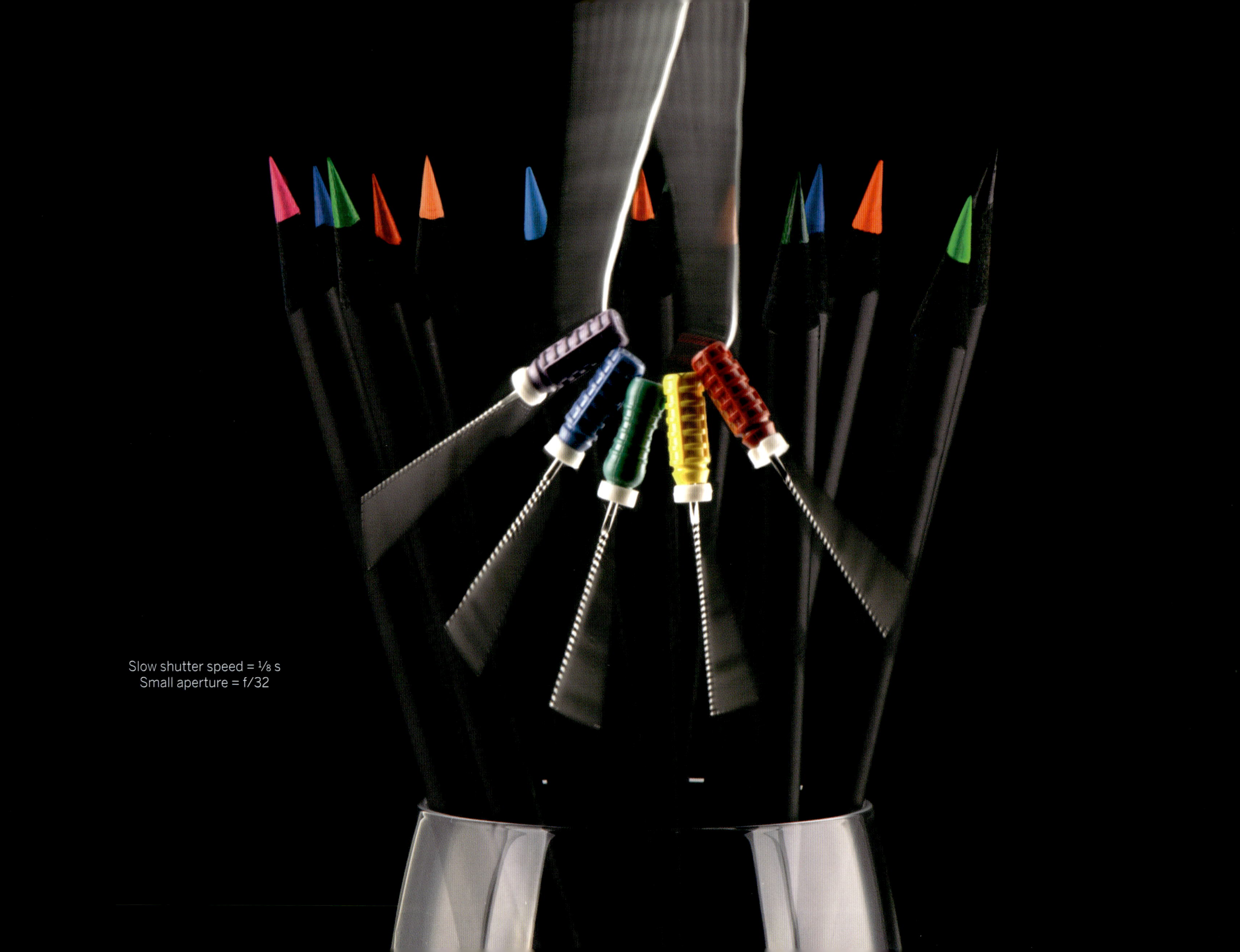

Slow shutter speed = 1/8 s
Small aperture = f/32

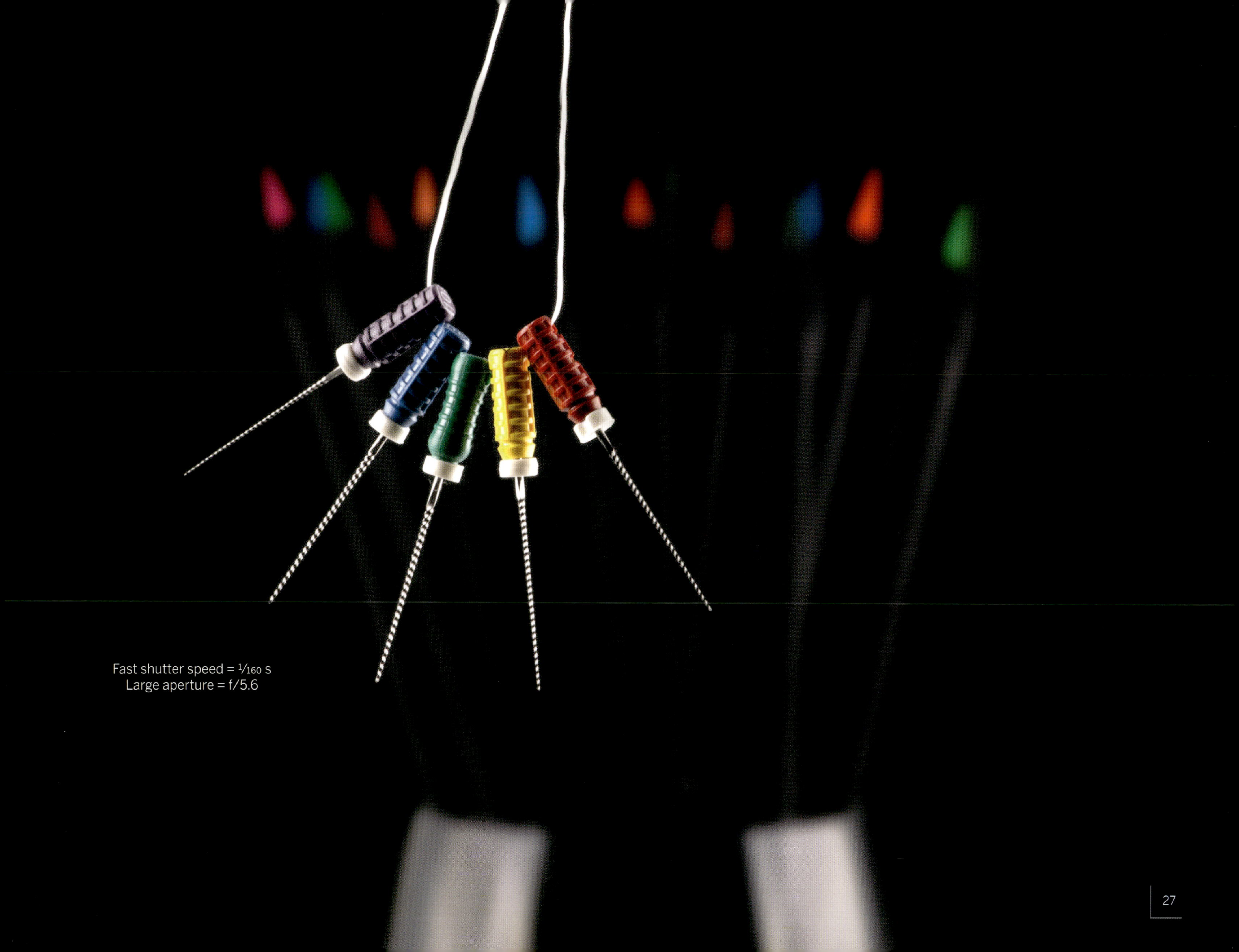

Fast shutter speed = 1⁄160 s
Large aperture = f/5.6

4/5: Depth of Field

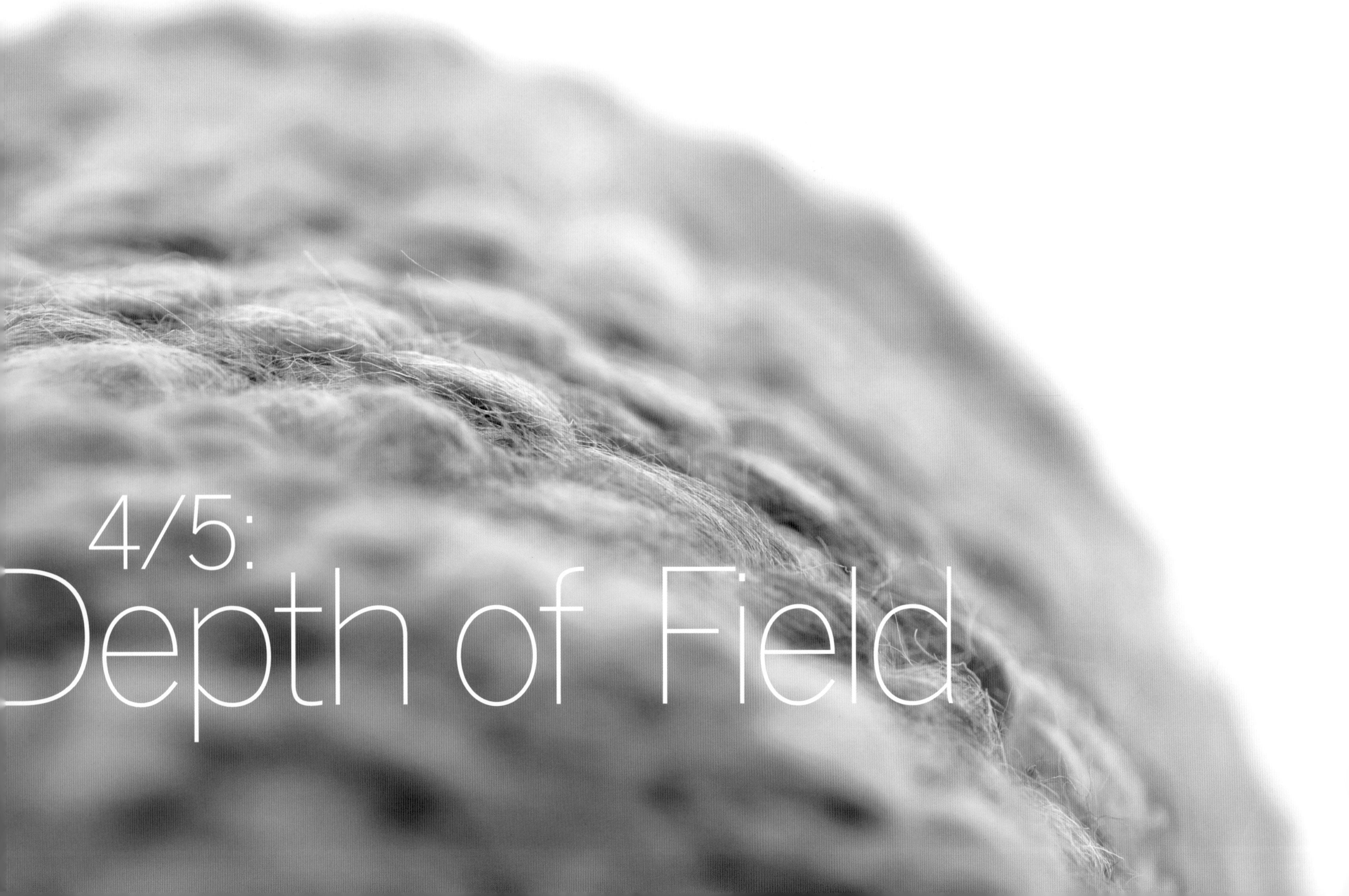

DEPTH OF FIELD

The **distance** between the closest and the furthest things in your photo that are seen to be in focus.

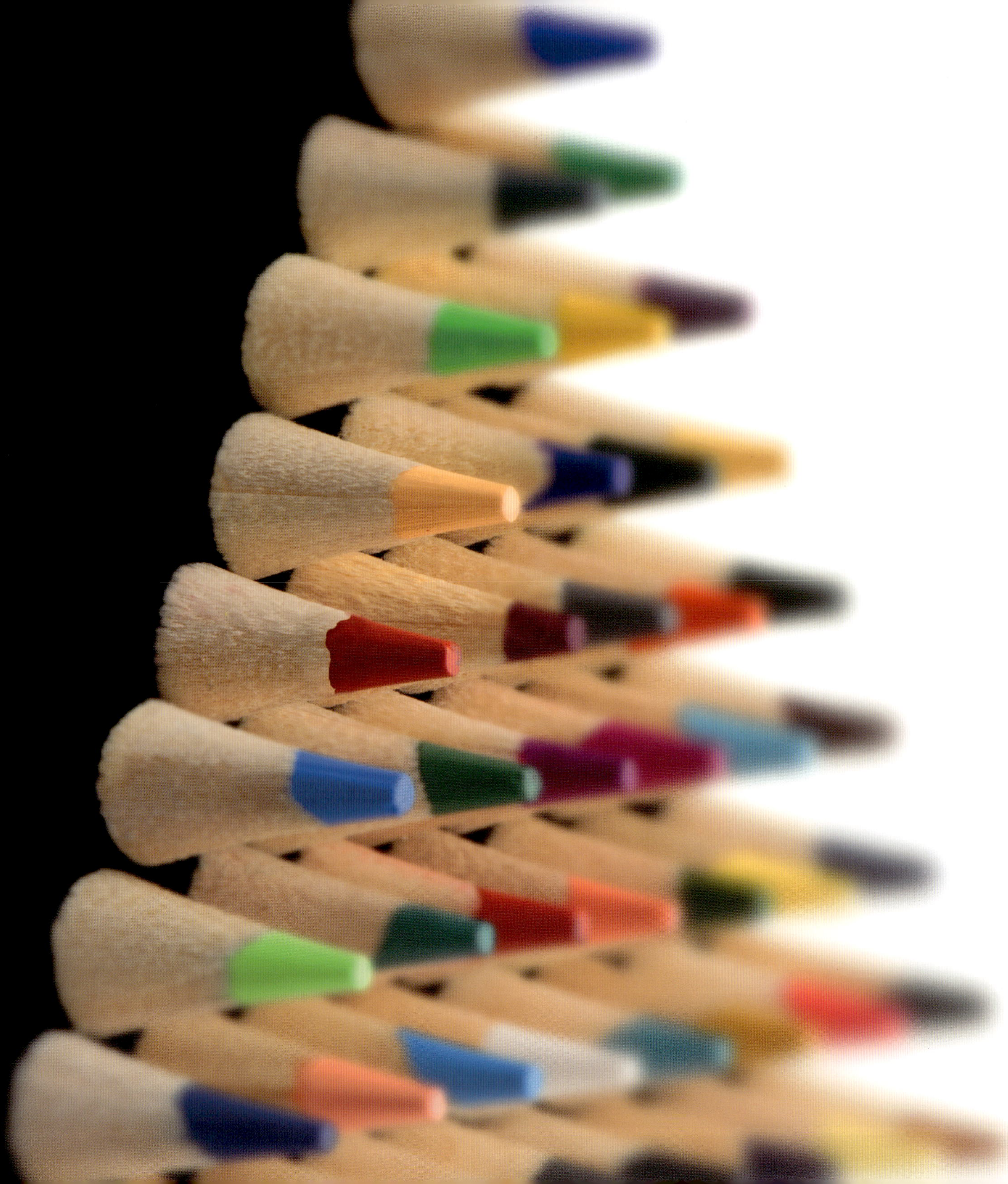

Narrow DOF
f/2.8

APERTURE CONTROLS THE DEPTH OF FIELD (DOF). THE HIGHER THE F-STOP, THE LARGER THE DOF AND THE MORE THINGS IN FOCUS.

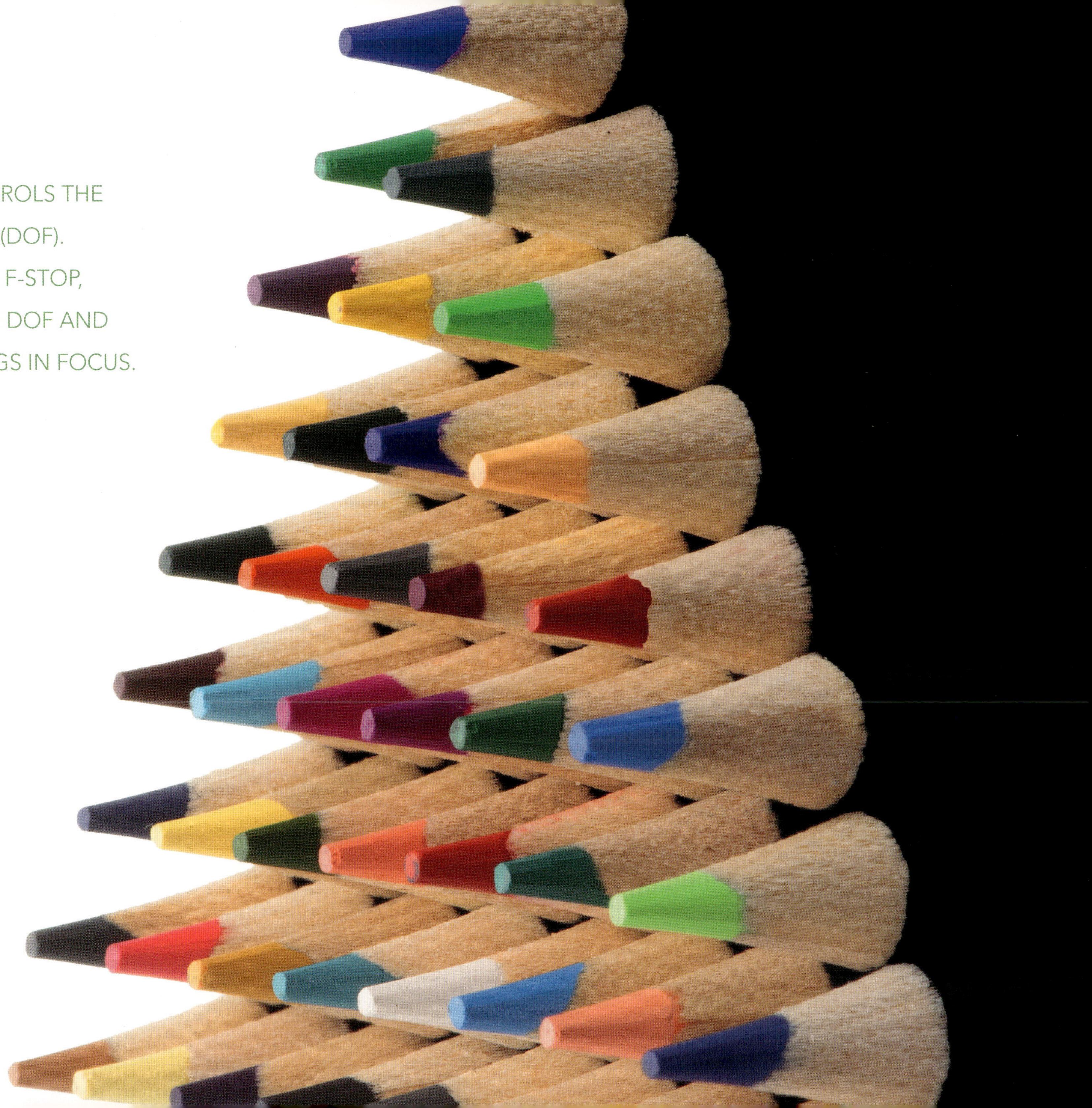

Wide DOF
f/32

DOF is related to focus. As with our own visual system where not everything is in focus all the time, our camera system has the same capabilities. If you pay close attention to what you are reading right now and keep your eyes right here—right on this sentence—you can appreciate that your peripheral world is not in focus. The areas all around you to your right and to your left, up and down, are a bit blurry. Hey hey hey!!! Keep your eyes HERE and pay attention to your surroundings; they are out of focus. The same happens to our photos. If we are not careful in selecting our focus point, we might get our subject out of focus—blurry. DSLR cameras, as many others, have the capability to automatically focus on a subject by pressing the shutter release button halfway down. It is done via a motor in the lens that moves the optical elements back and forth to achieve the desired result. Our body does this by the cornea and by stretching the lens behind the pupil with tiny muscles.

The lens gets thinner and thicker as the muscles pull and release, allowing the lens to change shape and focus on what we want to see. This is the why later at night, after a long day at work or school, the eye has trouble focusing on the page you are reading. Those tiny muscles get tired too.

In our camera lens, we don't get to stretch the glass, but we can move the glass back and forth to focus on a point in our scenery. When that point is in focus, we have created not a focus point but a focus plane, right in front of us. That plane has an area in front and an area behind that is also in focus, as far as our brain can tell. That distance—from the closest thing to you that is in focus to the farthest from you that is in focus—is called the *DOF*.

The DOF can be very narrow, meaning that only a bit of the scenery will be in focus and everything else in front or behind will be blurry (out of focus). Or it can be large, where most things in the frame are in focus. Guess what? We can control our DOF.

3 ways to change DOF

1 Distance from camera to subject

Even though camera to subject distance is used a lot in photography to change the DOF, we do not use it that much in dentistry. However, we do need to be aware of it at all times because we will move closer or farther from the patient frequently, altering the DOF. The distance between the patient and us is more or less always the same, when compared to most other forms of photography. In dentistry, if we want to change the DOF, we do not back away or move closer. We use other methods. What is important to remember is that the closer you get to the subject, the narrower the DOF becomes.

2 Focal length of the lens used

The focal length of the lens is the distance between the lens and the image sensor when the subject is in focus, usually stated in millimeters on the lens: 28 mm, 50 mm, 100 mm, etc. In the case of zoom lenses, both the minimum and maximum focal lengths are stated, for example 18 to 55 mm. As the focal length changes, so does the DOF. The larger the focal length, the narrower the DOF. In other words, as we zoom in, the DOF decreases. We use macro lenses of fixed focal length, and we are not going to change the lens if we need more or less DOF. This is why we do not use focal length as a tool to modify the DOF in dentistry.

3 Aperture settings

This *is* the way we modify our DOF in dental photography. Remember the aperture hole? The bigger the hole, the more light that will come through. The bigger the hole, the smaller the f-stop number. And the bigger the hole, the NARROWER the DOF. This means that if you want everything in your photo to be in focus, you need to have a large DOF. To have a large DOF, you need your aperture to be small. Small aperture, big f-stop. If you want all 32 teeth in focus, you need an f-stop of 32. As my friend and mentor Dr Carlos de Carvalho once stated, "How is that for simplicity?"

The inherent problem with having all 32 teeth in focus with an f-stop of 32 and higher is that our aperture is so little that barely any light comes through. So we might be tempted to reduce our shutter speed in order for light to have more time to come in. But if we have the shutter speed too slow, or open for too long, then we introduce blur that comes from our hand shaking. How do we solve this problem? Easy. We use flashes.

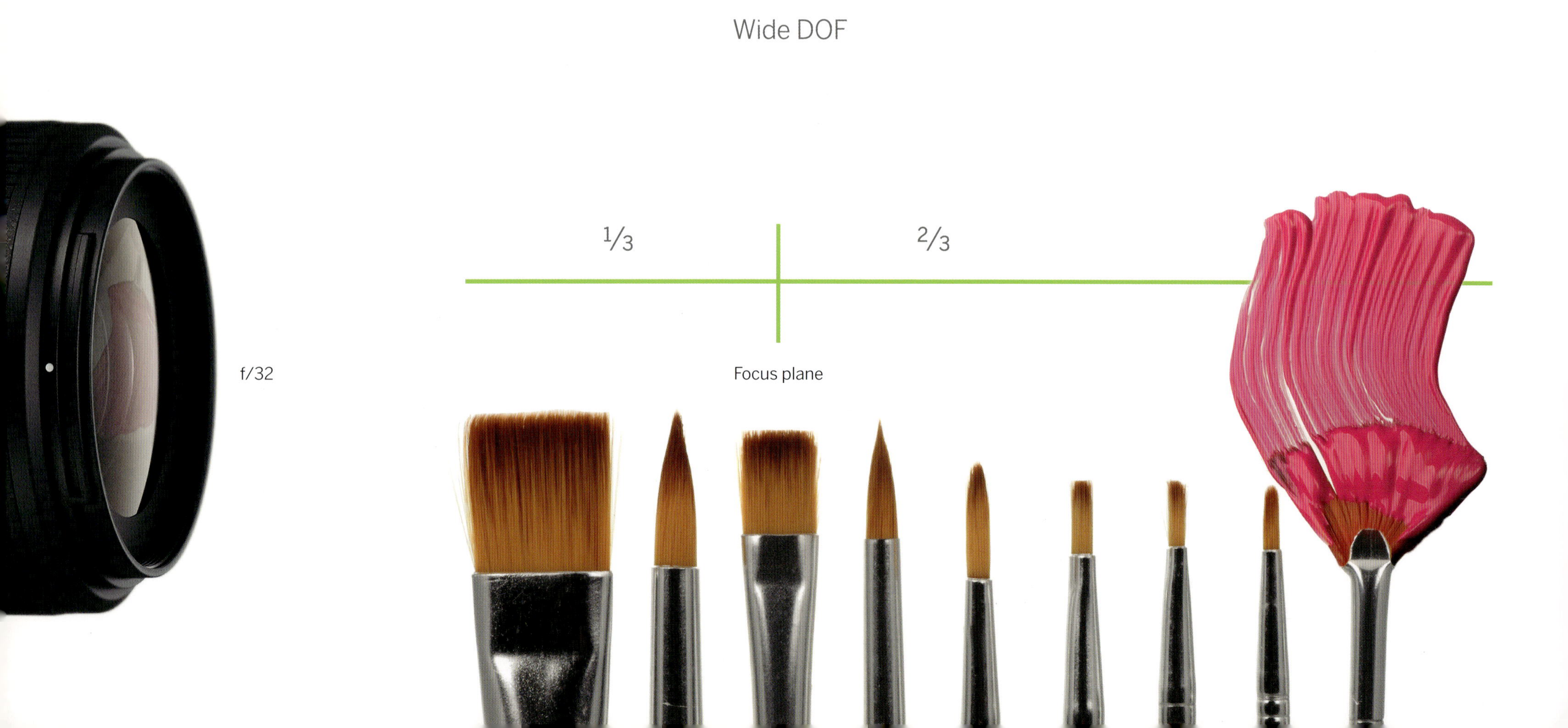
Wide DOF
1/3
2/3
f/32
Focus plane

Narrow DOF

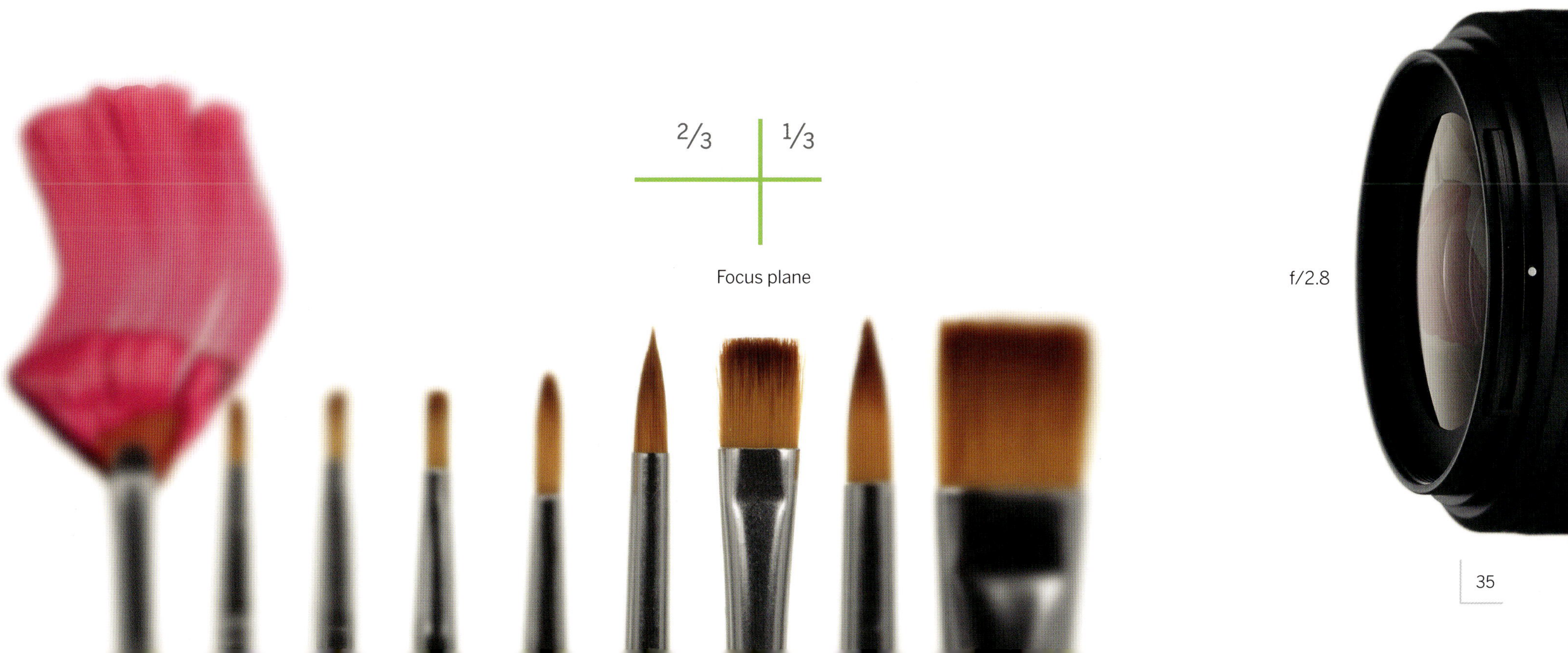

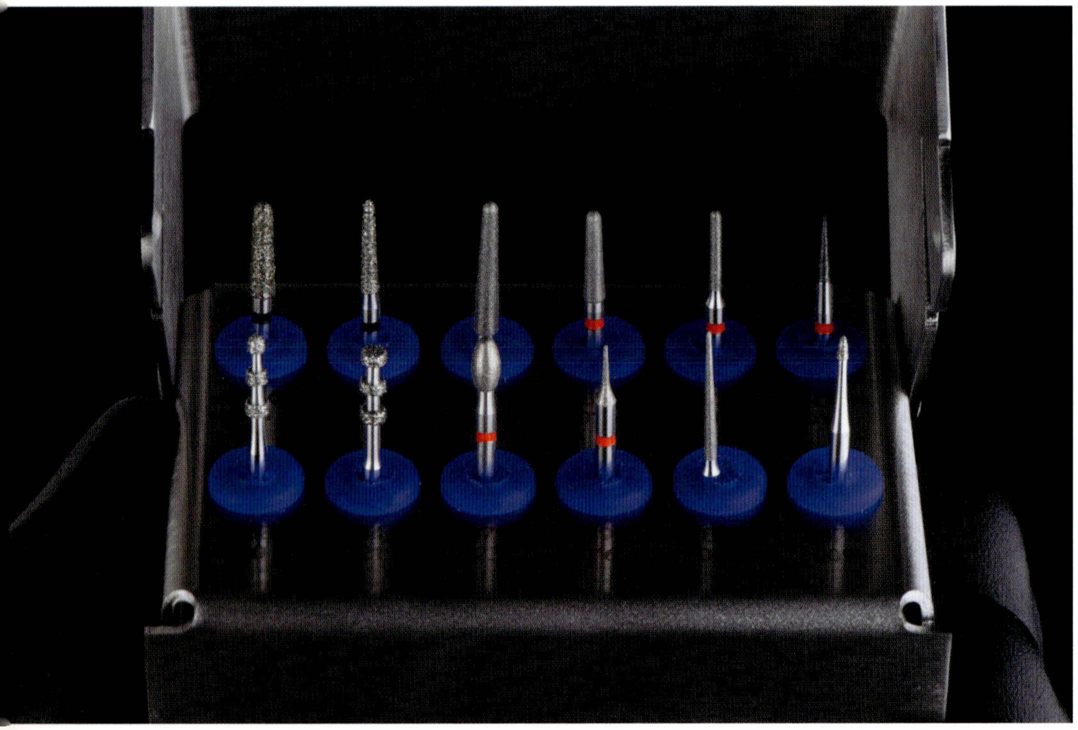

THE $\frac{1}{3}$, $\frac{2}{3}$ RULE:

$\frac{1}{3}$ IN FRONT, $\frac{2}{3}$ BEHIND

As you focus on your subject, whatever the DOF, $1/3$ of the DOF will happen in front of the focus plane and $2/3$ will occur behind it. This concept will become very relevant when we discuss how to choose our focus point during intraoral and extraoral protocols.

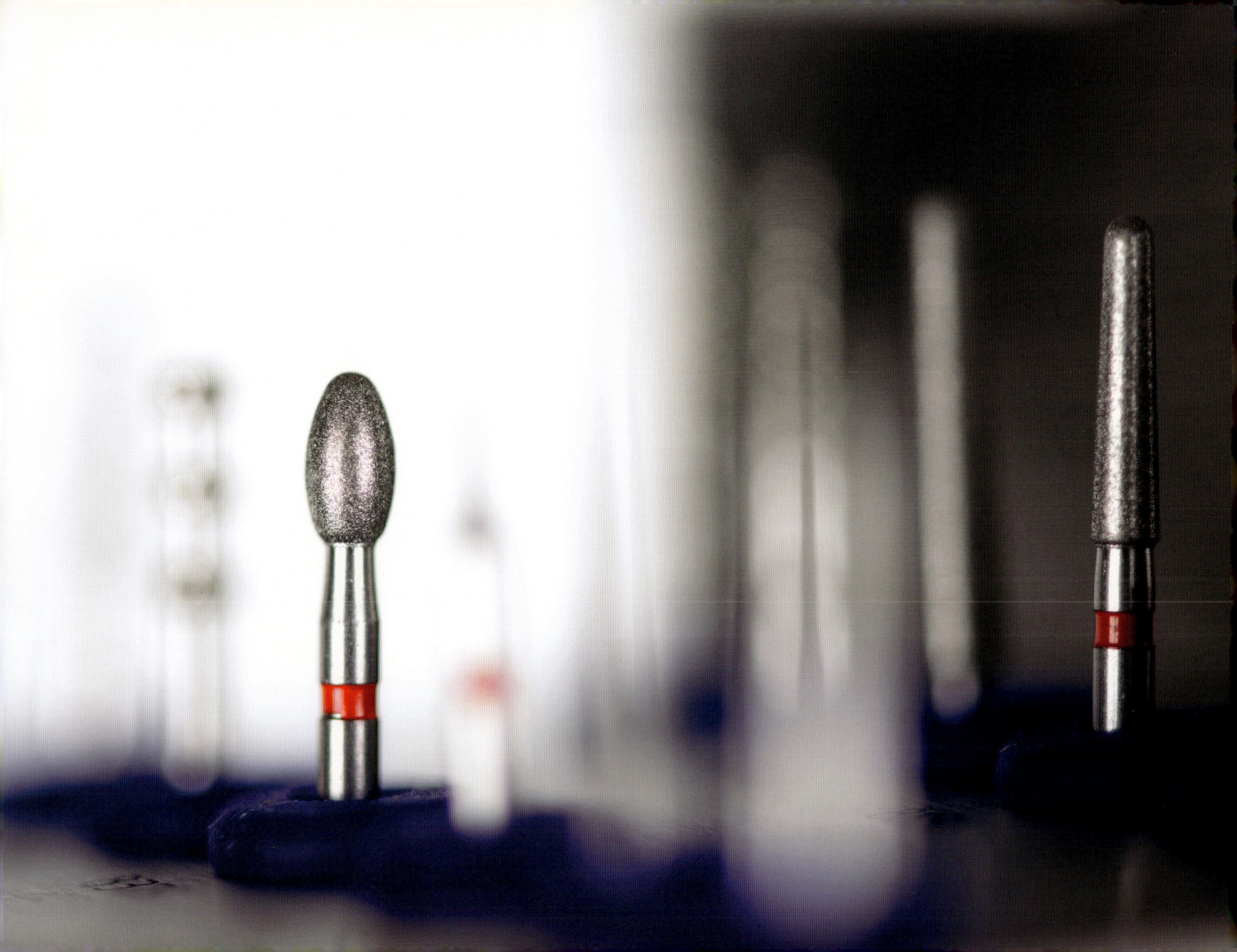

5/5: White Balance

It is all about the light temperature.

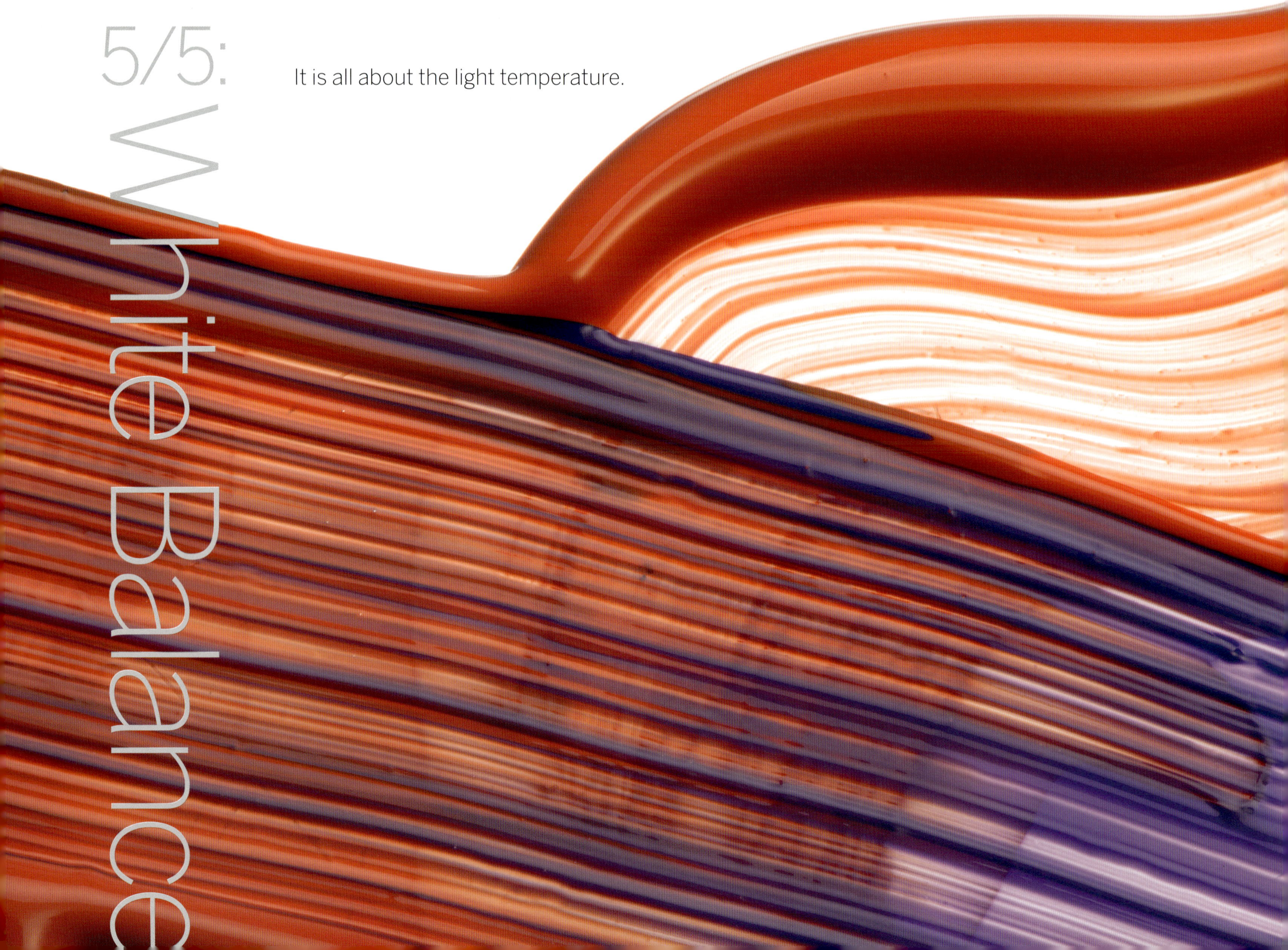

WHITE BALANCE

A way of telling your camera about the **quality/temperature** of the light in your environment so that it can adjust the photography accordingly.

Let's make this very clear. If you are taking pictures and the exposure is, as far as you can see, optimal, but the photo looks a little odd, then chances are that your white balance is set to the wrong parameter. White balance is the way our camera tries to compensate for what it thinks the quality of the light in the environment is. Wait, what? My camera thinks? Well not really. Let me back up a bit.

Light is made of wavelengths. White light is made of many different types of wavelengths. That light has, for the purpose of this discussion, all the colors of the rainbow in it. But not all colors are present in the same amount. For example, the light coming from a bonfire has a lot of red/orange in it. The light coming from our sky in the afternoon has a lot of blue in it. We don't see the difference as much because our brain can process the information about the light coming in and adjust the visual image to make it look "right" or color corrected.

This explains why indoor photos sometimes look orange, even if the walls look white to your eyes. Is your camera broken? The answer is no. The camera is probably showing you a more accurate representation of the environment than your eyes are. Your brain has manipulated the information to make you see white walls. It knows from experience the walls are white, so it acts on this information to make them look white. Yeah, I know, that's some wicked *Matrix* stuff right there. Just take the blue pill and move on, Remember, all I am offering you is the truth, nothing more, Neo.

So what is white balance then? *White balance* is a way of telling the camera about the quality of the light in which you are taking photos. The camera can then modify the image in post processing to make it look "right." Yes, the camera is the Matrix.

Every camera has a menu, or sometimes even a dedicated WB (white balance) button. In this place you can choose to have it in "auto" (let the camera decide what light is in the present environment) or several other predetermined settings, such as sunny day, cloudy day, shade, tungsten light, etc. The two settings that we care about in dental photography are "flash" and "custom." Remember when we said that if you want all of your teeth in focus you need an f-stop of 32? We also said that at this aperture value we limit the amount of light coming through so much that we need a flash system. The good thing about flash systems is that we know exactly what kind of light the flash emits. It is measured in Kelvins and it usually ranges from 5,200K to 5,600K. Check the manual for your flash to get the exact number and put it in your white balance custom setting. If you cannot find it, even in the era of Google, put your white balance on "flash." It will get you close enough. Later on, I will teach you to evaluate the color temperature of a flash light source, in case you want to have it set as precisely as possible. Even though we can find the color temperature of any flashes in their manuals, we will be putting diffuser filters in front of them and that itself changes the color temperature. Do not worry about it for now. That comes in later chapters.

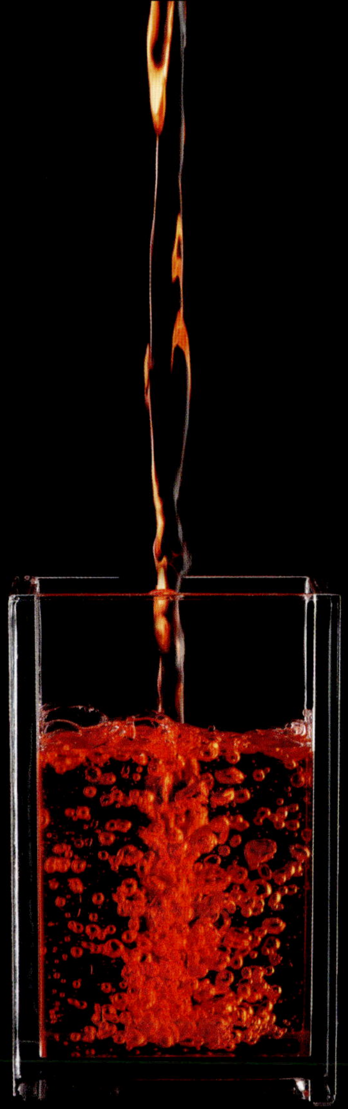

Warm light = Reddish photos
up to 5,000K

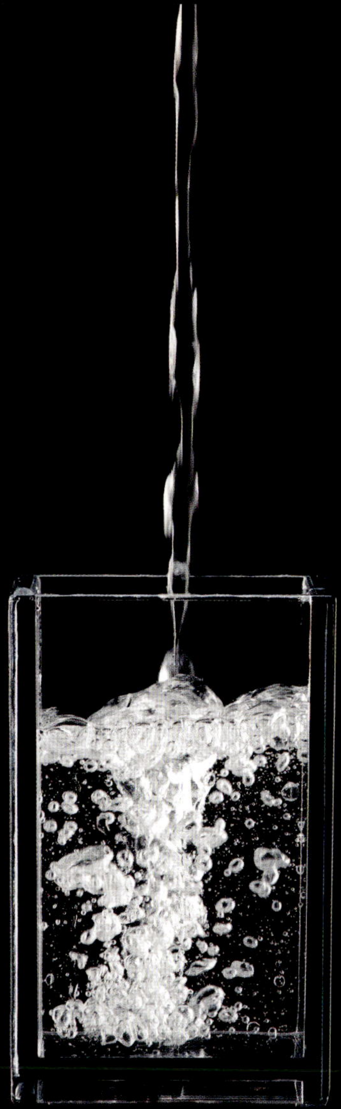

Color-calibrated light
5,000–6500K

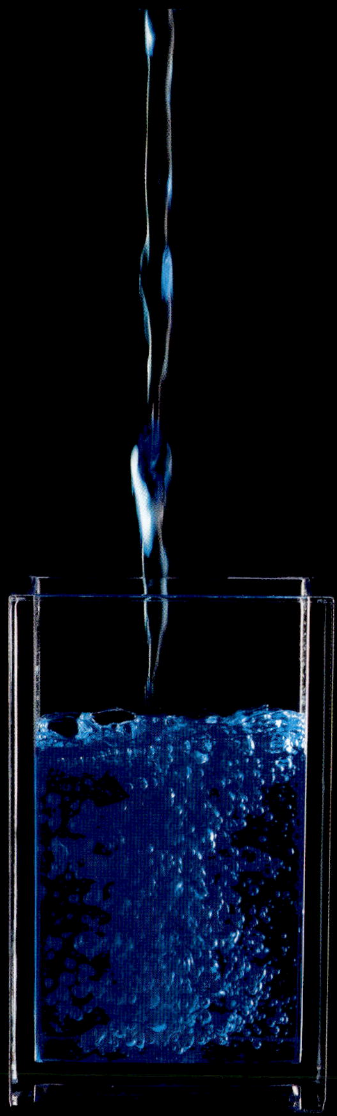

Cold light = Bluish photo
over 6,500K

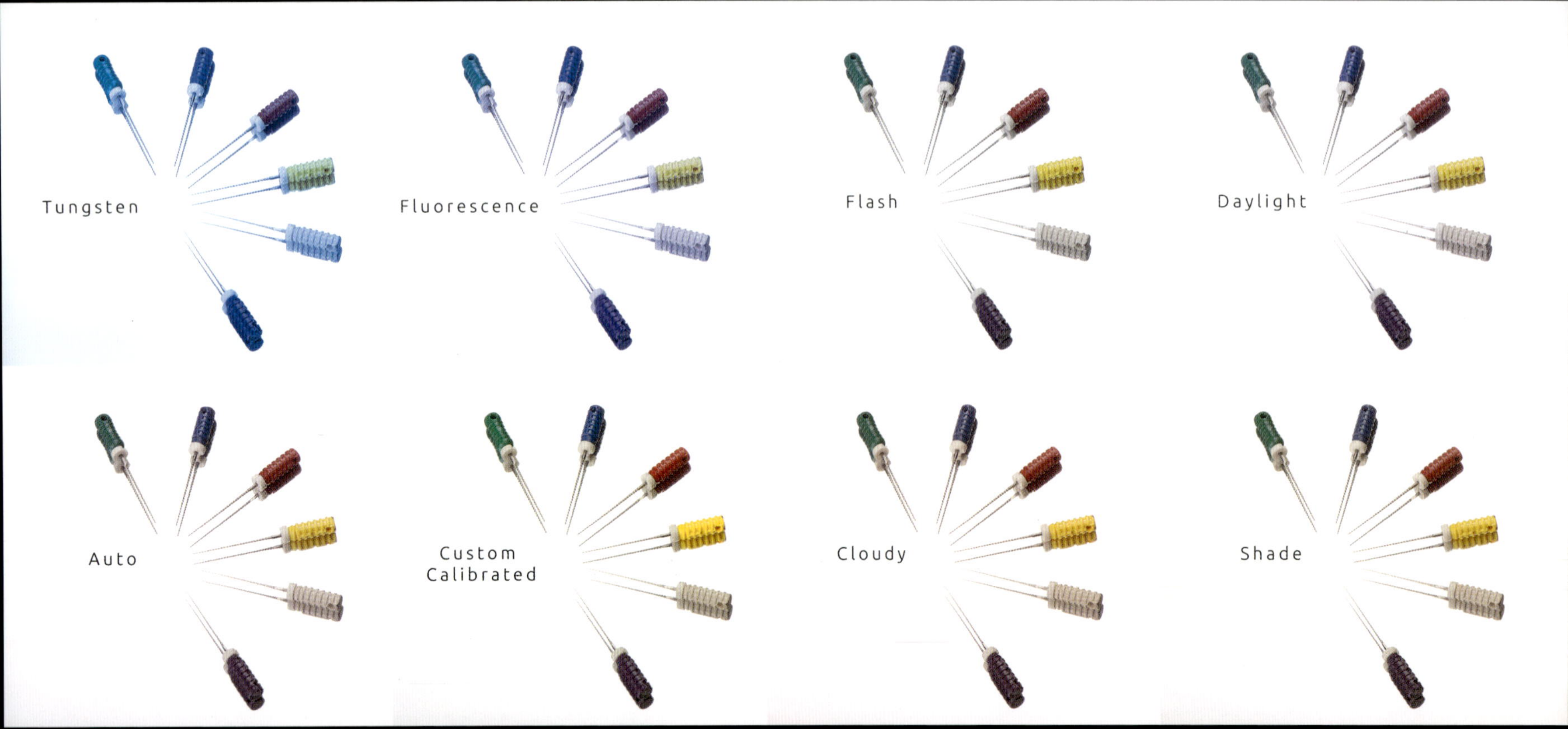

These photos were taken under the same lighting conditions, using a

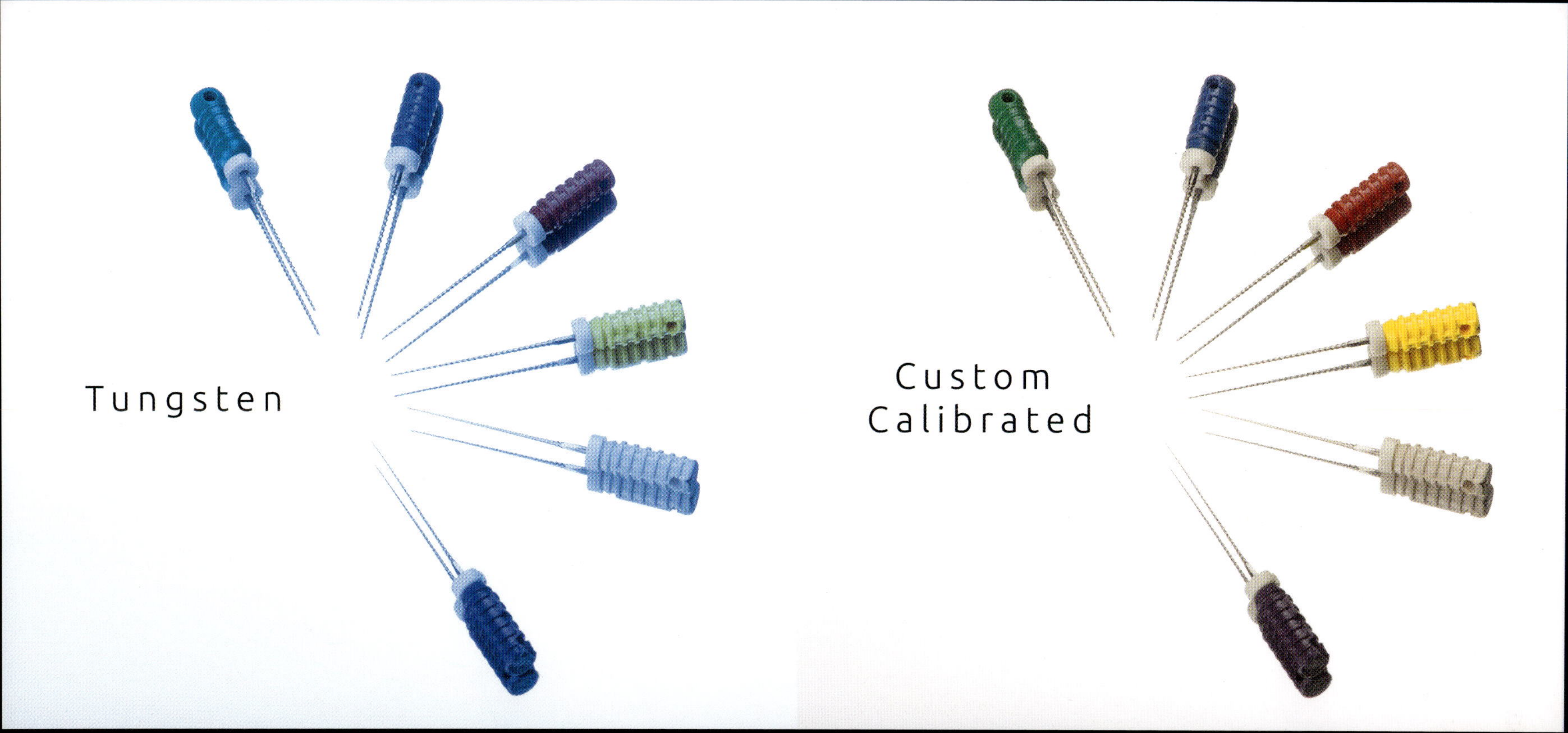

Same lighting conditions. The white balance setting on the camera was changed from

Advanced Tip

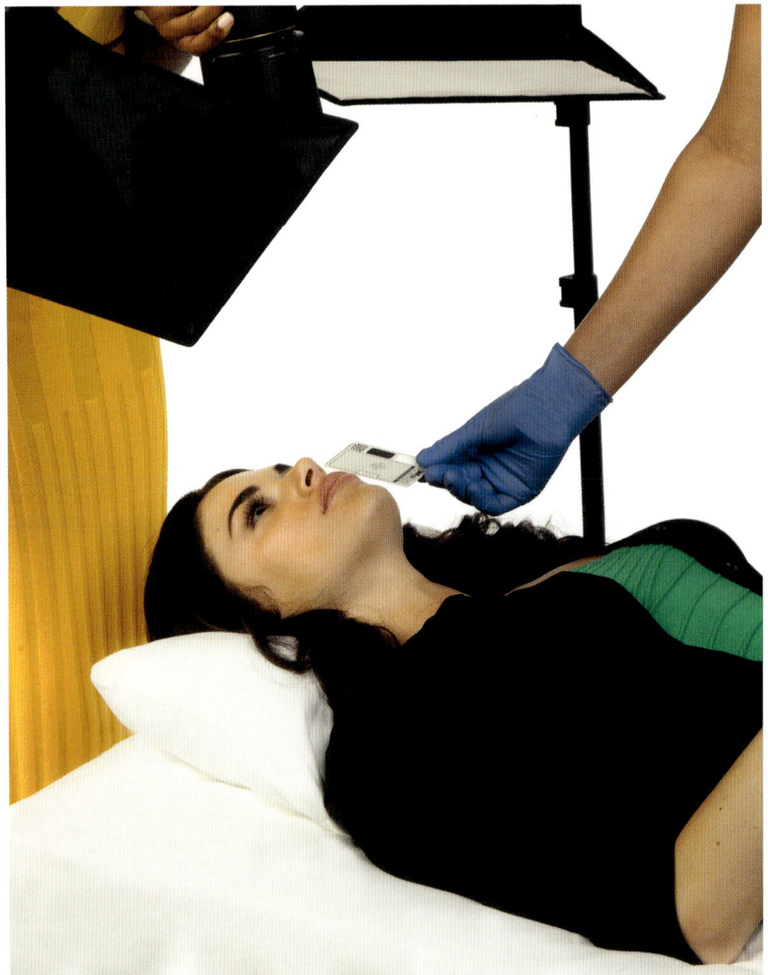

CUSTOM WHITE BALANCE

Take a photo of a gray card under your flash lighting conditions and your white balance set at 5,600K. Go into Photoshop and check the red, green, and blue (RGB) values on the card using the dropper function. If your photo has blue values higher than red and green, then your flash temperature is higher than 5,600K. That is why your picture has a blue tint to it. My flash/diffuser combos have a color temperature of 6,950K for example. Keep increasing your white balance settings to 5,700K, then 5,800K, etc, and taking the same photo with your gray card. When your RGB values are all the same, you have found the closest approximation of the real color temperature of your lighting conditions. Now, by placing this value in your camera's white balance setting, your photos will be as close to color balance as possible, as long as your lighting conditions do not change too much.

The camera can do this as well; it's called *custom white balance*.

The Big 5.

Master these and you will have mastered photography:

EXPOSURE

APERTURE

SHUTTER SPEED

DEPTH OF FIELD

WHITE BALANCE

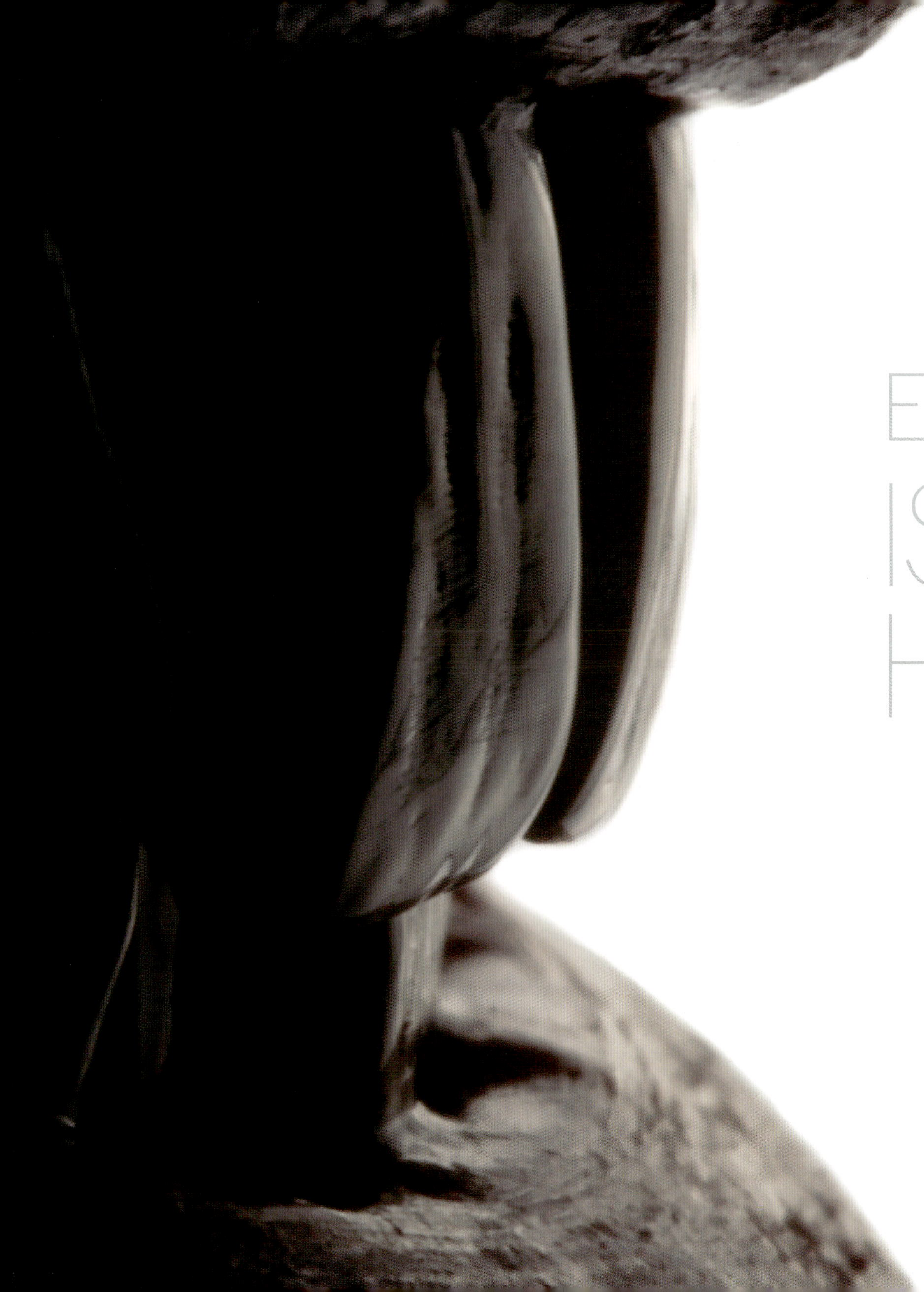

Encore: ISO and Histograms

The one that used to be: ISO

ISO used to be an important member of the Big 5. Now, slowly but surely, it has been losing its place, not because it is getting worse as a tool but because it is getting better. It is a bit like the planet Pluto. There I go again calling Pluto a planet. Sorry, I am so used to it. I do not know about you, but I talk about Pluto all the time, so it is hard to get used to a solar system with only 8 planets. Just like Pluto, ISO is losing relevance but for the better. ISO is related to the ability of the sensor to be sensitive to light. And who does not like a sensitive sensor? In the old days of film, we had the chance to pick what ISO number our film was. The common knowledge was that if you were shooting in low light conditions, you needed a film with ISO1600. If you were lucky enough to have the means you would buy ISO3200 films. These films were chemically different in a way that they could do more with less light reaching them. The negative trade-off was that the photo would incorporate noise in the form of graininess. Fortunately we can "ask" our digital sensors to be more sensitive to light by increasing the ISO number. Noise in the picture is once again the trade-off for increasing ISO. However, sensors are becoming so good that increasing ISO nowadays has almost no apparent noise. Increase your ISO once you have exhausted the limits of your settings for aperture and shutter speed. The higher the ISO number, the higher the exposure will be. Always do this by being aware of the limits of DOF and motion blur while modifying aperture and shutter speed. More about what those actual limits might be in dental photography will come later.

Question: I said before that as we increase the ISO, we increase the exposure of our photo. Was that a correct statement?
You might be thinking I am crazy right now. First I give you an explanation of ISO and then I ask you if my explanation is okay. That is nuts, right? Well, it is not that nuts, actually. I really want you to think about this for a second. What is the definition of *exposure* that we talked about in the first of the Big 5?

The definition of *exposure* has to do with the amount of light that reaches the sensor. If I take a photo and it is underexposed, then I increase my ISO and take the same photo, which is now exposed properly, did I increase the exposure? The answer is no. You did not increase the exposure because you did not get more light to that sensor. What you did was do more with the light you had by asking the sensor to be more sensitive to light. ISO does not change exposure; it changes "apparent exposure," which is a term I just made up. (So what? I can do that. I dare you to return this book when we are just getting started.)

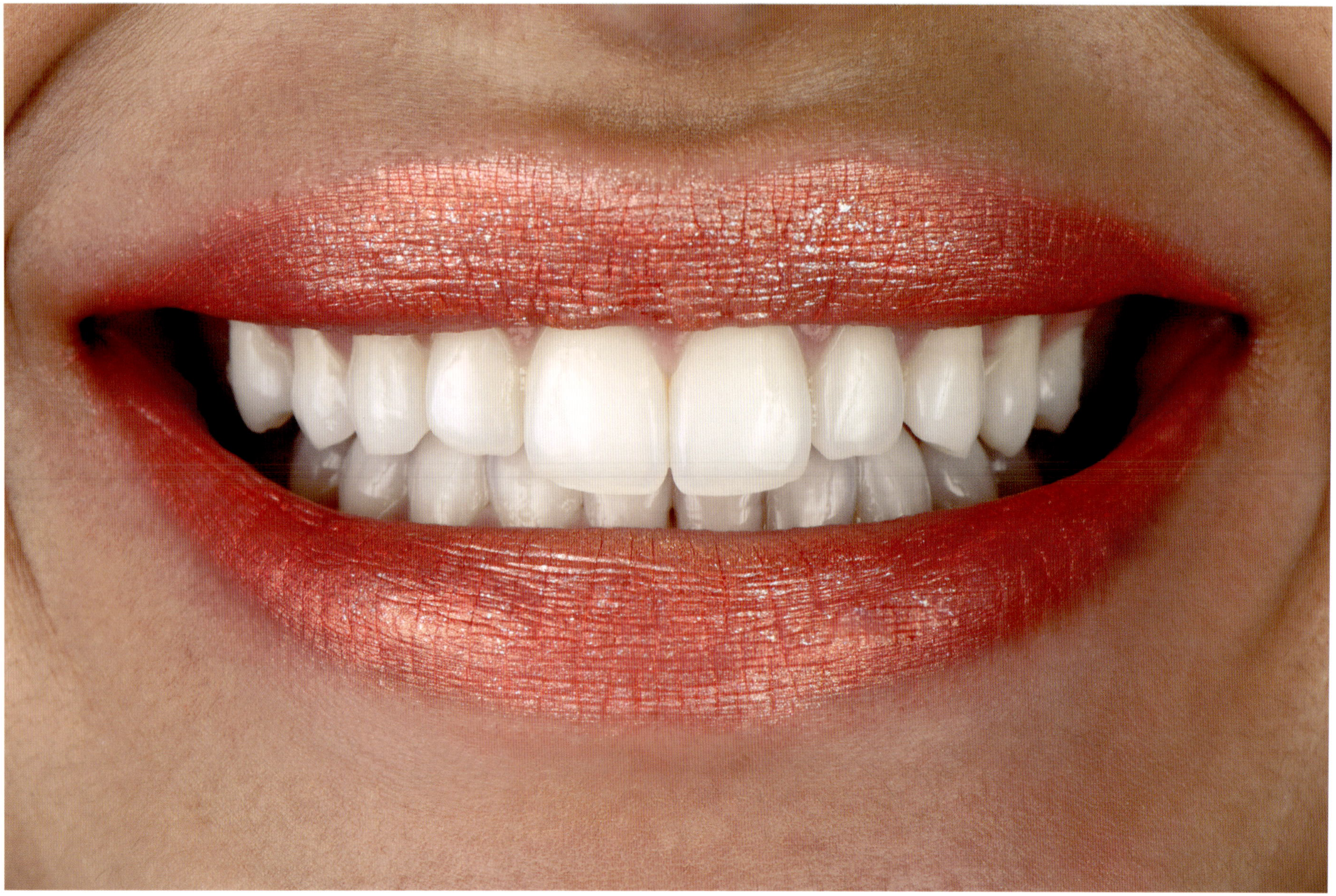

Optimal light
Low ISO

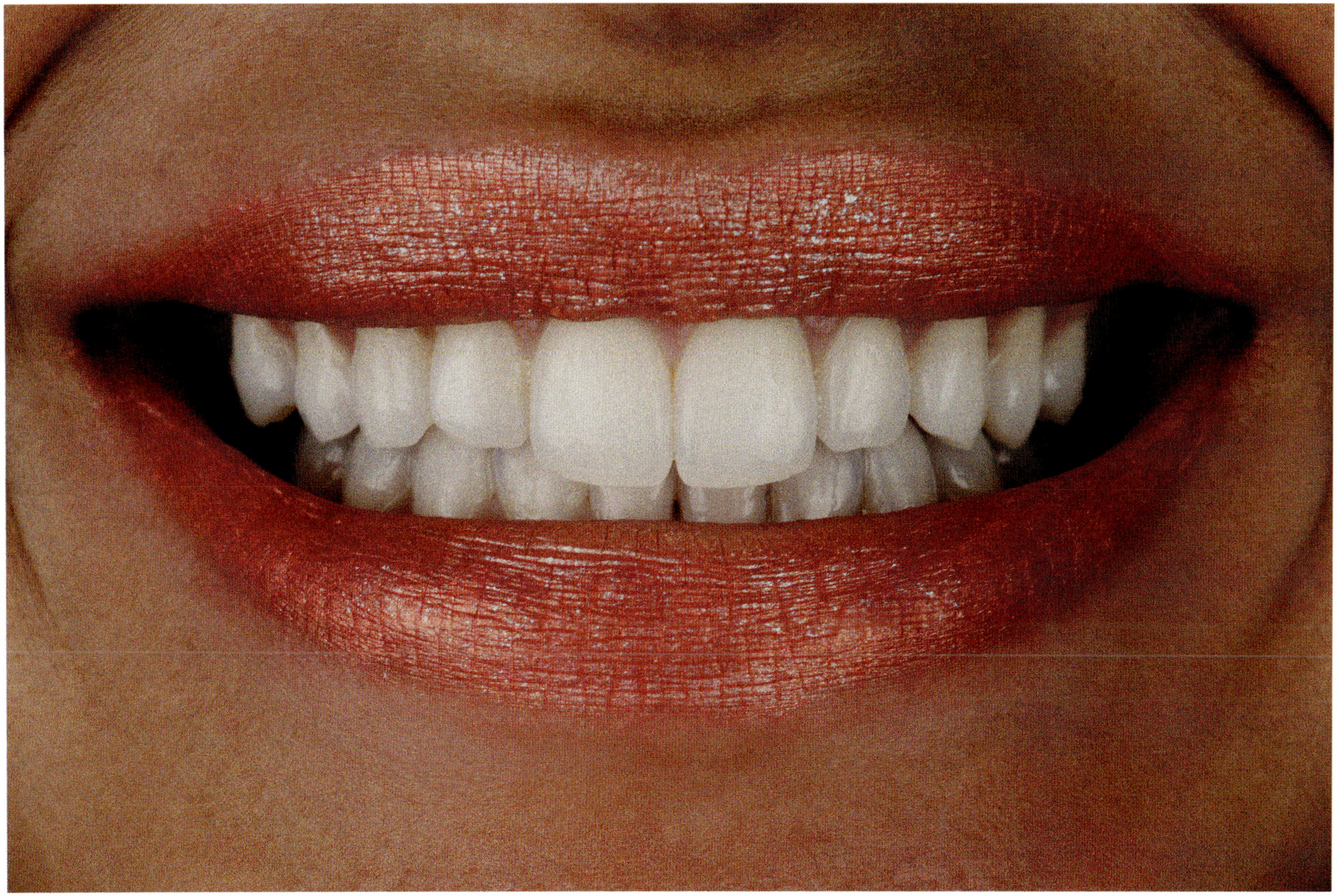

Low light
High ISO

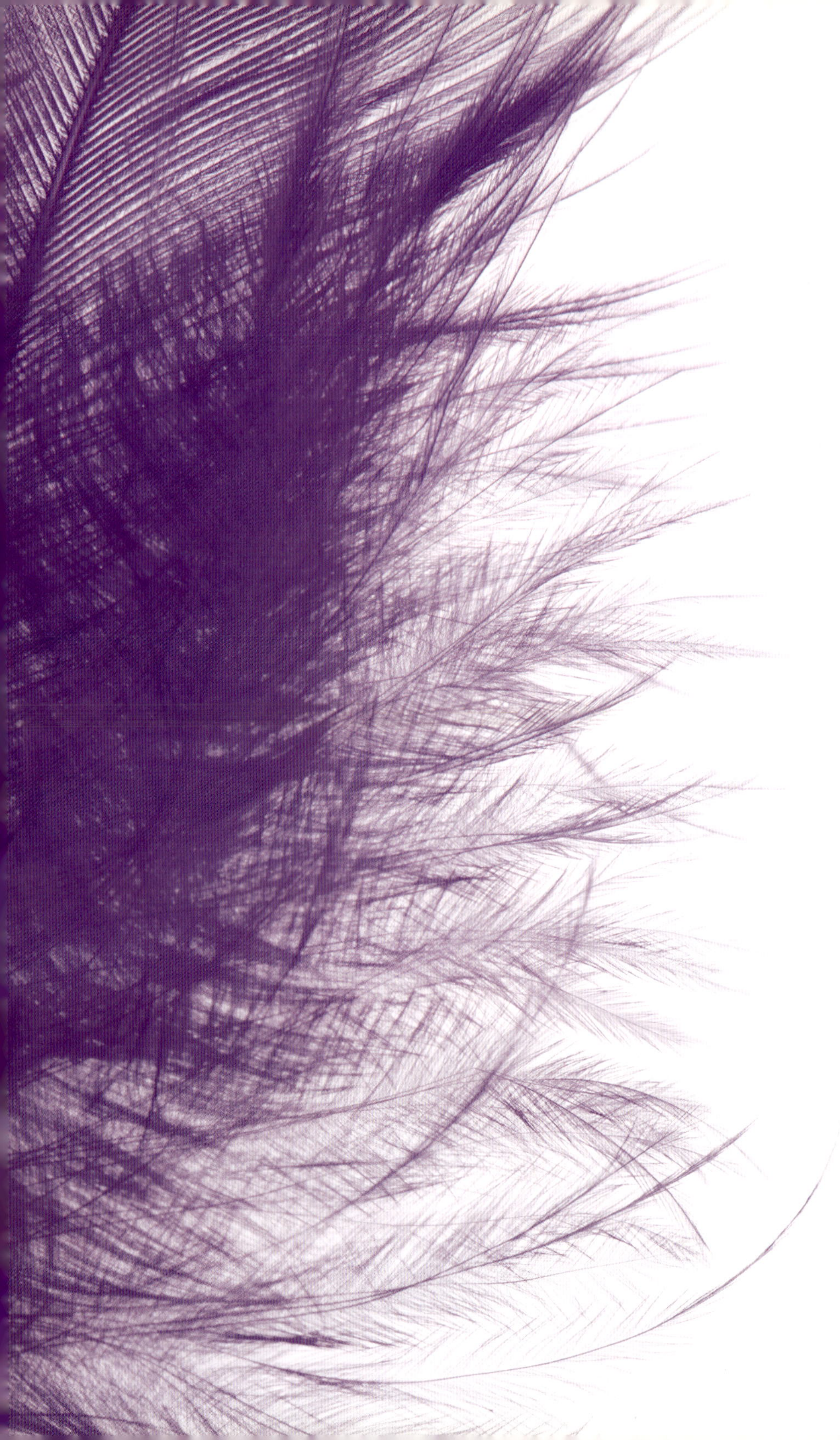

The histogram, not the Instagram

The *histogram* is a graphic representation of the amount of dark, medium, and light pixels found in your photo. It is a way of seeing, in a quantitative and visual manner, the amount of light versus dark present in your photo. It is presented on a graph with x and y axes. On the x-axis, we have a scale from 0 to 255. On the left, 0 depicts the darkest pixels—black pixels. On the right, 255 depicts the lightest pixels—white pixels. In between, we find the midtones, all the grays from dark to light. On the y-axis, we measure the number of such pixels as a relative amount.

The puzzle pixels

Imagine your photo is a jigsaw puzzle and each piece represents a pixel. Some are bright, some are dark, and some are shades of gray.

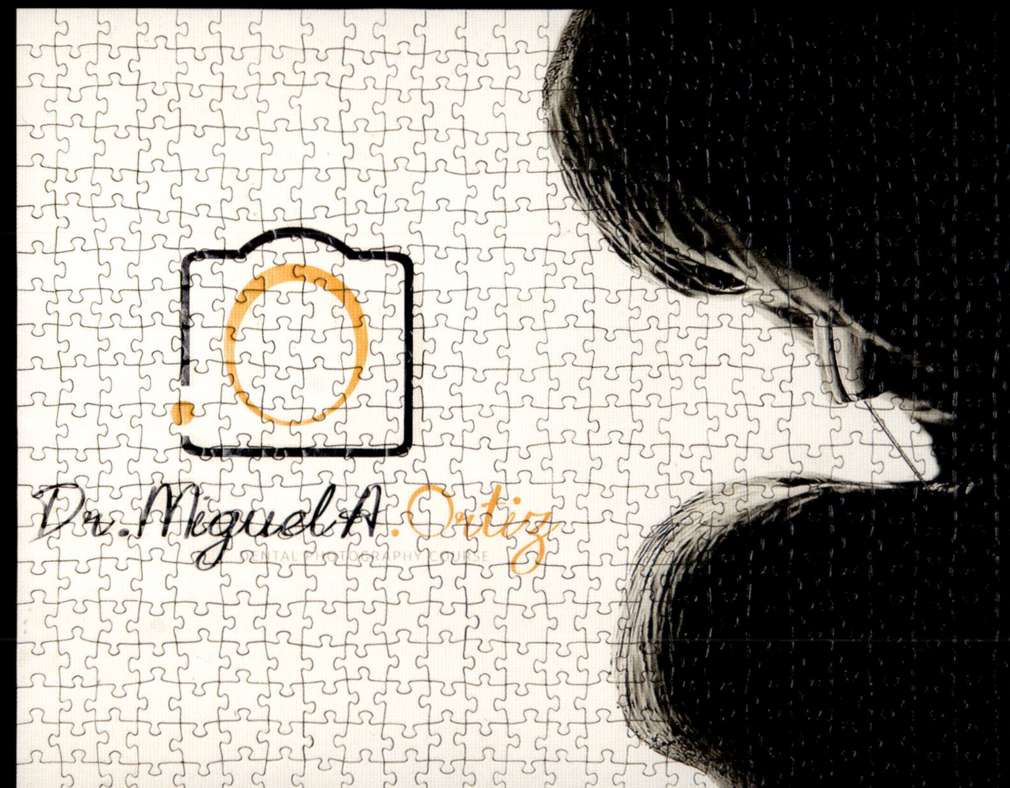

The puzzle pixel

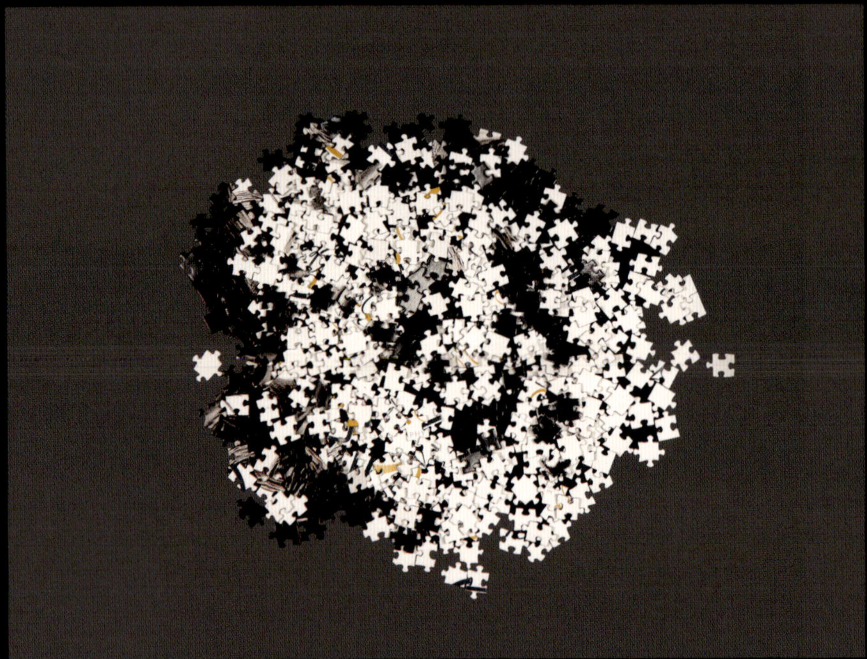

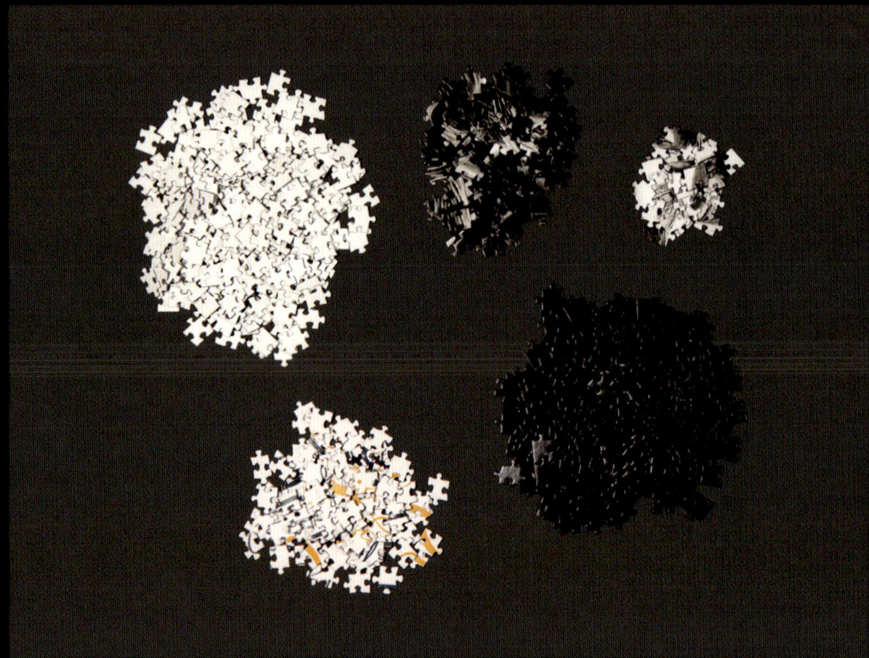

If you scramble all the pieces and separate them into piles by brightness—a pile of bright ones, a pile of dark ones—then you can count each pile and place the dark ones on the left and the other piles to the right, increasing in brightness.

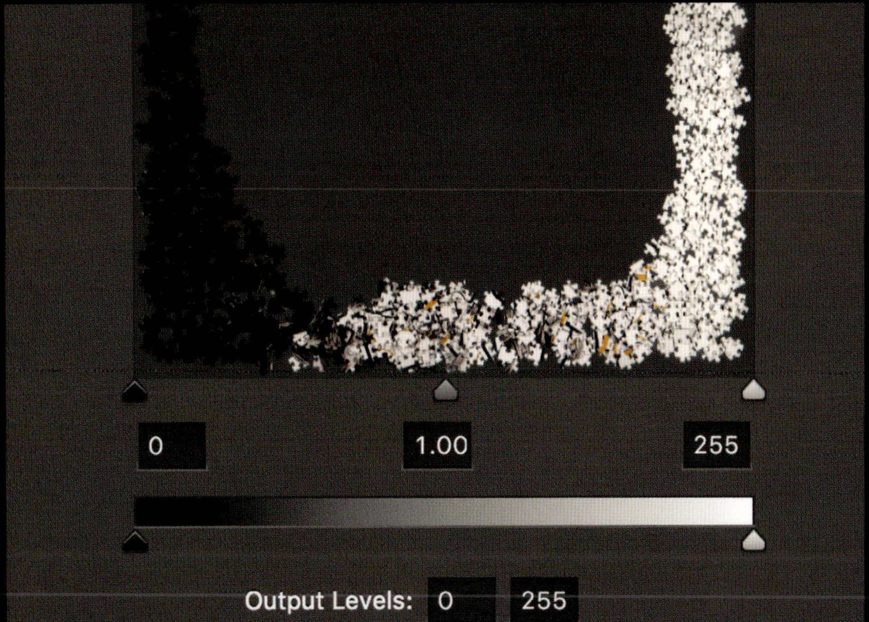
0
1.00
255
Output Levels: 0 255

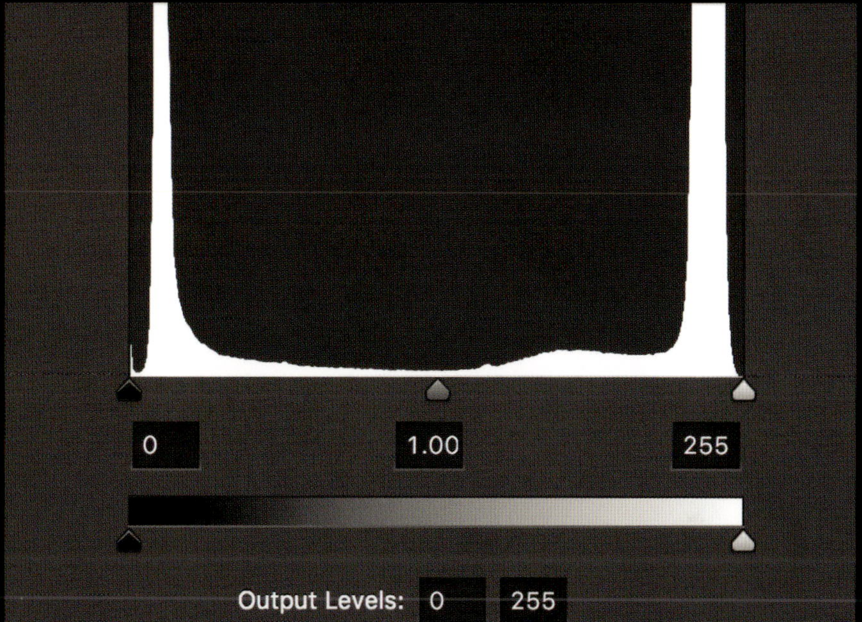
0
1.00
255
Output Levels: 0 255

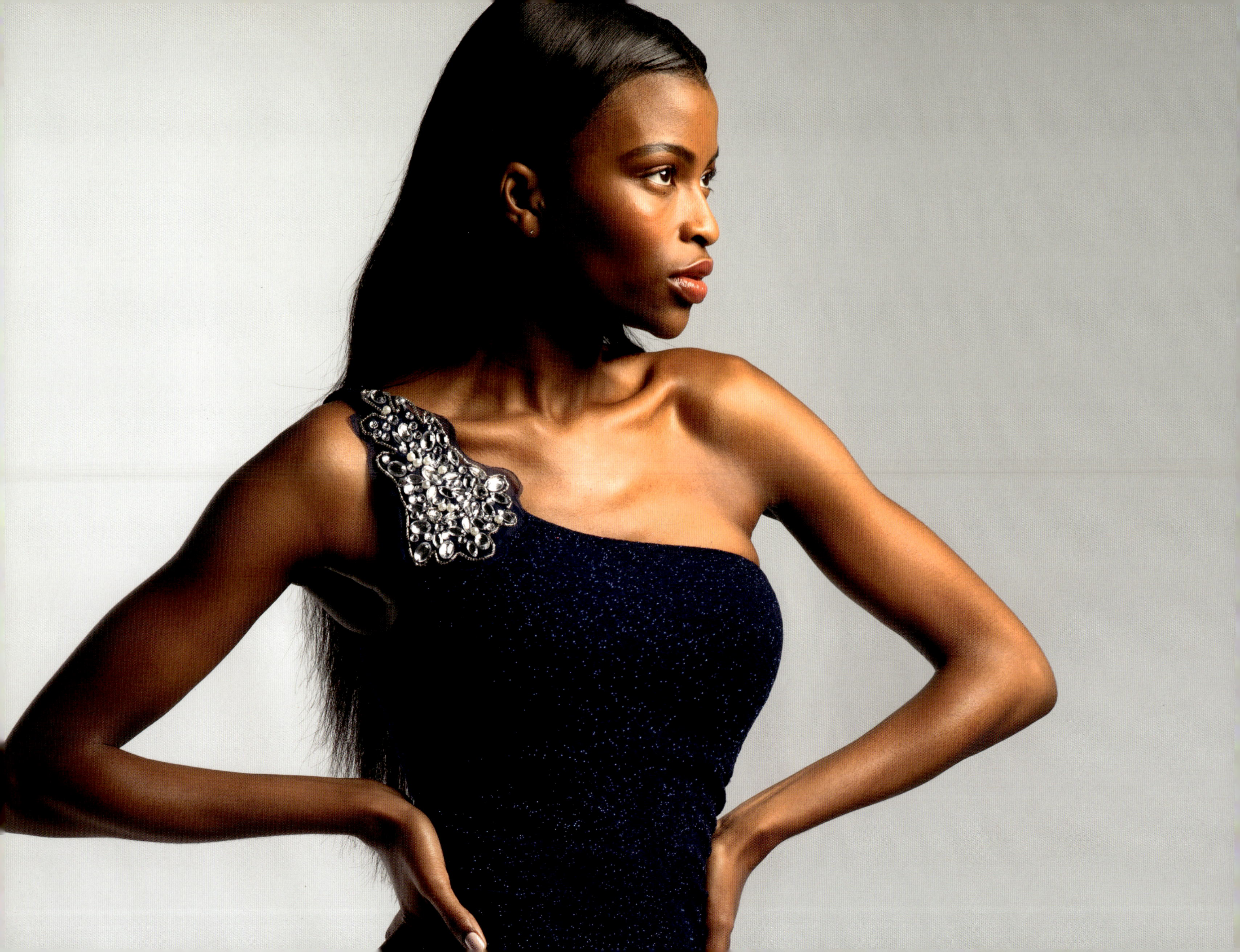

Sample histogram evaluation

A: The dark hair and dress

B: Skin tones

C: The light gray background

D: The lighter stones on the dress

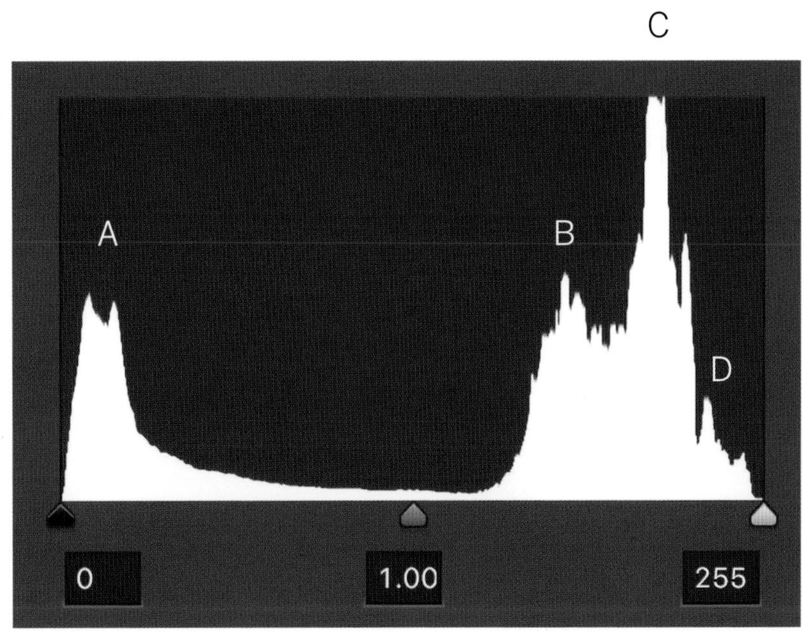

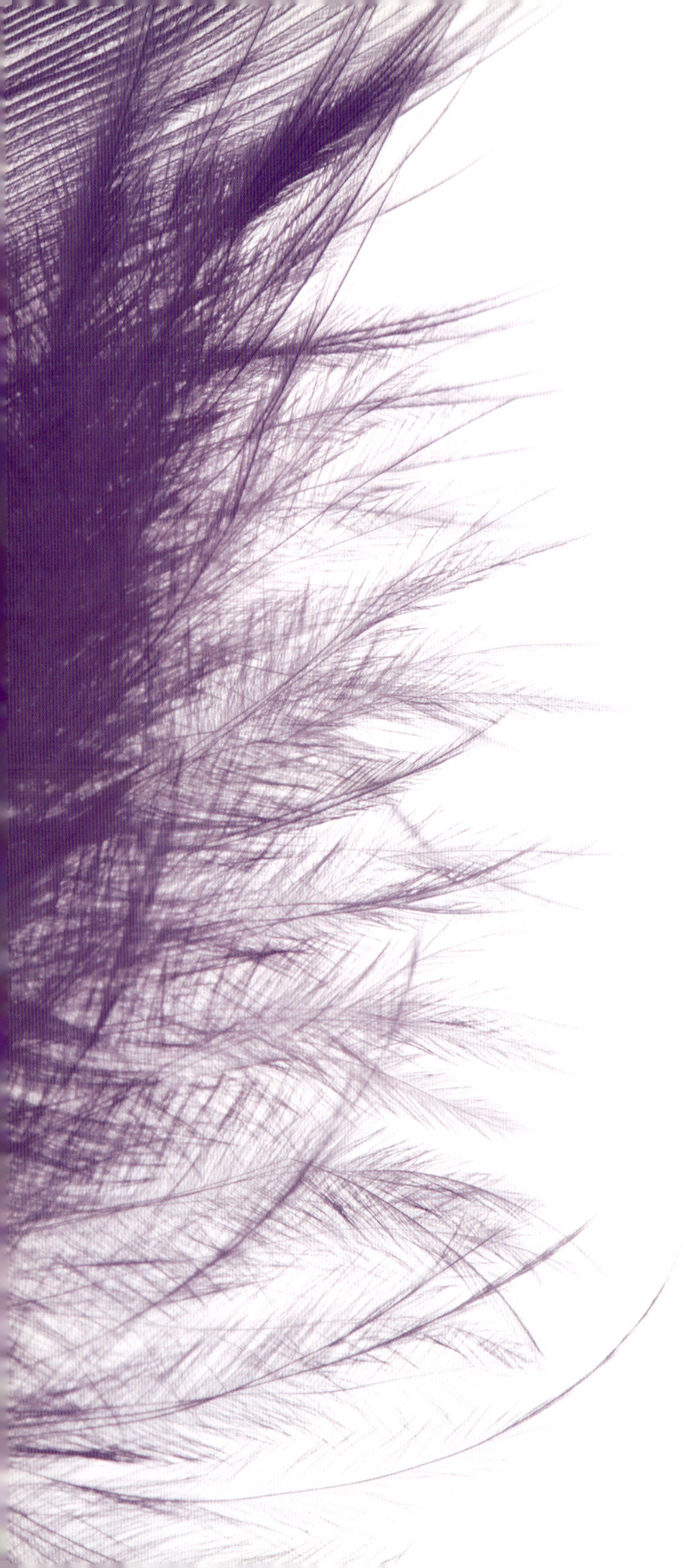

A valuable tool

The histogram can be set to appear on the camera screen, next to every photo we take. It is a tool to analyze exposure. If the graph looks one-sided to the left, it means there are a lot of dark pixels in that image. It might be okay if you are taking a picture of a black cat that occupies the whole frame. But if you are taking dental photographs, most of the time it indicates underexposure. The same applies for a heavily right-sided looking graph. Too many light pixels can often indicate that the photo is overexposed. I use the histogram for every photo. I barely look at my actual photos anymore. After I take a photo, my eye goes directly to the histogram and from there I can tell the quality of my exposure immediately.

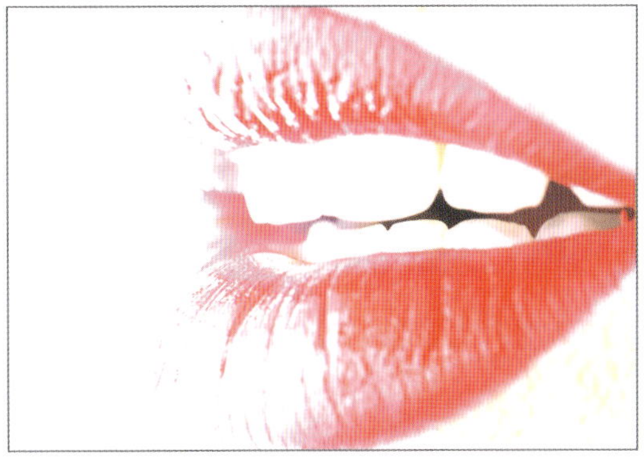

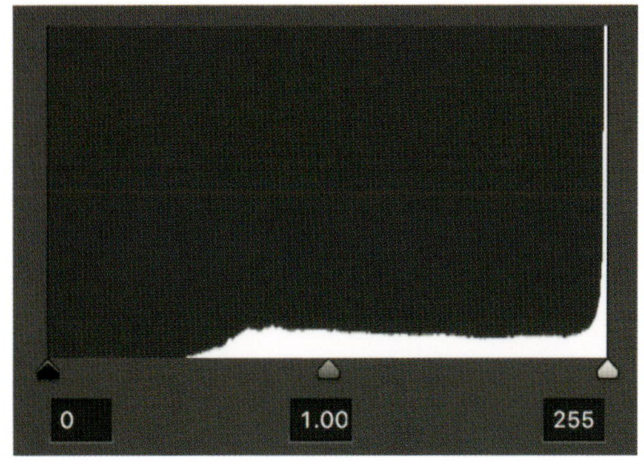

Overexposed = Right-sided histogram

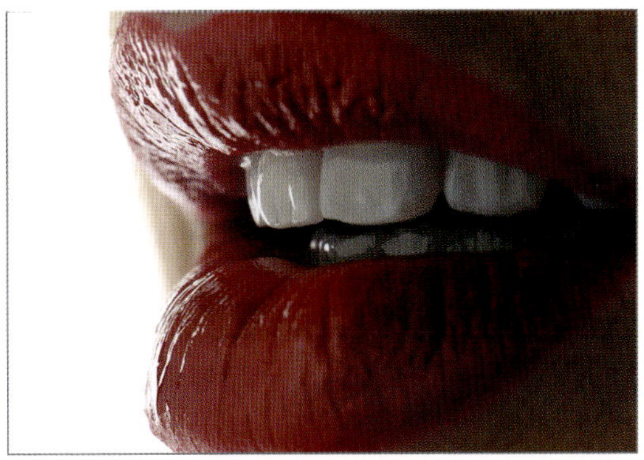

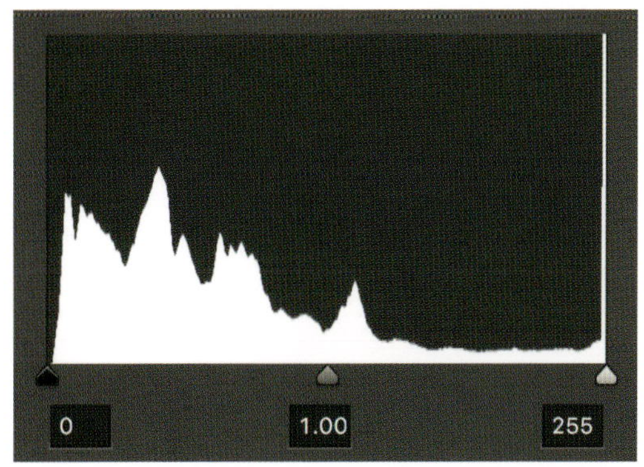

Desired exposure = Within the graph

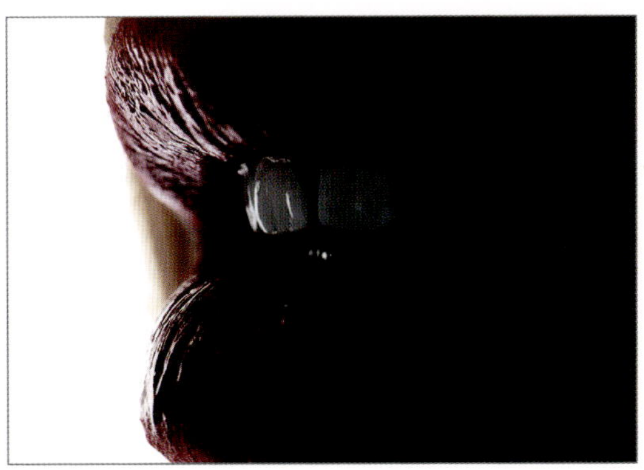

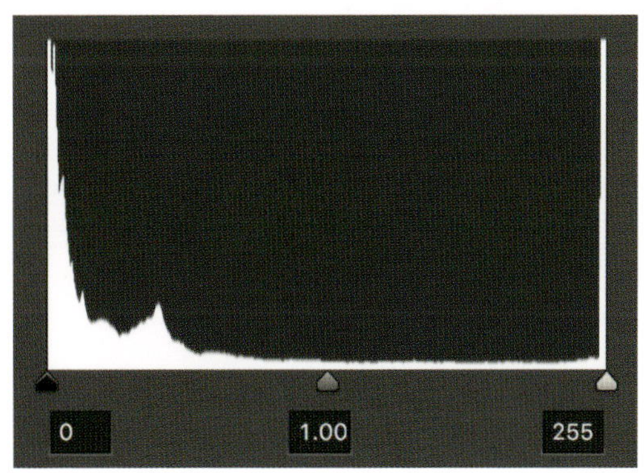

Underexposed = Left-sided histogram

Histogram of a smile

The classic histogram of a properly exposed photo of a smile has two main peaks:

A: In the middle, belonging to the skin and lips
B: To the right of the middle, belonging to the teeth

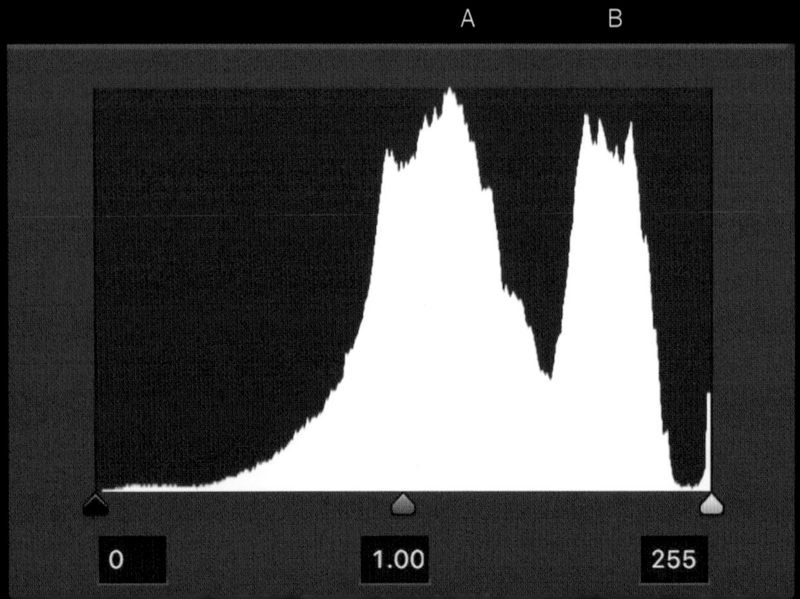

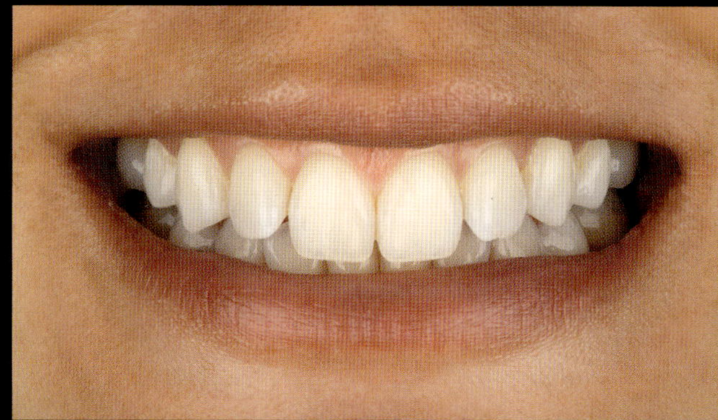

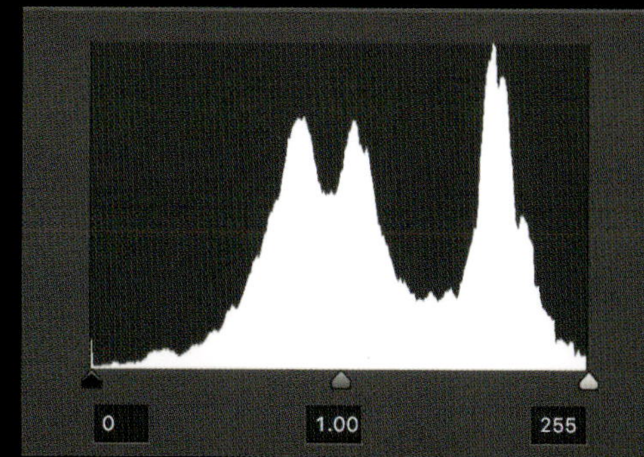
0
1.00
255

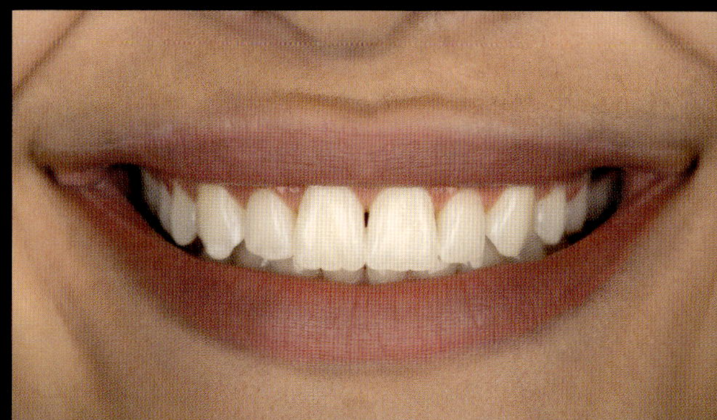

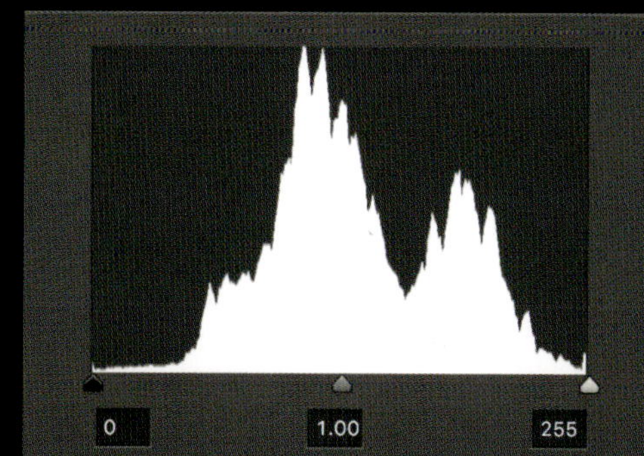
0
1.00
255

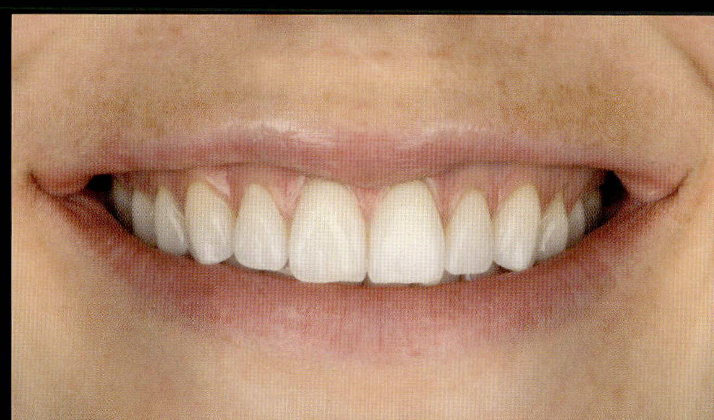

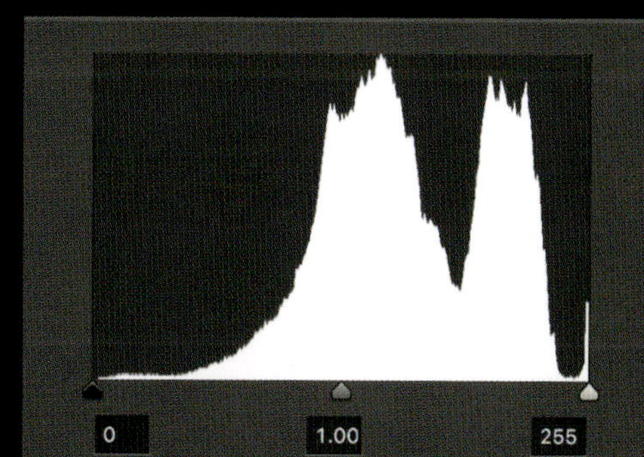
0
1.00
255

The Importance of Setting Limits

Aperture

Intraoral: Stay in between f/22 and f/36 to ensure proper DOF.
Portraits: f/16 to f/36

Shutter speed

Stay above 1/100 s to avoid motion blur and below 1/250 s to synchronize with your flashes. Never go above 1/250 s if you are using flashes.

ISO

Stay at 100, if possible, to avoid introducing noise.

Flashes

Always use full power and manual mode.

Dental Photography Equipment

The Main Items

Let's do a quick overview of the basic items you need to have. You do not have to break your piggy bank to get them.

- CAMERAS
- LENSES
- LIGHTING
- MIRRORS
- CONTRASTERS
- RETRACTORS

Cameras

The number one question I get from every beginner who wishes to take my courses is, "Which camera should I buy? Nikon or Canon?" If you are reading this book and you want to know which one is better, then I have an analogy for you. Imagine you are 16 years old and your parents are finally allowing you to learn how to drive. Not only that, you are lucky enough that they will buy you a brand new car. At this point, you ask your friend what you think is the most important question: "Which car should I buy: Mercedes Benz or BMW?" As you can see, I have come up with this bizarre analogy because I want to get a point across: It doesn't matter; you need to learn how to drive first. It doesn't matter if you get a Nikon or a Canon. They are both top-of-the-line equipment, just like Mercedes Benz or BMW. You just need to pick one. At the beginning, it might seem like an appropriate and important question, but the reality is that it is not. Once you buy an entry-level semiprofessional DSLR camera from either brand, you are equipped with all you need to succeed in dental photography. As I am writing this book, the Nikon D850 and D7200 are great options. The Canon EOS 5D Mark IV and EOS 80D are as well. When it comes to camera bodies, it is more important to know the difference between full-frame and cropped-sensor cameras.

Actual scene

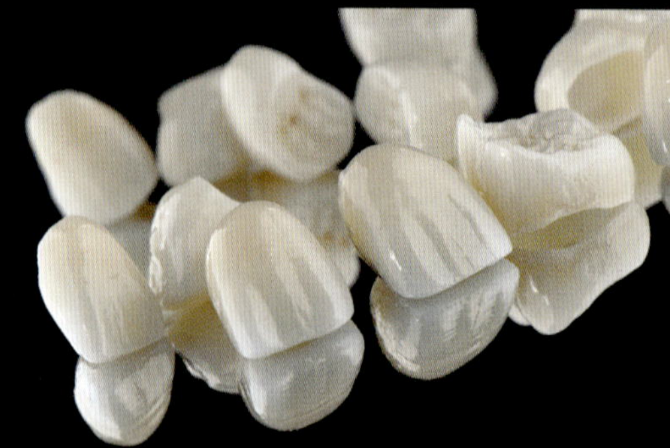

Light coming in the lens

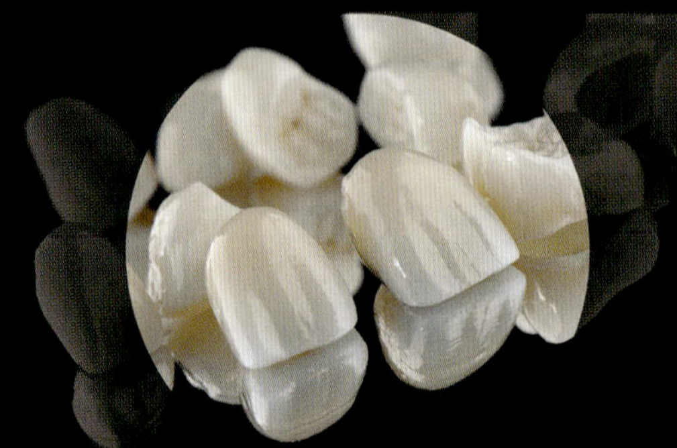

Light captured by full-frame sensor

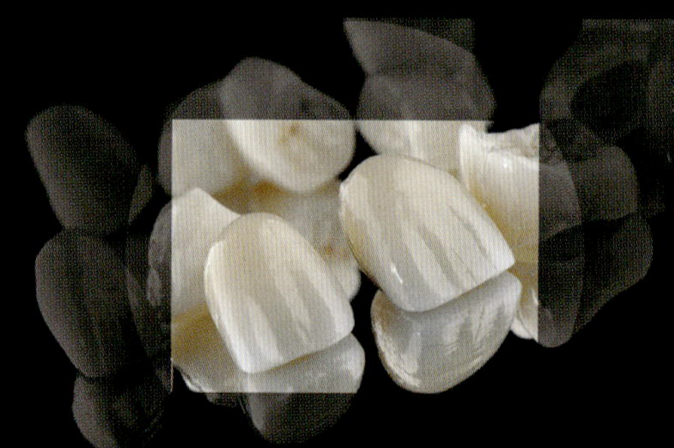

Light captured by cropped sensor

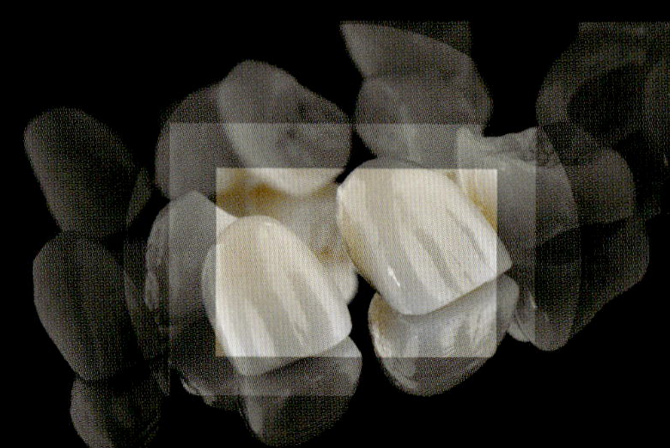

Cropped vs full frame

Full-frame cameras have a larger 35 mm sensor. Cropped-sensor cameras have a 24 (ish) mm sensor, creating a crop factor. The crop factor is about 1.5X. In plain language, when you use a cropped-sensor camera, you are zoomed in by 1.5X. Your 100 mm macro lens is actually a 150 mm lens.

You are zoomed in!

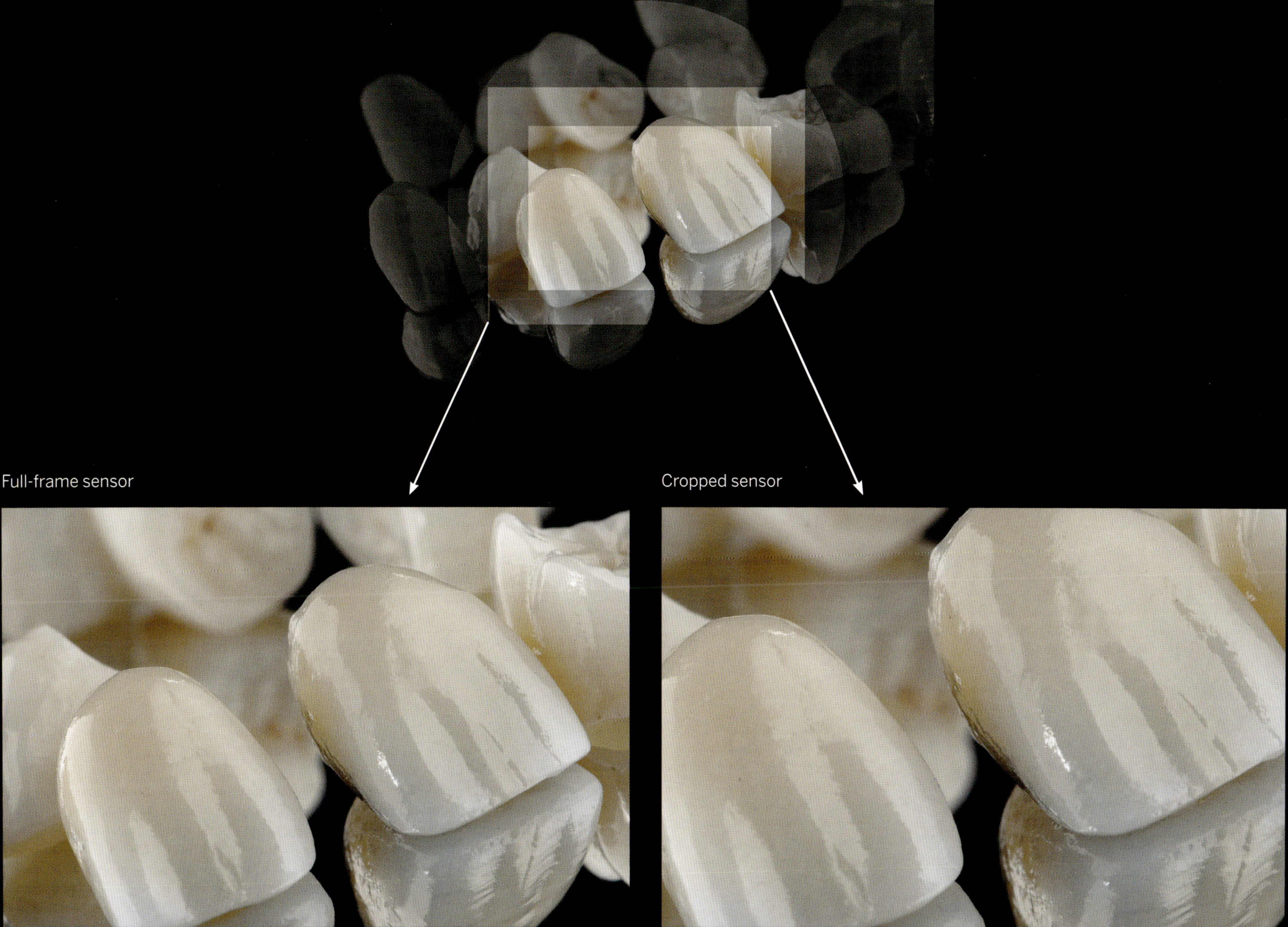
Full-frame sensor
Cropped sensor

Lenses

Lens selection is one of my favorite topics. I make a point in every course to ask the participants which focal length they think is the best for dental photography. My students have strong opinions about whether an 85 mm macro lens is better than a 100 mm, or even better, a 105 mm lens. There are always those who show up with a 60 mm macro lens and try to defend it, unsuccessfully.

Well let me tell you: You need a macro lens, that is for sure.

A macro lens allows for a reproduction ratio of 1:1 or larger, meaning that the subject size is reflected in the sensor at life size or larger. Macro lenses allow for the perfect working distance for dental photography at the highest image quality possible. Just like everyone in my courses, I have a strong opinion about which lens is better for dental photography as well. But people tend to get surprised about the reasoning behind it. Most people will respond when asked that a 100 mm or 105 mm is the best macro lens in dental photography. However, they cannot explain why. If a good answer is given, the same people fail to explain why their answer holds true for the 85 mm lens or a 90 mm lens also.

So why do most dentists use a 100 mm or 105 mm macro lens?

I think the answer is because they were told to do it. Those who told them to do it were, in turn, told by somebody else to do it. That is it and that is all. There is no scientific explanation for why a 100 mm or 105 mm is better than a 90 mm or 85 mm macro lens. However, I can give you a rational argument why 100 mm and 105 mm macro lenses are NOT better than an 85 mm macro lens. If you are reading this book and you are no taller than 5′10″ and you own a 105 mm lens, you might find the following scenario familiar.

Have you ever tried to take an intraoral photo using your 105 mm macro lens at the same time that you were holding the retractor or the intraoral mirror? If you have, have you ever wished your arms were longer? Or have you ever taken an intraoral or extraoral photo of a patient's smile, with the patient in the supine position where you are located behind the patient's head, and you found yourself on your tippy toes? Or have you ever tried to take a portrait of a patient with your 105 mm macro lens with a flash that is attached to your camera and the photo is repeatedly underexposed as if your flash was not working?

If you have encountered these scenarios yourself, you might suffer from "large-focal-length-for-no-reason" syndrome. This is a syndrome, that I just named, in which people buy 100 mm or 105 mm macro lenses because they were told to do it, and then they defend that choice while ignoring its limitations. How can we cure the syndrome, you might ask? Easily. You use an 85 mm macro lens. It is cheaper and lighter and has a shorter working distance, which allows you to stay off your tippy toes and not wish for longer arms or to be taller than average. When taking portraits, it positions you closer to the patient, allowing you to make better use of your flash, if it is attached to your camera. All of that and you get the same quality photos. To me, it is a no-brainer. However, I have to say, this only applies to cropped-sensor cameras. In a full-frame camera, I am okay having a 105 mm macro lens.

Lastly, should you buy lenses from the same manufacturer as your camera or can you buy lenses from a third-party manufacturer? The answer is both. Third-party lenses, such as Sigma, Tokima, and Zeiss, have achieved great quality and perform at a level of those from camera manufacturers.

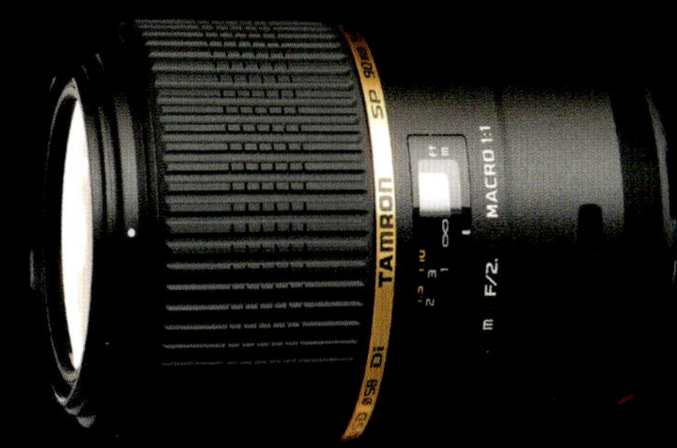

Tamron 90 mm

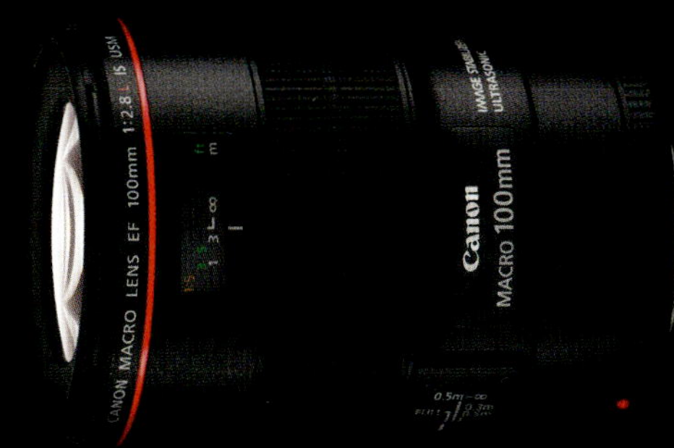

Canon 100 mm

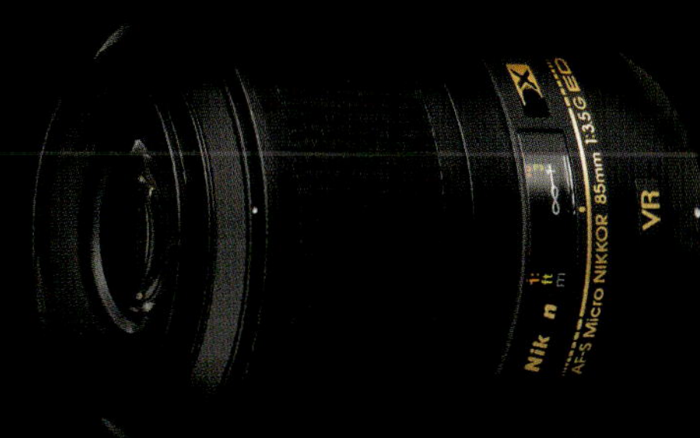

Nikon 85 mm

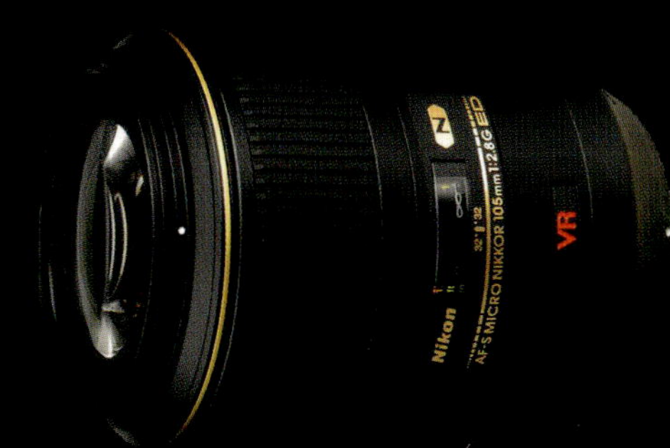

Nikon 105 mm

Large-focal-length-for-no-reason syndrome

Prevalence: Almost 50% of dentists suffer from this condition. It affects mostly people shorter than 5'10" who bought a Canon with a 100 mm lens or a Nikon with a 105 mm macro lens, just because they were told to do so. The crop factor puts them in a ZOOMED-in position equivalent to a 150 or 160 mm lens. People who are taller than this also forget their assistants might not be.

Symptoms: The classic tiptoe dancing behind the patient in order to get the entire smile in frame; stretching the arms to infinity to hold any appliance while taking the photo themselves; and walking backward about a mile to be able to take a portrait.

Treatment: Consider an off-brand 70 to 90 mm macro lens or the Nikon 85 mm Micro.

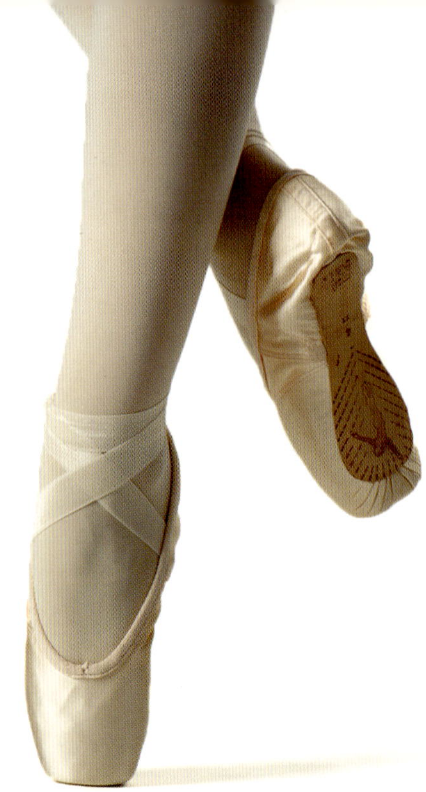

We have come to the most underestimated aspect of dental photography, or possibly any kind of photography: lighting. We must remember that photography is nothing but light hitting a sensor. Without light, photography will not exist. So let us dive into the different kinds of light and light modifiers that allow for all the magic to happen.

For the purpose of dental photography, there are two types of light sources: continuous light and flashes.

Continuous light is a light that is always on. These types of light sources are mostly used for video recording. If you think of the news anchors on television, they are under large high-intensity, continuous light, such as spotlights. These lights are great because they allow the scene to be evaluated and modified based on what it looks like in the present time. The person behind the camera knows if more or less light is needed before recording or taking the photograph. However, continuous light has some serious drawbacks. They are large, expensive, and hard to mobilize. They consume lots and lots of energy, and they can become extremely hot after being on for some time. In the dental arena, they are not practical. So we do not use them in clinic at all.

Flashes, on the other hand, have most of the qualities we need. They are small, inexpensive, and portable, and they do not tend to get hot. The most common is the on-camera flash—that useless little pop-up thing on the top of your camera. Do me a favor: If you have made it this far in the book, it means that you care about the kind of photography you want to take. In that case, **do not ever use the on-camera flash**. I believe this so strongly that I do not want to give that flash any part in this book. Just do not use it.

There are several types of real flashes. I will review the general characteristics of the following: ring flash, dual flashes, speedlights, and strobes.

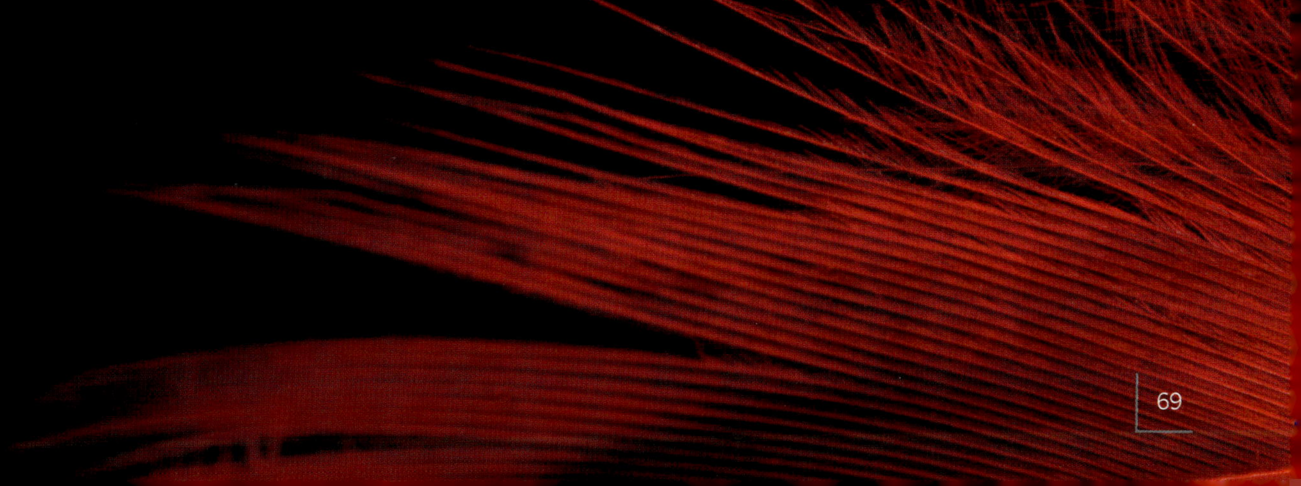

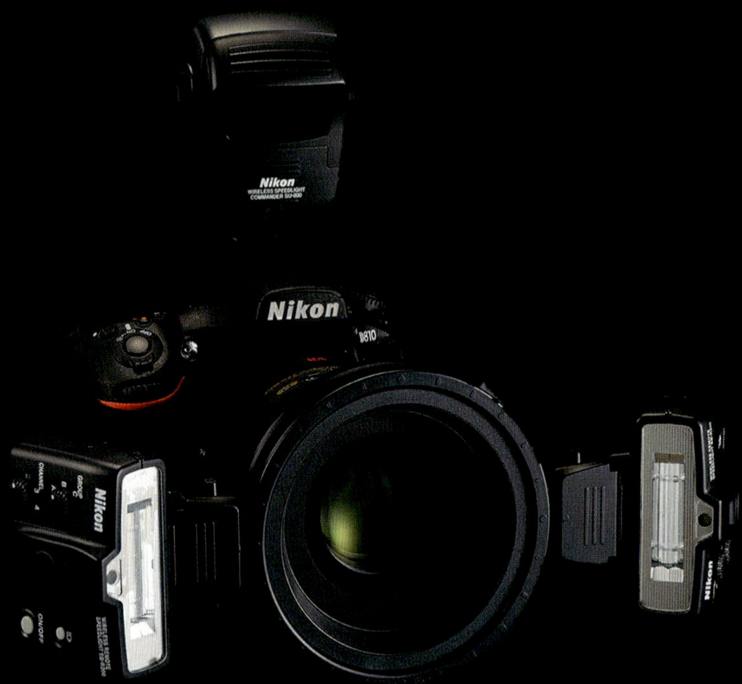

Nikon R1C1 dual flash system

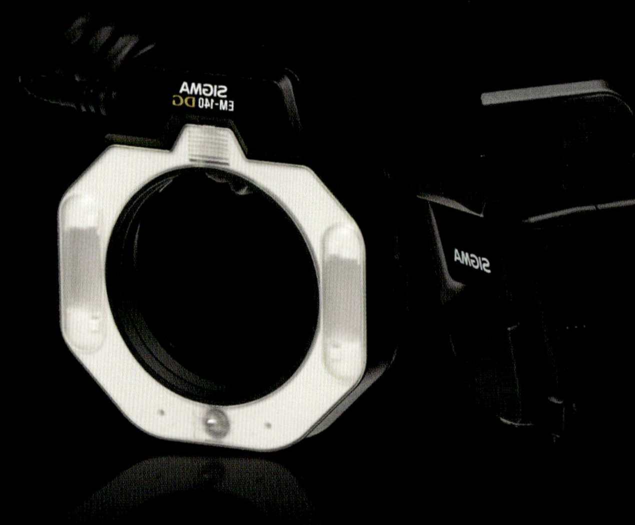

Sigma ring flash

Ring flash

The ring flash continues to be the number one dental photography flash for most dental offices. For those who do not have the time, space, or expertise to manage a dual-flash system, the ring flash will deliver properly exposed photos on most, if not all, intraoral protocols. Its closeness to the subject and the lens itself allows it to illuminate the farthest and trickiest places in the oral cavity. However, when it comes to that outstanding and breathtaking fine dental photography that we all love to see, the ring flash falls short. Its burst of light creates an aura of high intensity in the center of the frame. As we move outward, the light diminishes sometimes to a point of underexposure, all within the same image. The resulting photo presents with a lack of depth and character. It is flat and with minimal texture.

It is at this point that we need to talk about detaching the flashes from the camera to achieve more pleasant photos.

Dual flashes

Dual flashes are becoming more and more common in dental photography. With the introduction of the Nikon R1C1 system, the dual-flash system became one of the most desirable sets of flashes to own. However, as those who own one know, they are not as easy to use as they might seem. In order to really take advantage of these kinds of flashes, they must be able to be placed far from the lens itself. Having the capacity to reposition these flashes is what allows a photographer to fully explore lighting like never before. The problem is that, in the dental setting, it requires either a second person holding the flashes or the use of wings/brackets. These wings/brackets are terribly hard to master, and they increase the weight of the camera substantially. It also requires the photographer to constantly reposition the flashes to avoid unintended shadows in the picture. Fortunately, the positives outweigh the negatives when it comes to dual flashes. They allow for light effects and modification that cover the range of almost everything that is possible. They are small and can be used for all kinds of macro photography. In our field, they are great for tabletop laboratory-type photography as well.

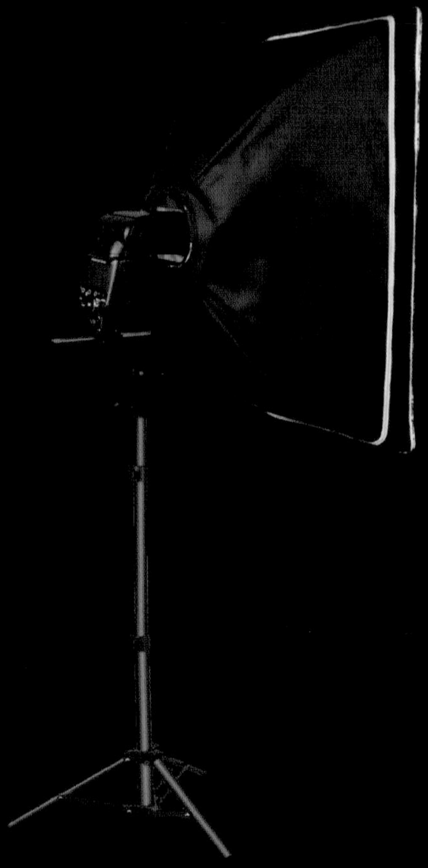

Speedlight mounted on softbox

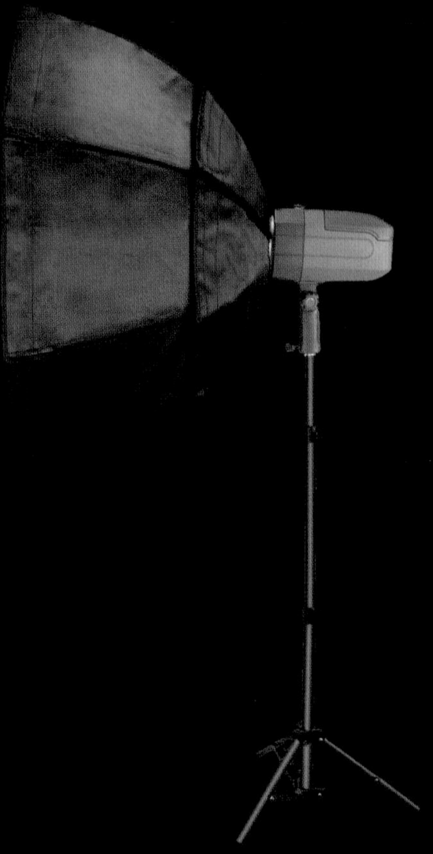

Strobe mounted on softbox

Speedlights

In my opinion, speedlights are the best thing that could have happened to dental photography. In recent years, a new wave of fully loaded speedlights have come out at a price that was a dream only a few years back. They are small, portable, inexpensive, powerful, and reliable. They can be used in as many ways as the dual flashes but at a tenth of the cost. They possess a greater battery life and higher intensity light than dual flashes as well as an immense capacity to be the subjects of light modifiers. Speedlights are what will separate you from the average dental photographer.

There are many ways to go about speedlights. You can buy the expensive but super reliable Nikon or Canon units. You will pay the price, but the result is guaranteed. You can also go with the off-brand speedlights. They are very affordable but do not have a strong brand behind them in case anything happens to them. The versatility of speedlights is what makes them perfect for dental photography. You will be using them off your camera with a commander. You can have a small diffuser on them, a large diffuser, an umbrella, a softbox, etc. You decide. One thing is for sure: Be ready to buy a large set of rechargeable batteries.

Strobes

Strobes are the number one tool of a studio photographer. They emit a large and powerful burst of light (just like flashes). Strobes are ideal when a designated area is set apart for taking photos. Strobes are not ideal if you have to move them a lot. They are bulky, pricey, and delicate. They require more room to maneuver. However, the positives are very enticing. They can generate high-intensity light in a fast, repetitive manner (fast recycle time). What this means is that you can take several photos back to back in fast succession and the strobes are going to keep firing. All other flashes discussed already have trouble with that. Strobes tend to be plugged into the wall, which means you do not have to worry about changing batteries. They are great but not practical around the dental chair. They also come with a continuous light that is helpful for pre-illumination and focusing. It allows you to see your photographic composition better than a flash.

We will discuss the use and results of each of these lighting systems in the next chapters, where portrait, clinical, laboratory, and artistic photography will be demonstrated in depth.

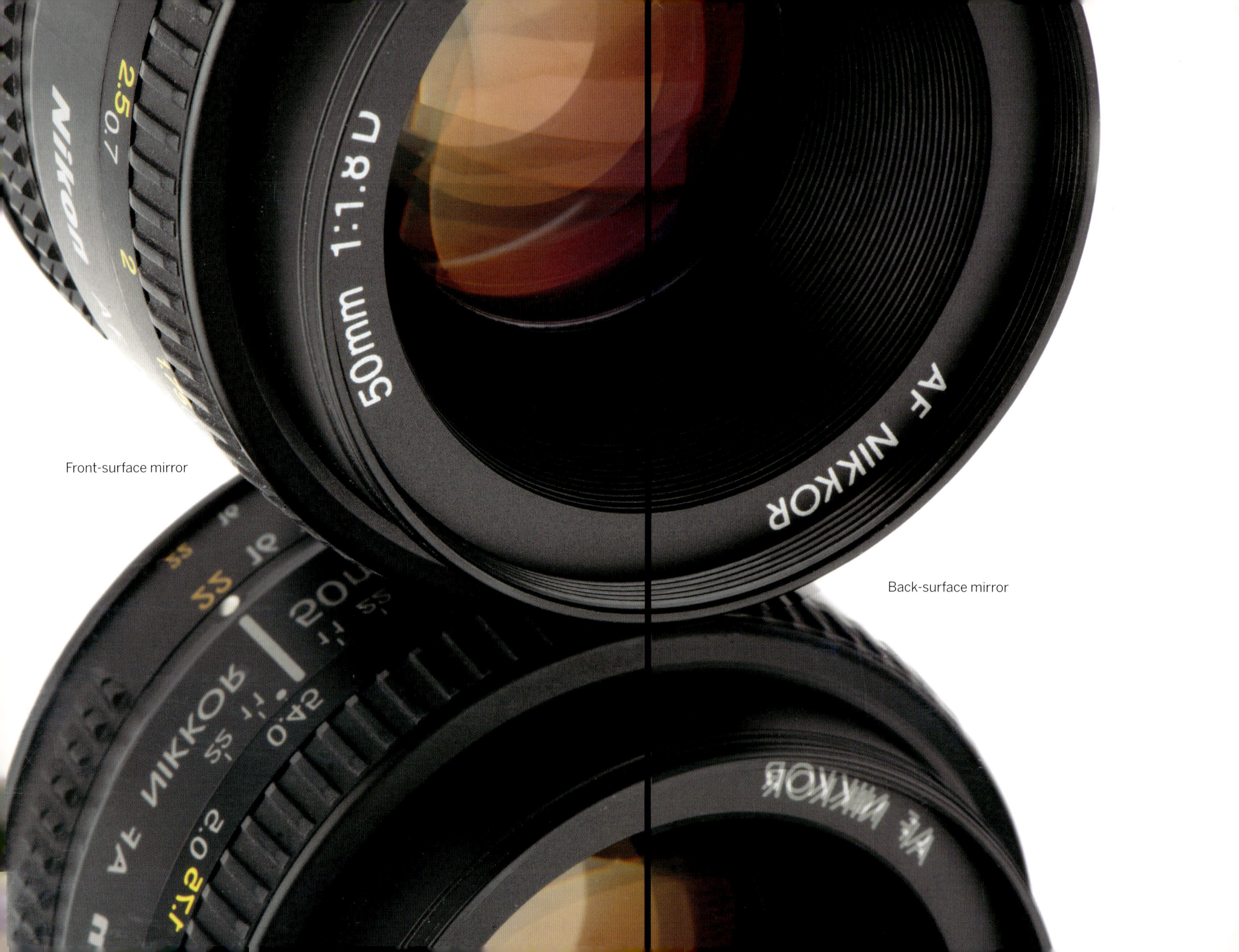
50mm 1:1.8 D
AF NIKKOR
Nikon
Front-surface mirror
Back-surface mirror

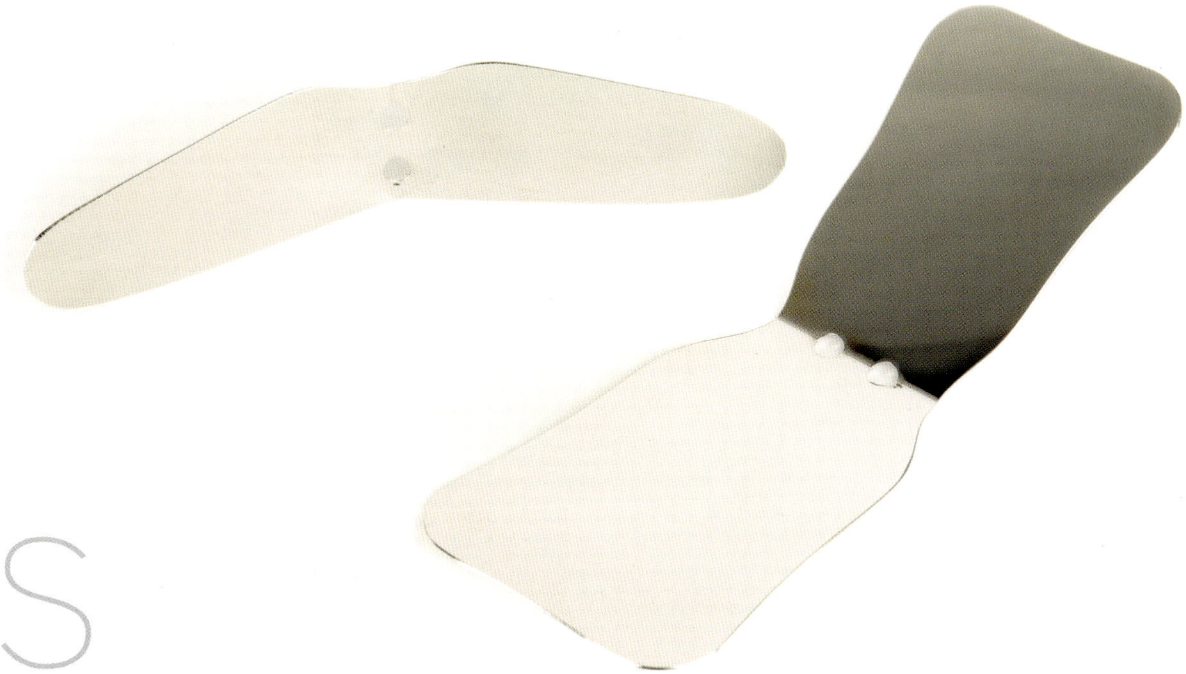

Mirrors

If we choose a glass-based mirror, we must understand the difference between a front-surface mirror and a back-surface mirror. A front-surface mirror has its reflective coating on the front of the glass element. This allows for an image with no ghost counterpart. A back-surface mirror has the reflective coating on the back of the glass element. When the light travels through the glass on a back-surface mirror, it reflects on the back coating and it comes back as a mirror reflection. However, some of the light does not make it through the glass, and it reflects on the front surface of the clear glass, creating a double image.

By any means, a crisp image without a double image is always desired. You might ask, "Why wouldn't we always use front-surface mirrors?" The answer is money, mostly. They are more expensive. At the same time, front-surface mirrors are much easier to scratch than back-surface mirrors. We all know that scratched mirrors are common in a dental office.

Metal mirrors are by definition front-surface mirrors. If the reflective surface is obtained by finely polishing the metal only (no coating present), then these mirrors tend to be a bit more scratch-resistant than coated ones. I personally like metal mirrors. I find them reliable, thin, and easy to use.

Contrasters

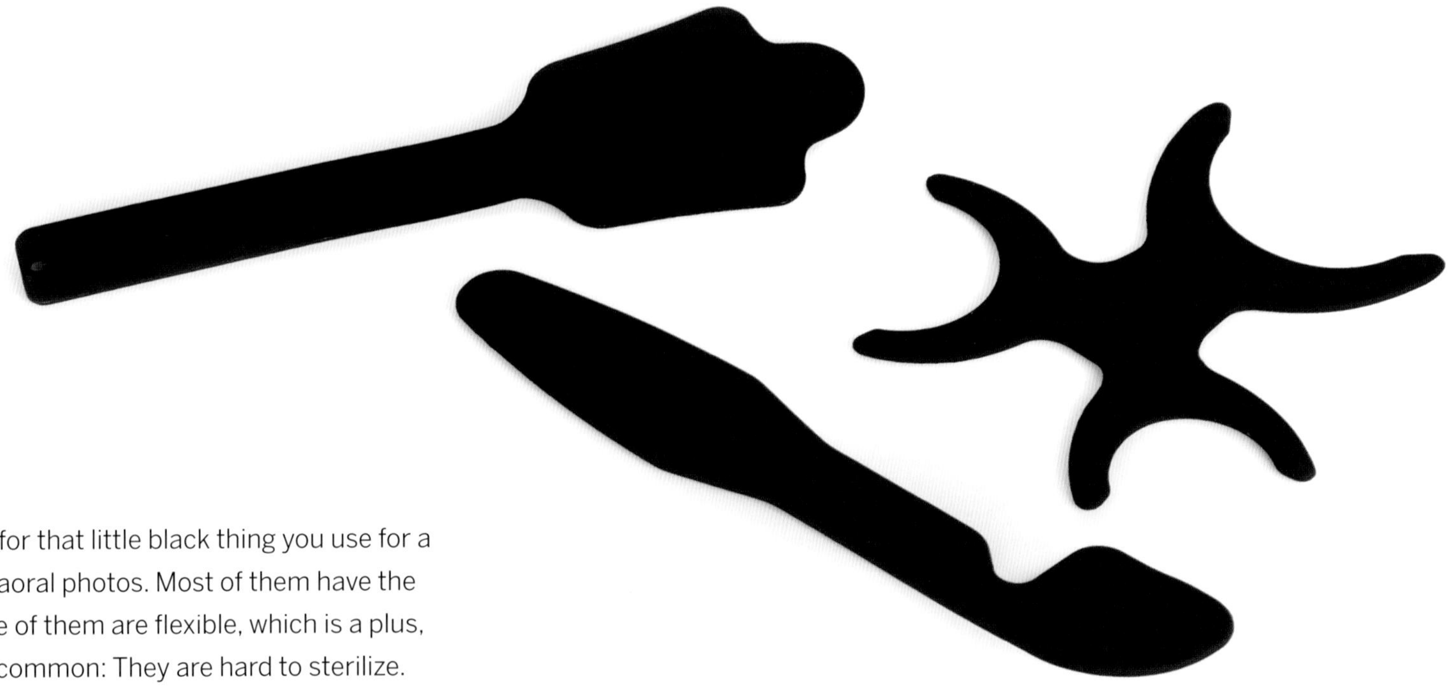

Contraster is the fancy name for that little black thing you use for a black background in your intraoral photos. Most of them have the same set of shapes, and some of them are flexible, which is a plus, but they all have one thing in common: They are hard to sterilize. No matter how you sterilize them, they seem to get gray or degrade with time. There are several brands available. You can find the ones that are made out of pure metal that have been painted black. There are also those that have a rubbery coating, creating a more light-absorbing surface. These last ones also have the capacity to be bent if necessary, which sometimes comes in handy.

Retractors

There are many types of retractors out there. I find that the metal wire retractors work best for me. Other clinicians like to use V-shaped plastic retractors. There are those who like to use C-shaped plastic retractors. You should use what works for you.

In any case, here is another tip: If you take two C-shaped retractors and cut one end off each retractor and polish it, you will be able to more easily position the contraster and occlusal mirror without interference from the retractors. I rarely have a problem with the wire retractors, so I use them for all situations. But cutting your plastic retractors is something to consider.

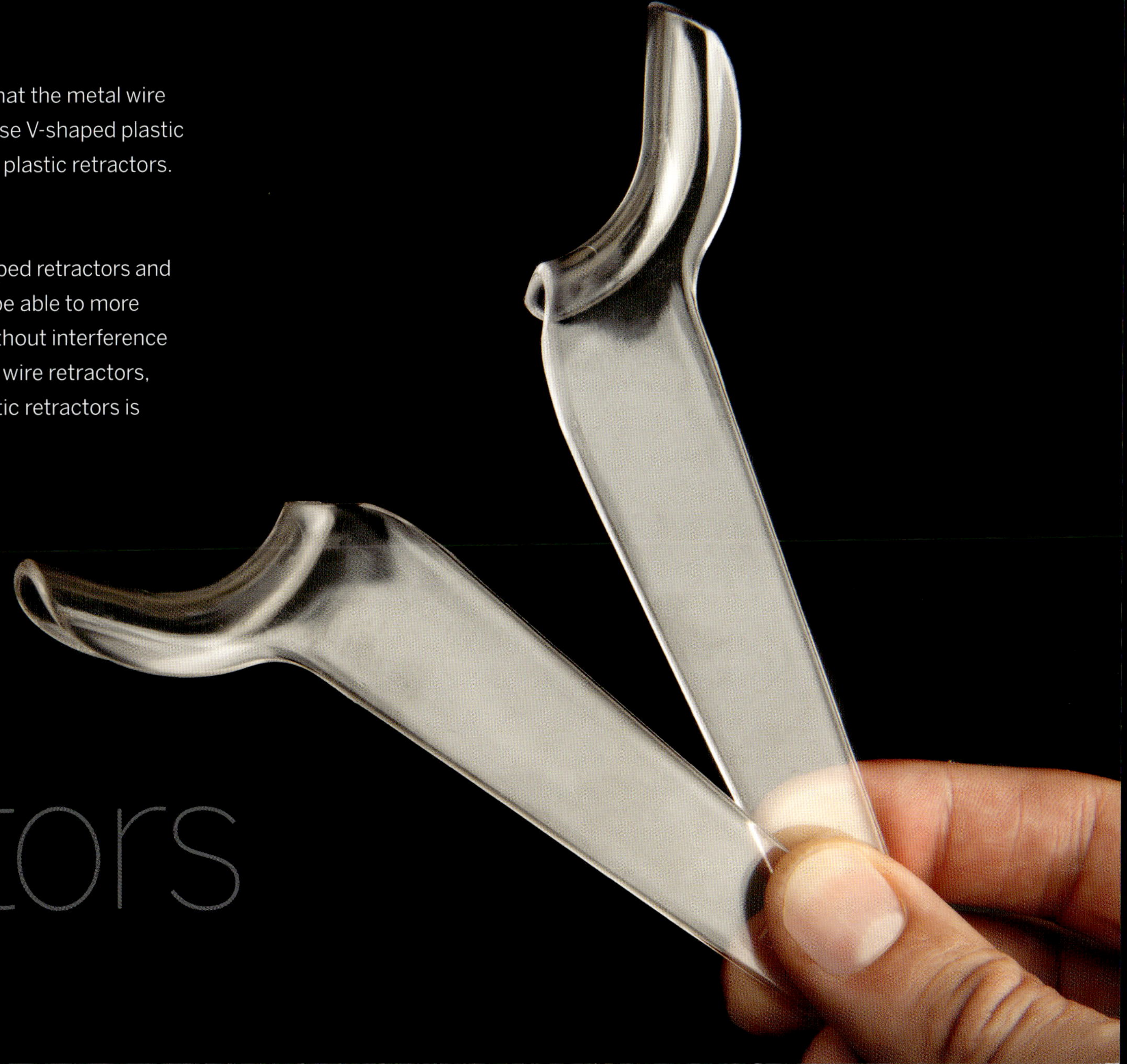

3

Portrait Photography

Portrait photography is an essential part of dentistry. As interest in digital dentistry and Digital Smile Design continues to grow, the need for adequate and pleasing portraits has become a reality. Fortunately, if you are serious about your intraoral photography, you already own most of the gear that is needed to take stunning portraits. In this chapter, we will discuss all the benefits and limitations of the different lighting settings for shooting portraits. Once again, it is all about lighting. We are also going to cover some of the normal complications that arise when trying to have a pure black or white background. But first, let me get something off my chest.

When taking portraits of your patients, there is one golden rule that I like to set for photographers: Do not take your portrait photos with the patient in the clinical chair. Just do not do it. It is not ideal in any aspect. I know that many of you feel like closing the book right now, thinking, "Well Miguel, how the heck am I supposed to take photos if not in my chair?" I understand that many of us do not have room in our clinics to have a designated area for portraits. Unfortunately, if you want to take great portraits, some minimal space is needed. It can be a hallway or the waiting area. You might have to get creative. In any case, your portraits will benefit from it greatly.

The first thing to consider is that we are shooting with a macro lens—hopefully an 85 mm macro lens. These lenses are great for portrait photography. The only issue is that in order to get a portrait, we will need to back up a bit. Depending on the lens, you will have to back up 3 to 6 ft. Hallways are great for this.

You want to have the patient in a relaxed position. Most patients cannot do this standing up. Sitting your patient down on a chair is the best option, but it is only half of the equation. You have to sit down as well. As we all know, patients come in different sizes, some of them tall and some of them short. If both of you are standing up and there is an obvious height discrepancy, it will be reflected in your photo. Your shot might be from a low or high angle, creating distortion. So, back up, sit down, and enjoy the session.

Next, let's break it down by lighting systems, choice of background, flash position, and some other tips.

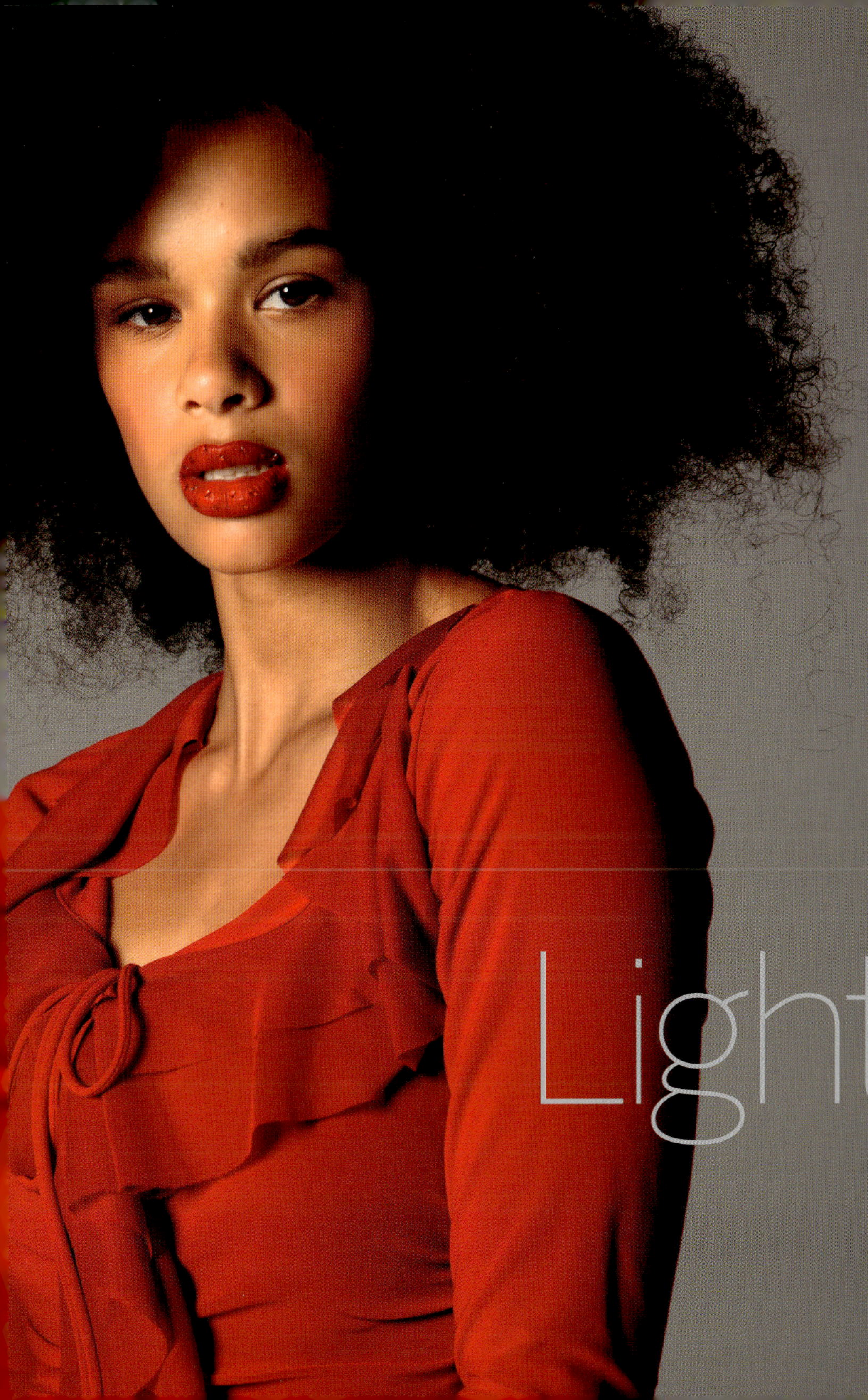

Lighting Systems

It is time to discuss some of the lighting systems you might be using for your portrait photography and the different results we get from them. We will focus on the following groups:

- Ring flash
- Dual flashes
- Speedlights
- Strobes

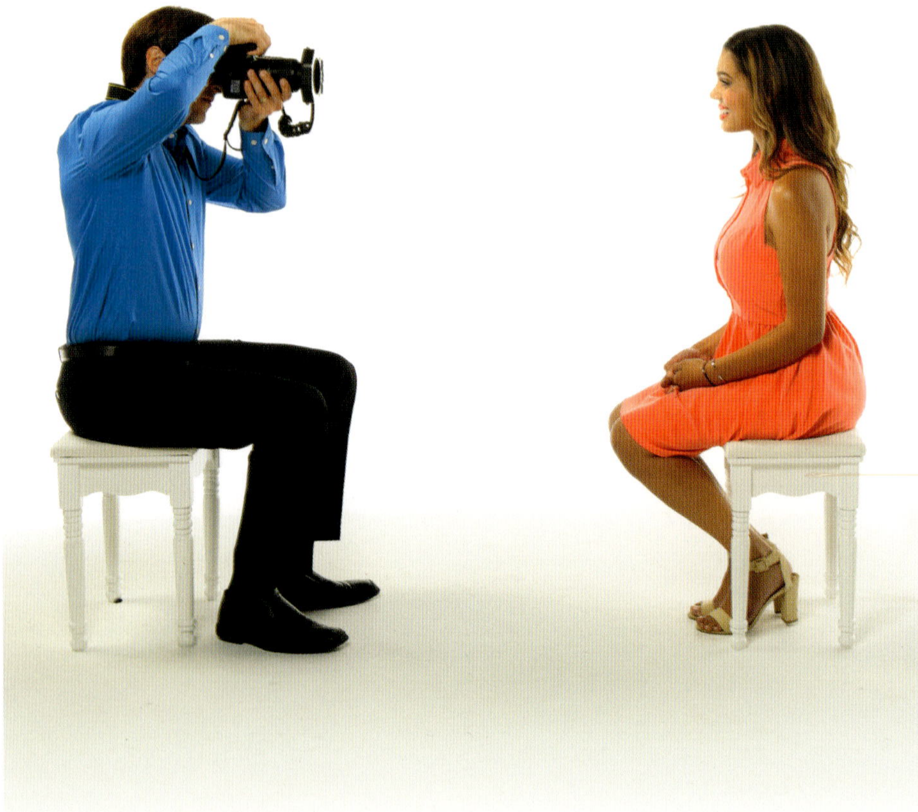

Ring flash

Ring flashes are great for intraoral photography in tight corners of the mouth. However, they are not good when it comes to obtaining beautiful and esthetic photos. Having said that, if you are using your ring flash to take your portrait, you will find yourself underexposed. The reason is simply distance. You have increased the distance to your subject by several feet. Light intensity will decrease to the square of the distance. So, if your distance to the patient doubles, the light intensity will decrease by 4. If your distance triples, your light intensity will decrease by 9.

At this point you will have to reduce your f-stop to somewhere around 13. Do not go lower than that or your DOF will suffer and you might have part of the patient out of focus. You will also have to reduce your shutter speed to about 1⁄100 s. Do not go below that or else you might introduce blurriness in the photo. It is very likely that you will still be underexposed. You will have to increase you ISO to about 400 to 800. With all of those adjustments, you might be able to take a well-exposed portrait with your ring flash. However, it will still be an ugly photo with high-intensity lighting on the center of the photo and decreasing light toward the edges. If you do not believe me, see the next page. No matter how beautiful your patients are, you can always make them a bit less attractive by using a ring flash.

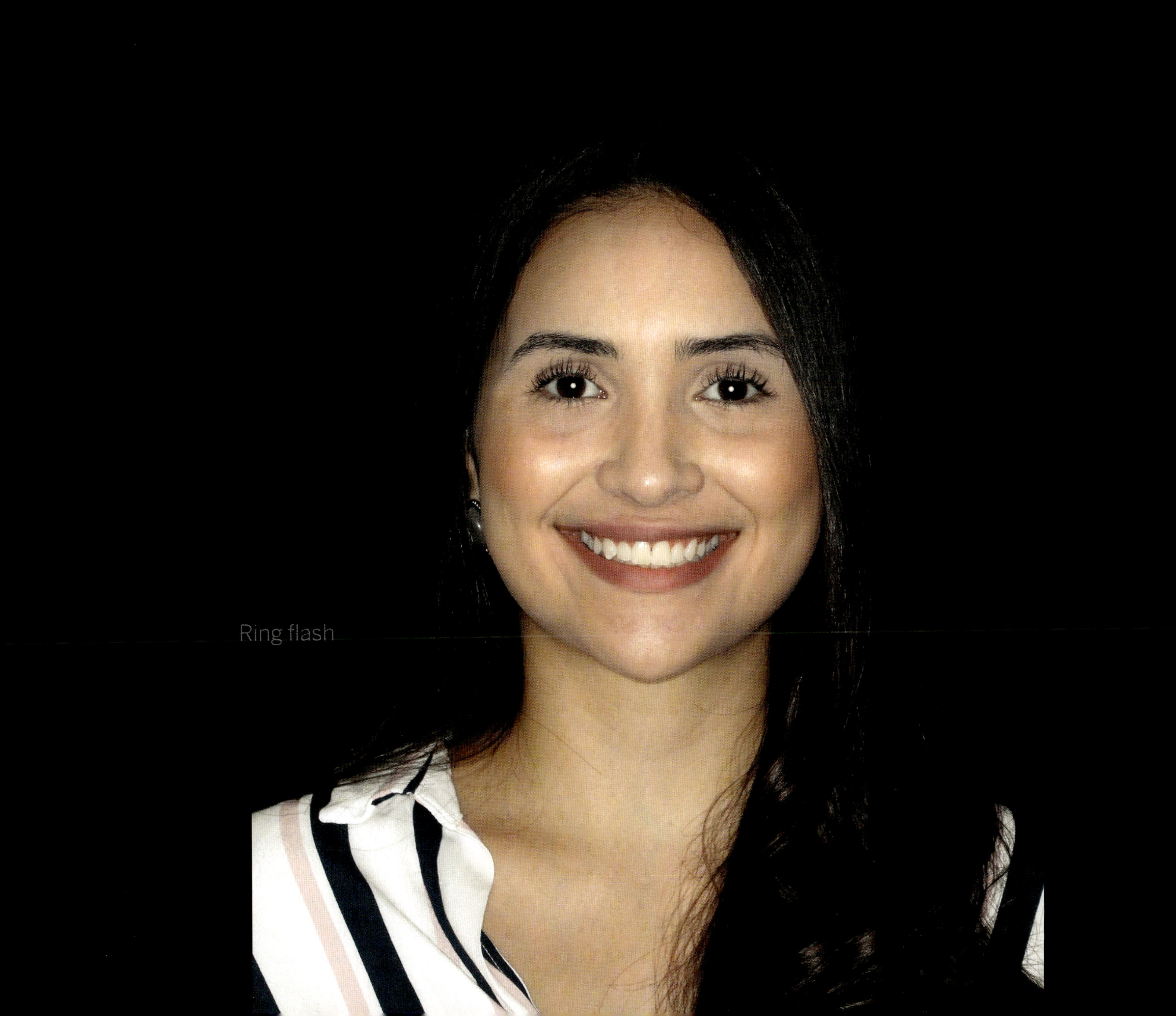

Ring flash

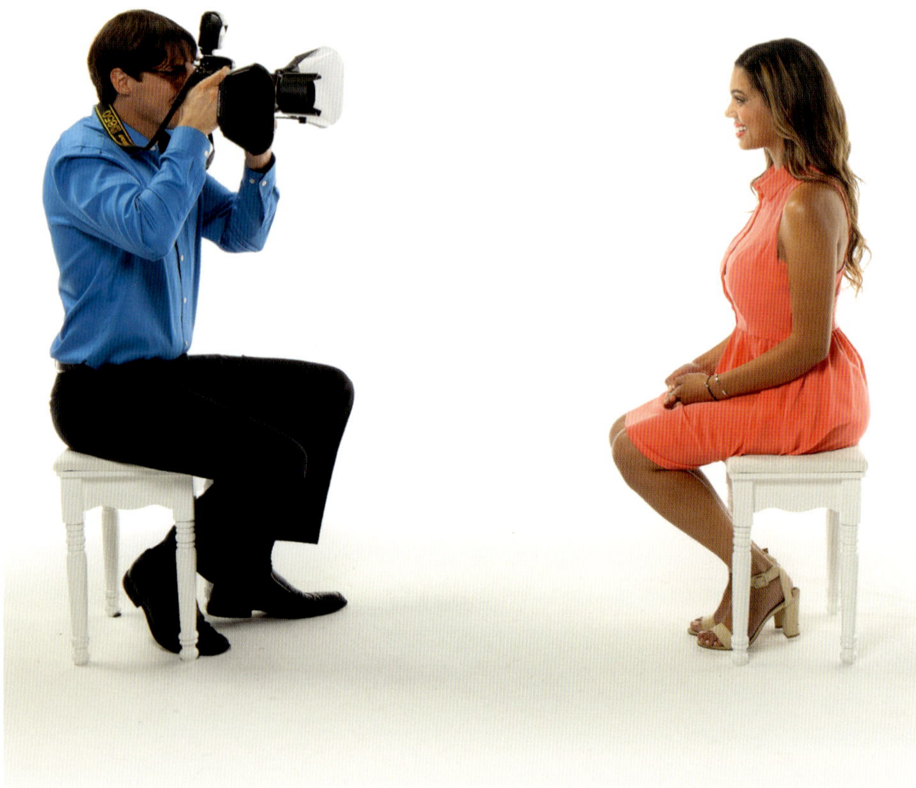

Dual flashes

A dual-flash system is a significant improvement from the ring flash setup. If you have the R1C1 from Nikon, then you are in luck. They are wireless. If you use the ring adapter that comes with the set, you will basically be taking a more expensive ring flash photo. The important thing to do with the dual-flash system is to get the flashes out from the camera. The R1C1 flashes are wireless; the Canon MT-26EX RT flashes are wired, but they can be separated quite a bit.

The key is to spread and diffuse the light coming from them. Most dental photographers have been going to third-party diffusers, such as those sold by LumiQuest. The LumiQuest UltraSoft with UltraStrap are the best bouncers in the market right now for dental purposes. Using a bracket helps. It gets the flashes away from the lens for a better-looking photo.

Ideally, the flashes can be mounted on two simple tripods, freeing your camera from the bulk of the bracket and flash combination. You can also ask for help and have somebody hold them. This setup allows you to obtain nice portraits, where the light is well balanced and the texture of the subject is optimally represented. It also allows for freedom of movement while ensuring the light conditions are stable. Unfortunately, there are several drawbacks of using the dual flashes this way, such as the Canon MT-26EX RT and its wires, or the Nikon R1C1 and its battery life.

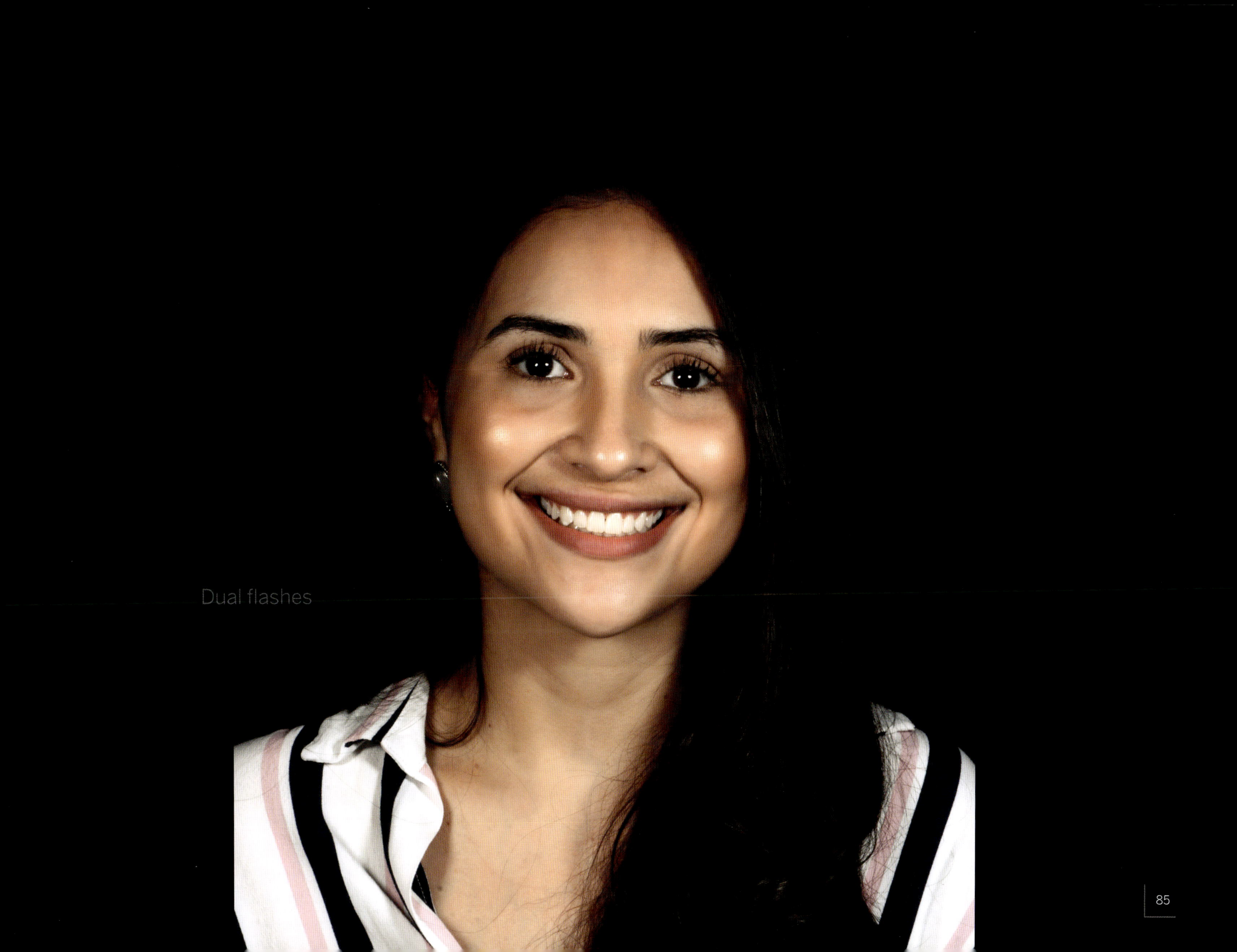

Dual flashes

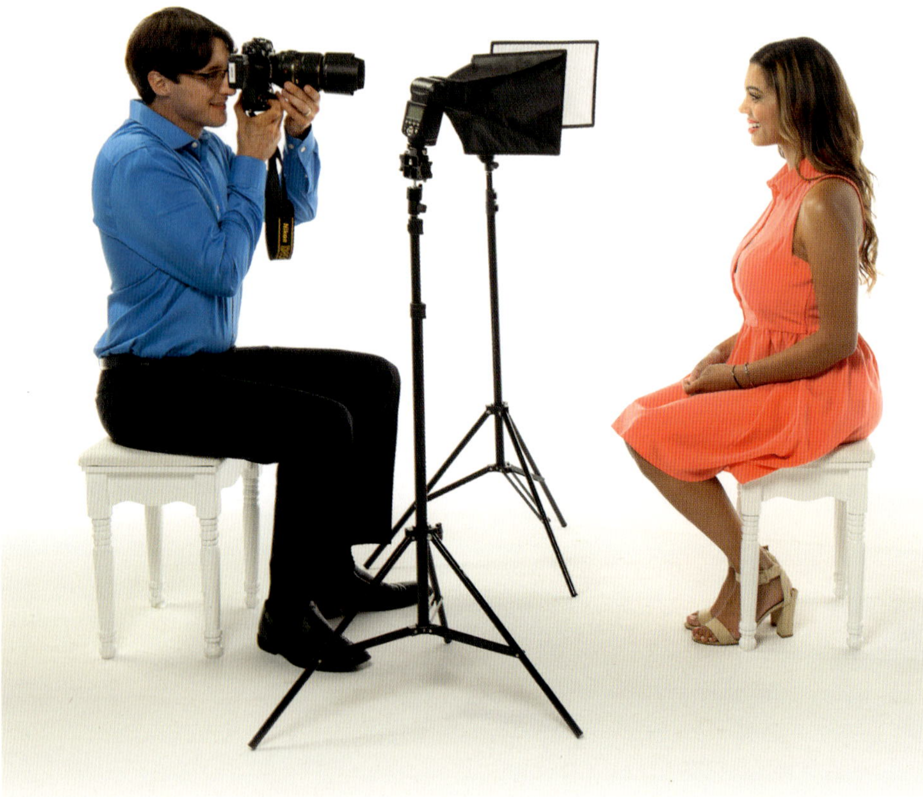

Speedlights

Speedlights give you the perfect balance of performance, budget, and versatility. Having two or three inexpensive speedlights and a commander will allow you to elevate your portrait photography significantly. With three speedlights set on simple tripods, you will be able to take beautiful photographs with crisp washed-out or stunning pure black backgrounds.

What makes speedlights preferable in dental photography is the ability to remove the flash from the camera. This not only makes your camera lighter (bye bye, ugly brackets) and more comfortable to handle, but it also allows for lighting compositions and angles of approach where the light is not always coming from your camera.

Battery life is another great advantage of speedlights when compared to dual-flash systems. With 4 AA batteries on each speedlight, you will be able to have a faster recycle time and more shots than with a dual-flash system.

They also have a wide range of diffuser options, from small diffusers all the way to large softboxes. The larger the diffuser placed on the speedlights, the better and softer your portraits will look. The setup is the same as before. One speedlight with its diffuser is placed in front of the patient on each side at about 45 degrees. The closer they are, the better. We will discuss the reasons why light distance matters in later chapters.

Speedlights have become relatively inexpensive in the last 5 years. Accessories such as tripods, brackets, umbrellas, and softboxes have also come down in price significantly. Being able to create a lighting set that is appropriate to your office needs, affordable, and multipurpose is what matters the most. Speedlights allow you to do exactly that. They are light, easy to set up, and simple to store.

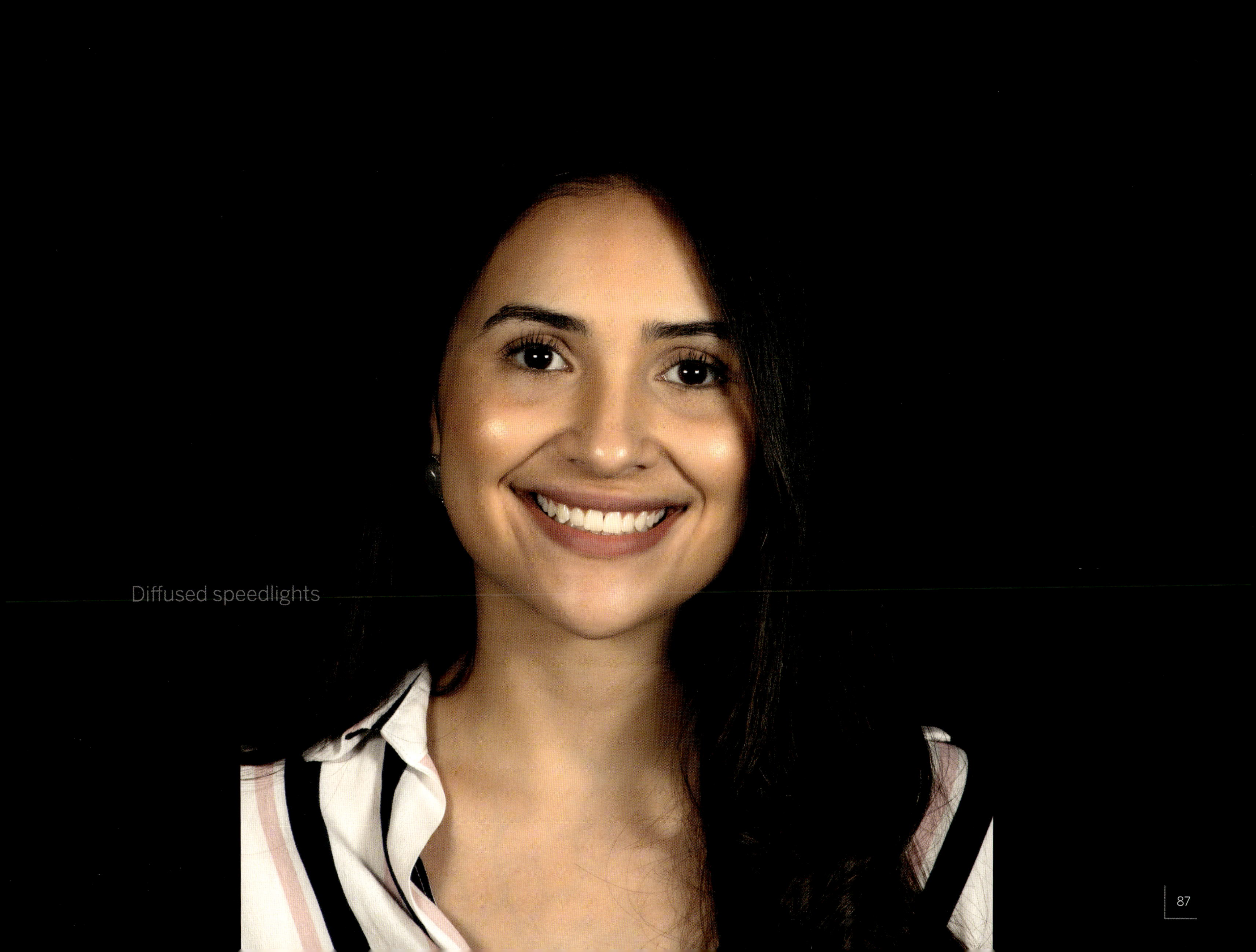

Diffused speedlights

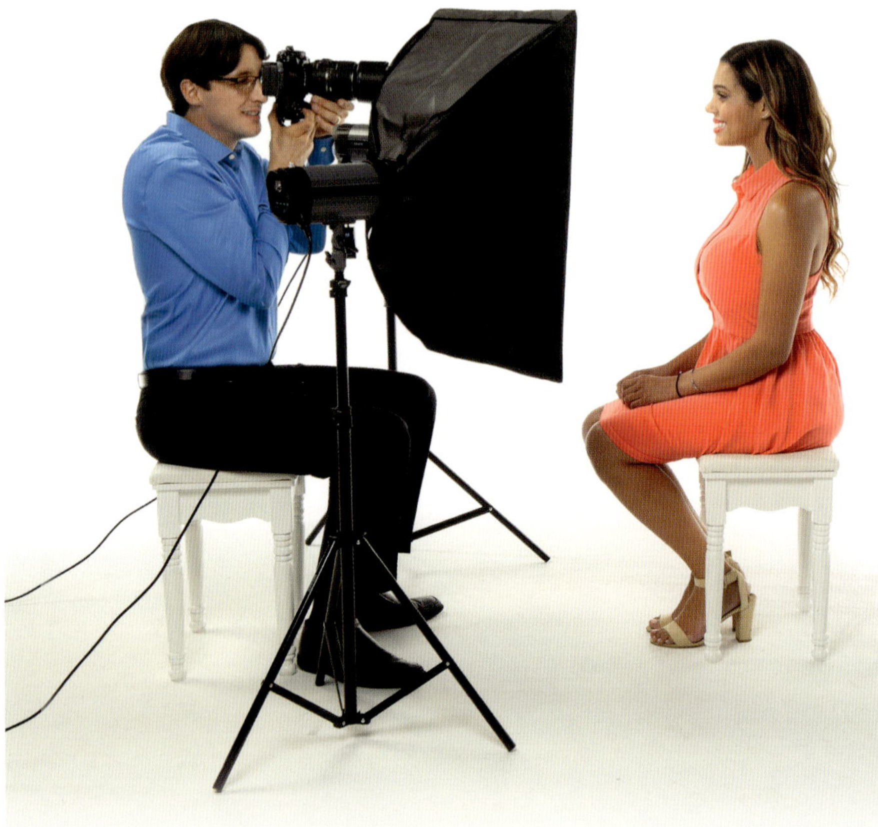

A set of strobes with softboxes

The best photographic result from the setups we have discussed so far.

Strobes

Strobes are also a good thing to consider, if you have a dedicated space to take your photos. They allow for better recycle time, meaning you can take back-to-back photos quicker, without having to wait for the flash to recharge. Strobes also have a great array of bouncer/diffuser types that can be mounted on them to modify and improve the light that is emitted. Softboxes and umbrellas of all types are bouncer/diffusers that we typically use with strobes.

However, they are harder to set up and store, as well as more bulky and difficult to move around. Strobes come with delicate lightbulbs, and special care should be taken not to accidentally drop them. Traveling with strobes can be quite a hassle. So if your setup has to be moved between offices, they are not ideal.

Depending on the size and weight of the strobe, the tripod can become large as well. Repositioning them from shot to shot is trickier than the other options we have discussed. Tripping on the cords is a known issue with them as well.

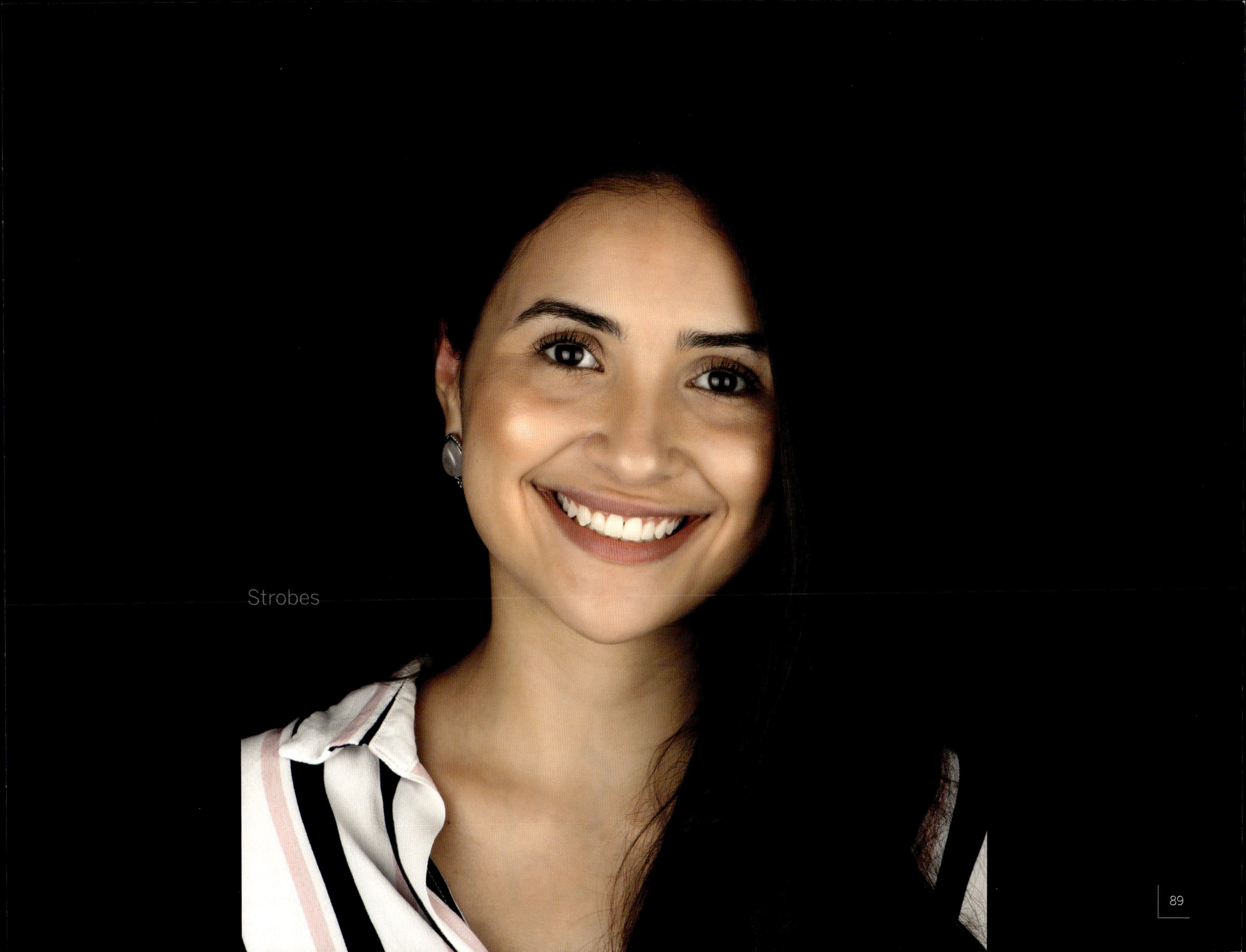

Strobes

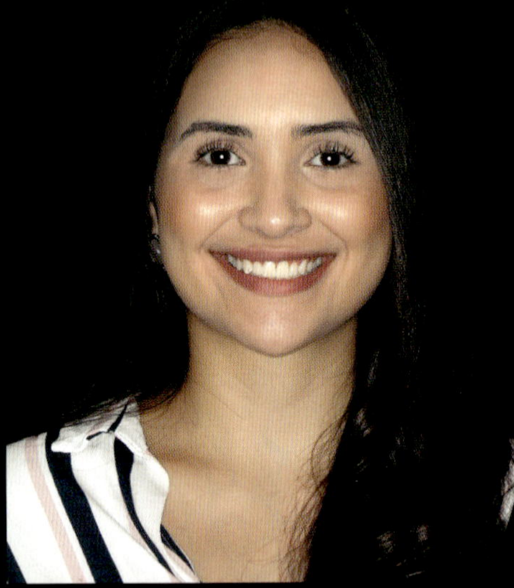
Ring flash

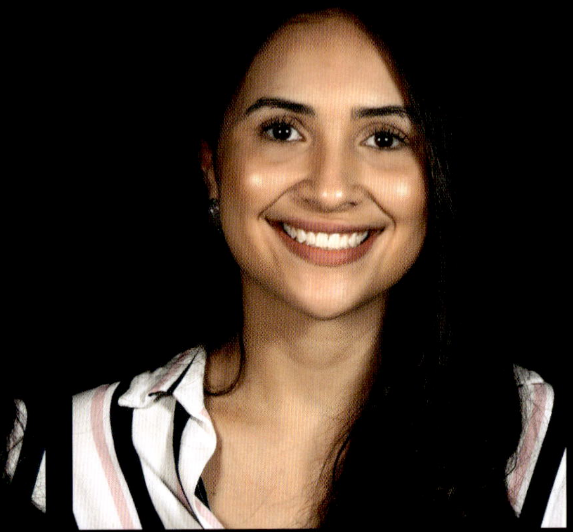
Dual flashes

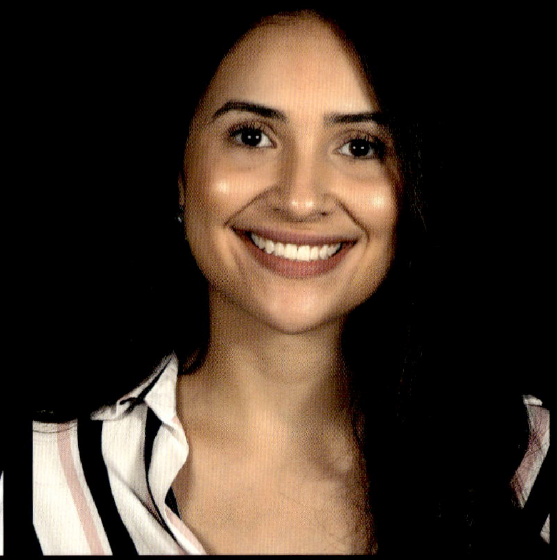
Speedlights

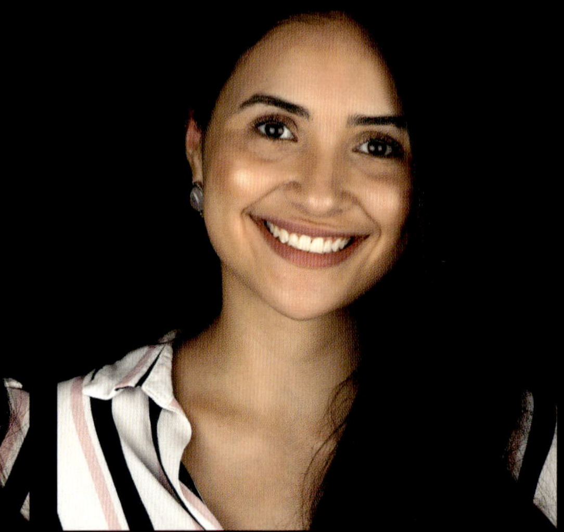
Strobes

Advanced Tip

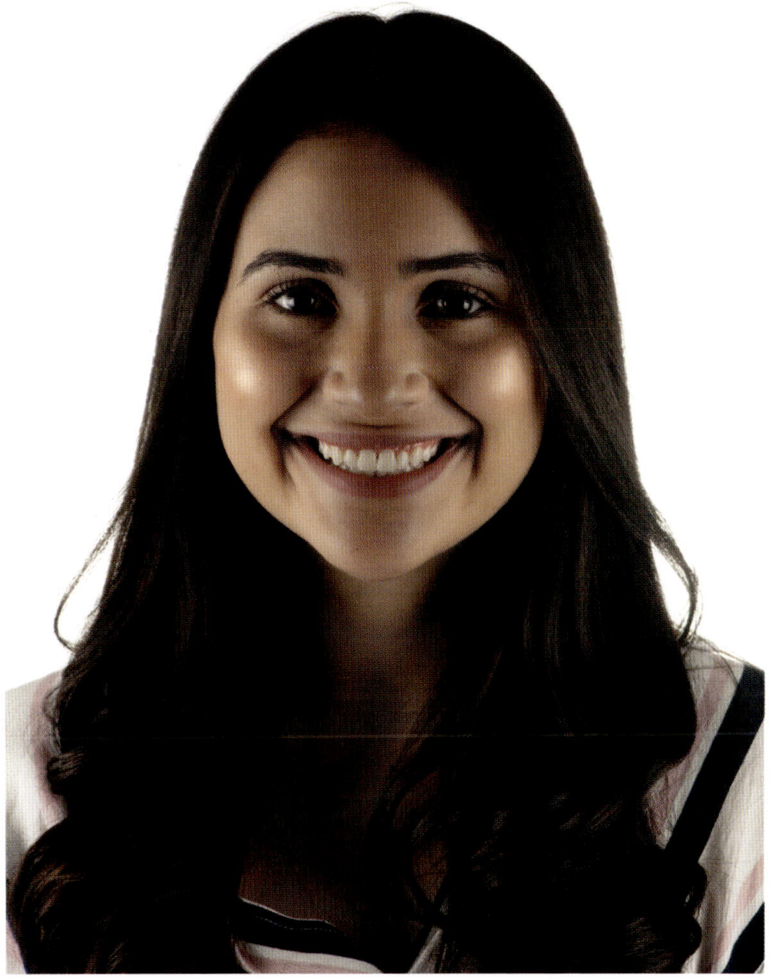

Flashes too wide on each side

FLASH POSITIONING

If the position of your flashes is too far on each side of the patient, resembling more of a 180-degree angle rather than the optimal 45 degrees, you will create dark shadows vertically in the midface area.

A diffuser will scatter the light to make it more diffuse. It is usually something that you place in front of your flash in order for the light to go through it. This scattering technique softens the light. If at the same time you capture the redirected, scattered light and bounce it back to the subject, you can achieve a full effect of light modification and softening. You can do that by having a wall or a ceiling near your flash and diffuser combo, which will redirect the scattered light onto your subject.

A bouncer is a reflecting material that is placed in front of the flash to redirect the light. The purpose of the bouncer is to create a source of light that is larger than the flash itself. You can buy bouncers or you can use readily available items as bouncers—a plain piece of white paper, a wall, a ceiling, etc. Making the light source larger will result in a softer and more spread-out illumination.

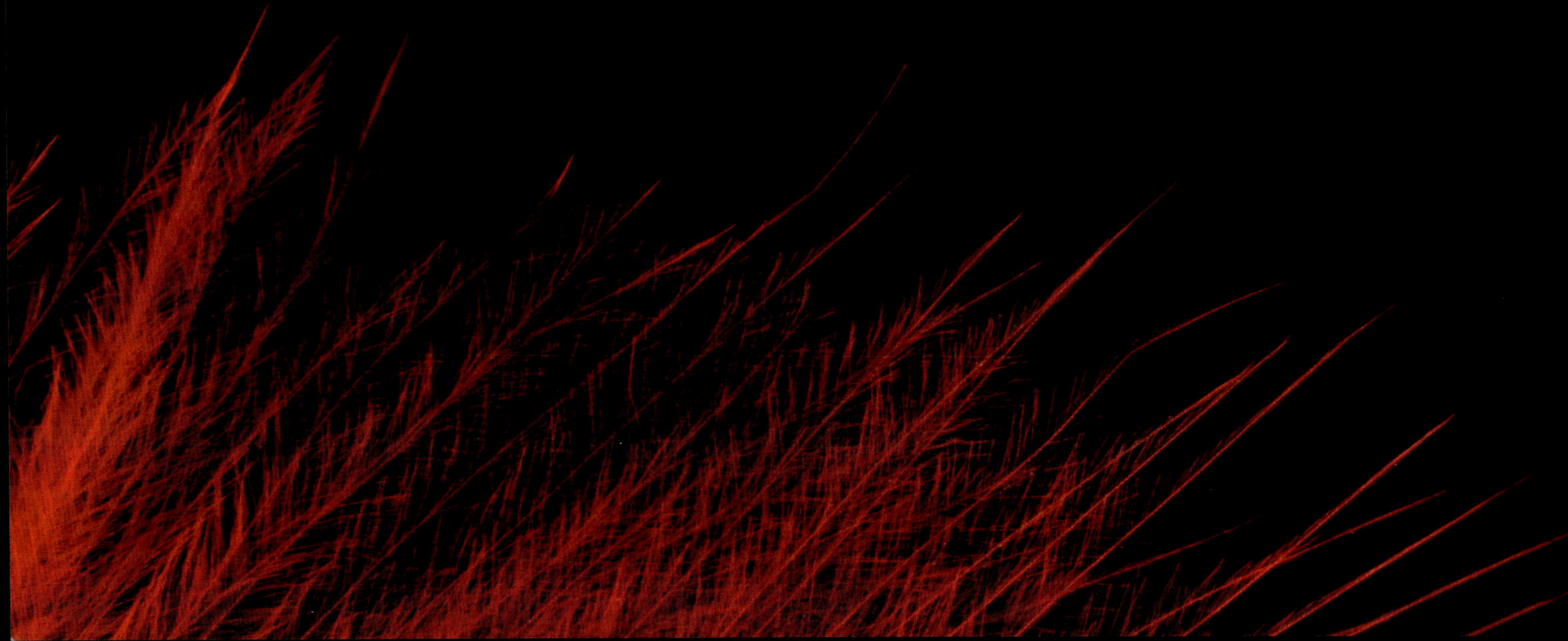

Simple and inexpensive setup for small offices

Here I will show you one of many setups that you should consider for your office, especially if space is limited. All you need is 3 tripods, 3 speedlights, 2 diffusers, batteries, and maybe a background if a wall is not available.

Leave the tripod, diffuser, and speedlight together. Just close your tripod, collapse the diffuser, and store it behind any door. Softboxes on speedlights are better, but they are bulkier and hard to set up and store in small offices.

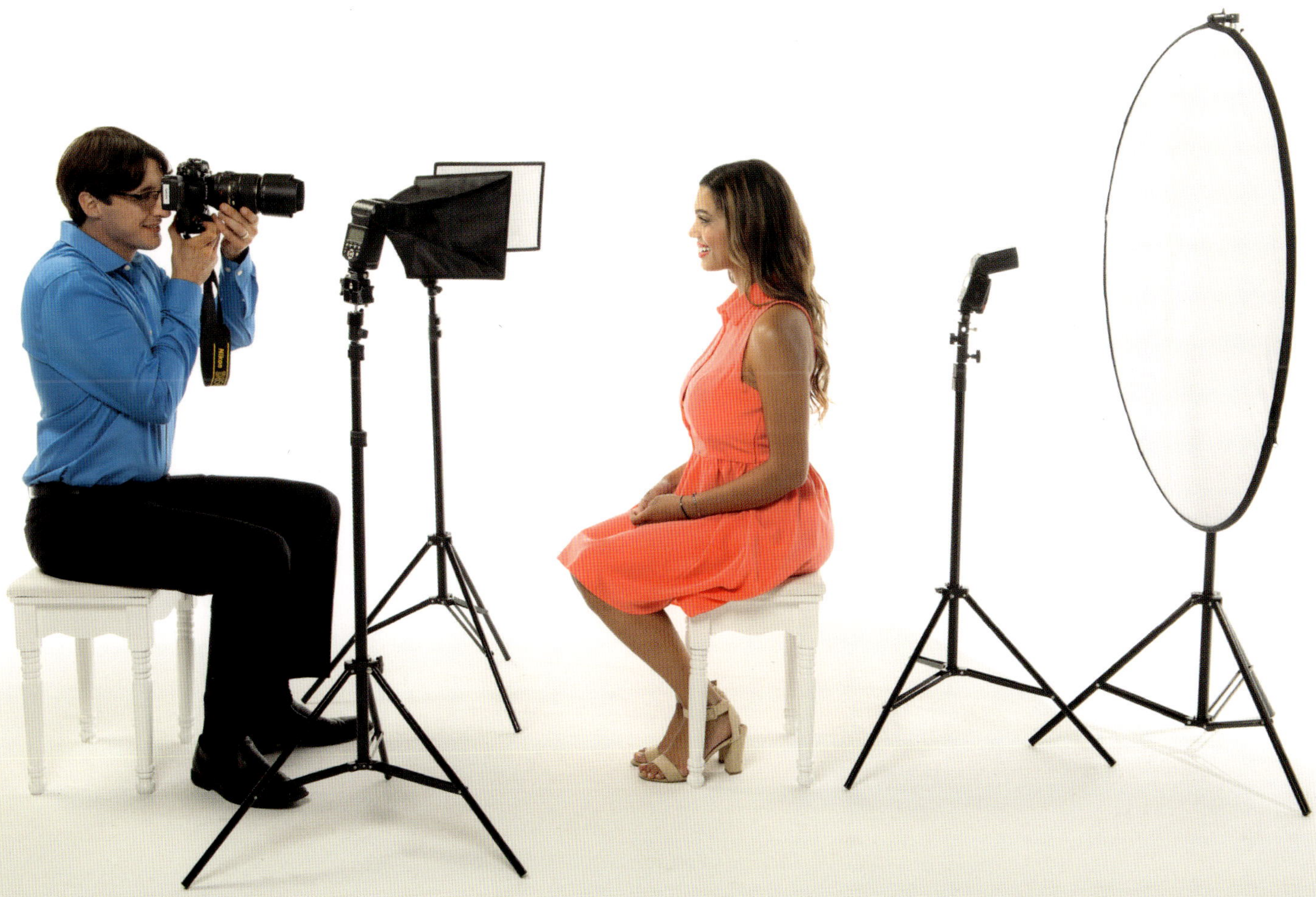

Black

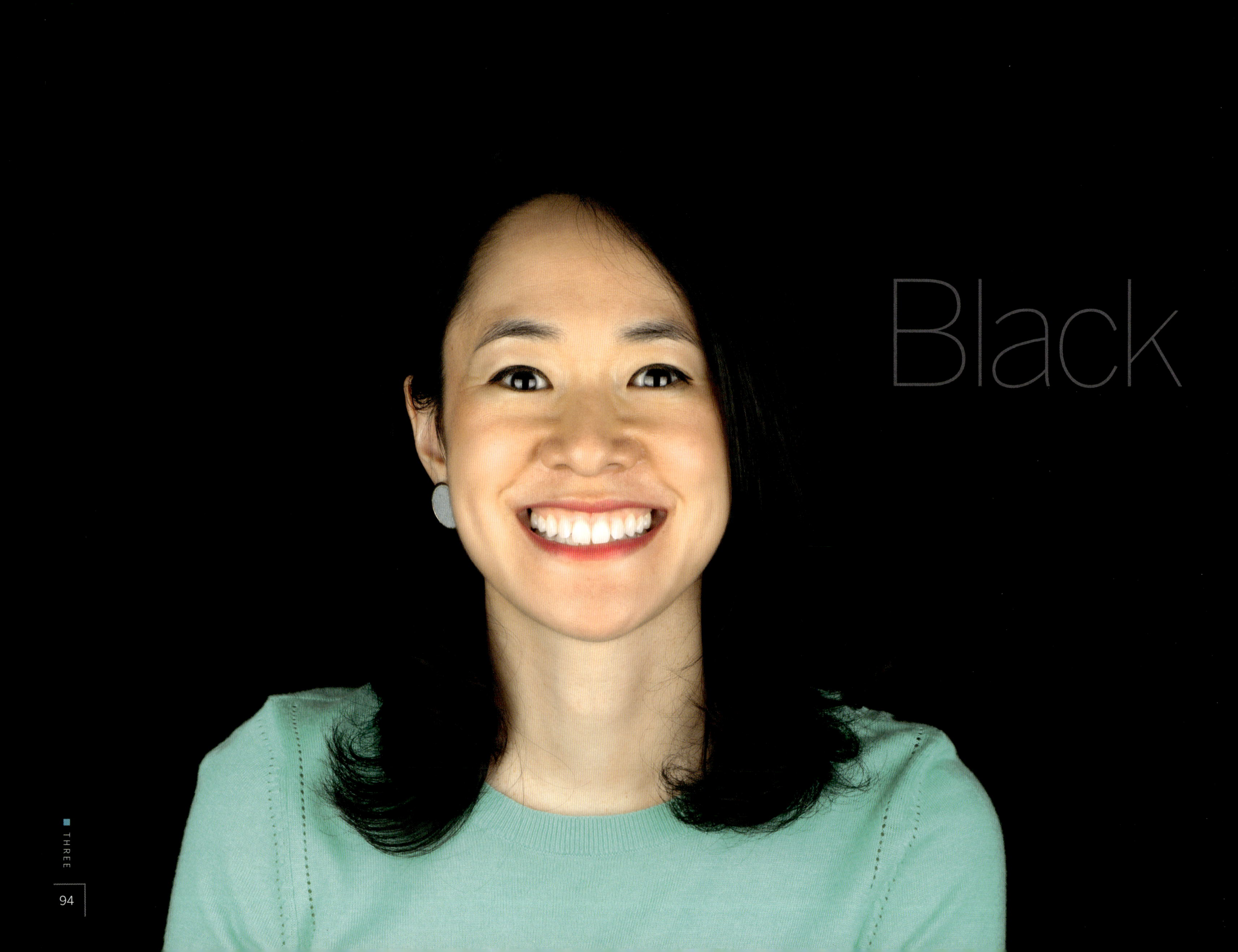

Background

Pure black backgrounds are challenging. Many shots will result in a gray or textured background instead of pure black. Choose a fabric that is nonreflective, and separate the patient from the background as much as possible. In cases where you do not have enough room to separate the subject from the background, use a higher f-stop if possible. Higher f-stops have a greater relative effect on the background than on the subjects. The higher f-stop will make your background darker. Use changes to shutter speed, ISO, or flash distance to compensate for the lower exposure.

With a black background, you might notice that darker tones of hair color will blend with the background. In order to overcome this, you might want to consider having a third light source high up behind the subject. This light should be positioned at 10 o'clock and should be directed at a 45-degree angle pointing down at the patient's head. This light should not be at full power; the sweet spot is somewhere between ¼ and ⅛ power, depending on the distance to the subject. This light will illuminate the subject's head to create tridimensionality and separation with the dark background. A separating light is not a requirement, however.

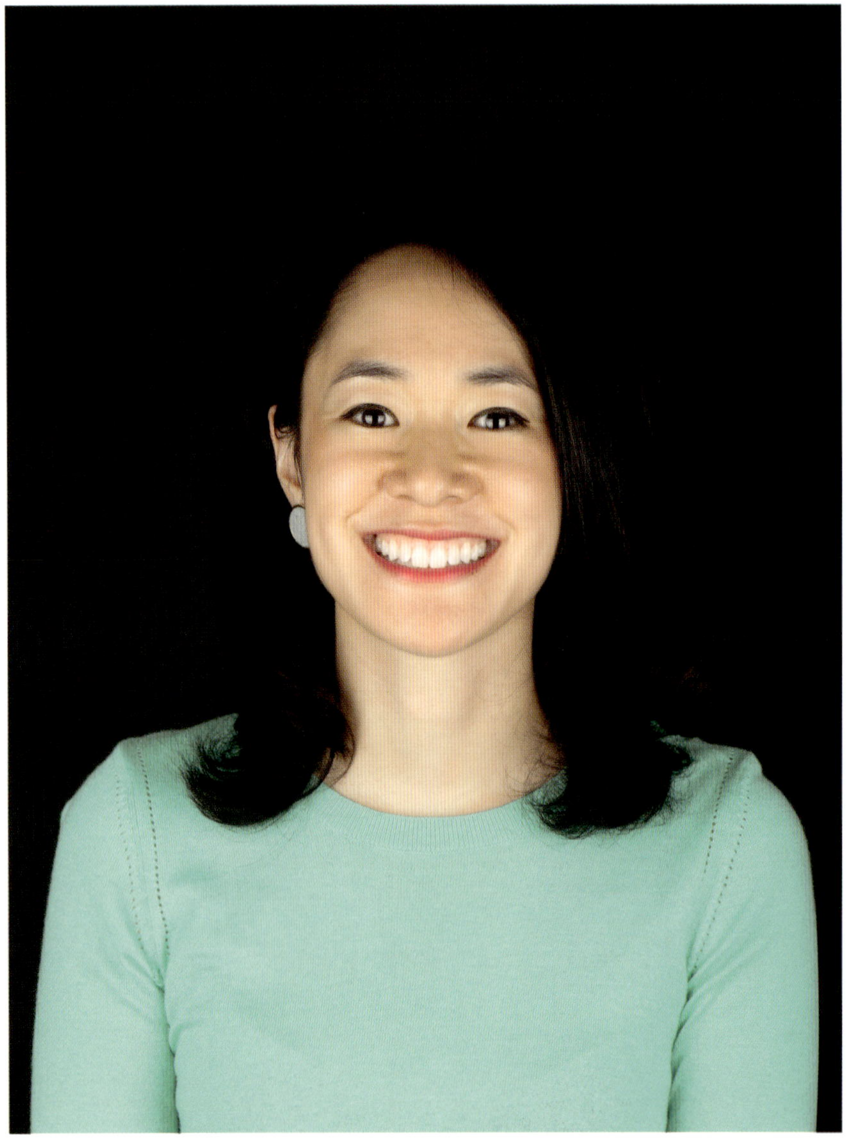

Patient too close to the background

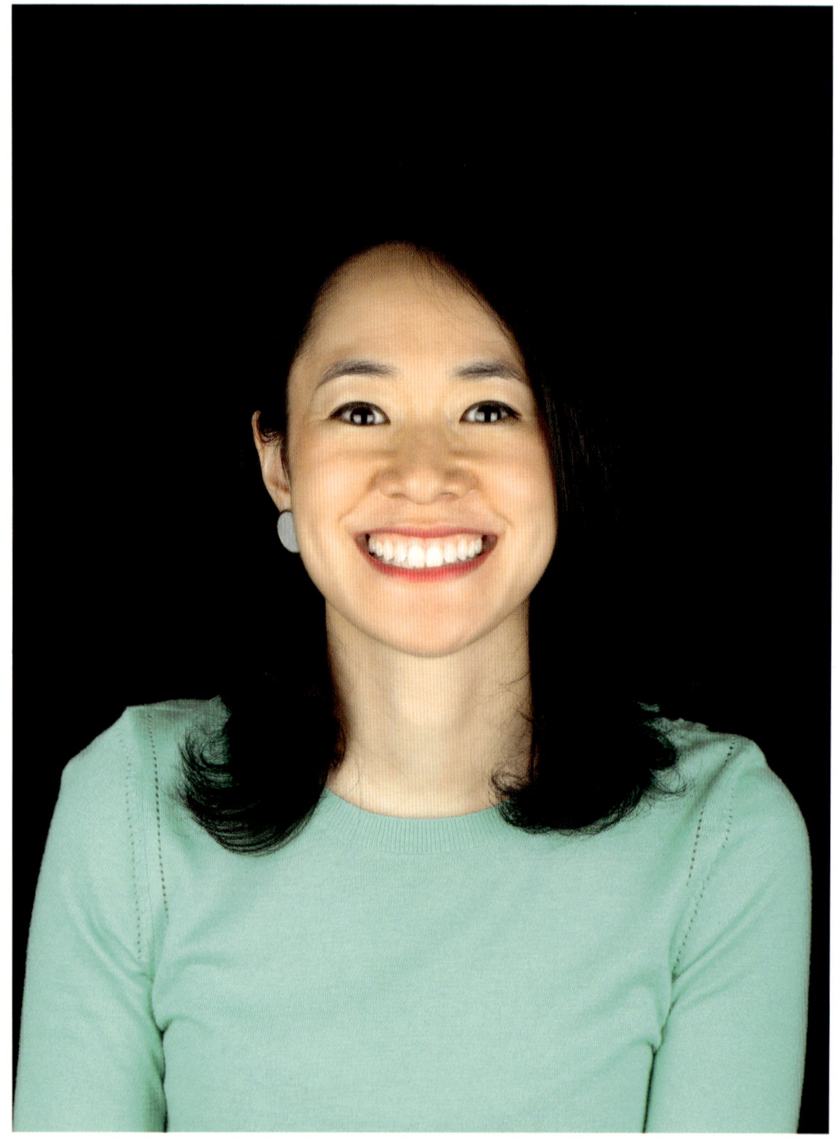

Patient moved away from the background

Black background too close

It might show as gray in your photo. Things you can do:

- Move the patient away from the background
- Turn the background or patient so the background is not perpendicular to the direction of shooting
- Increase the f-stop (aperture)

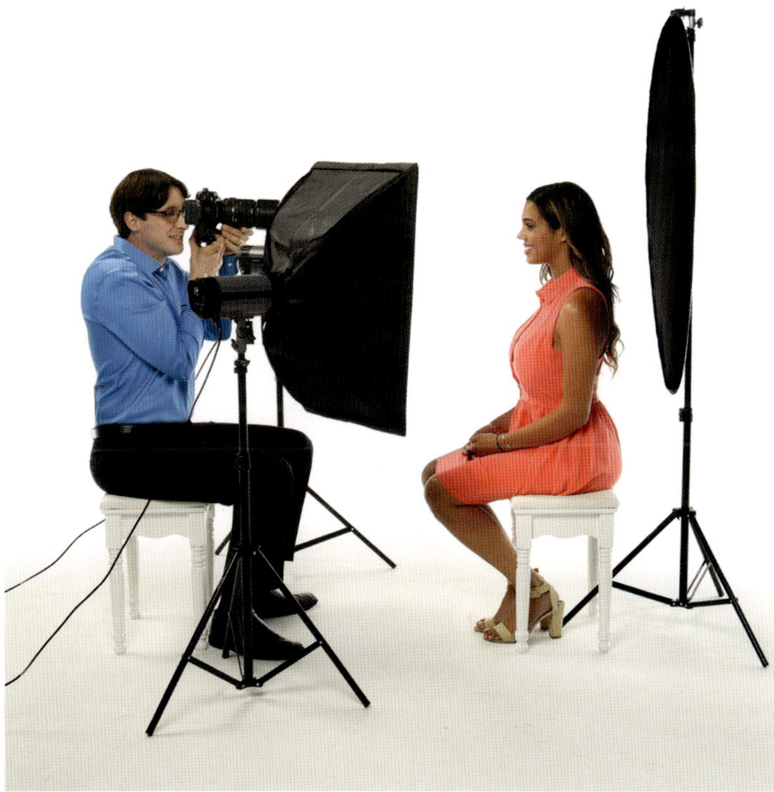

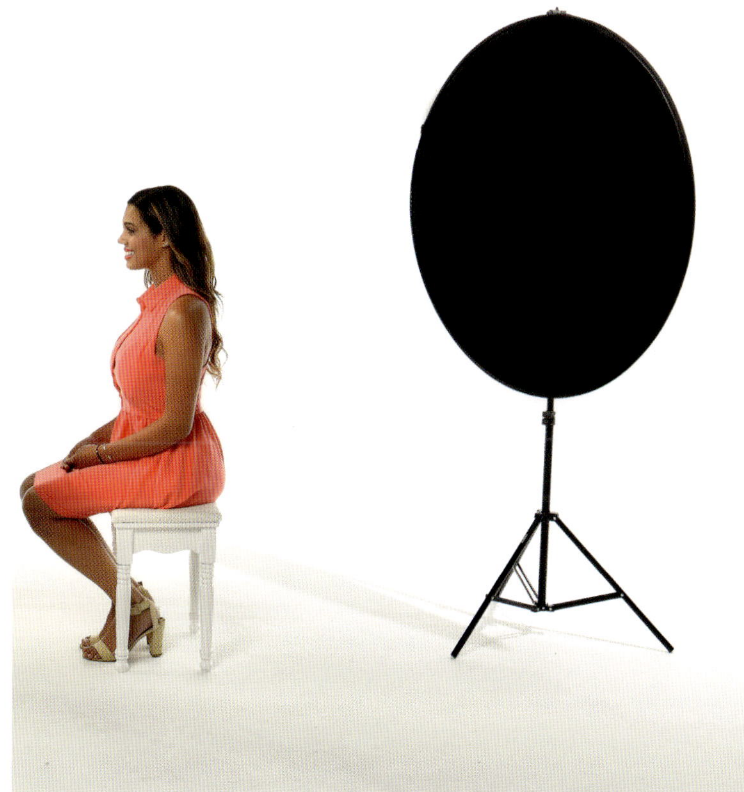

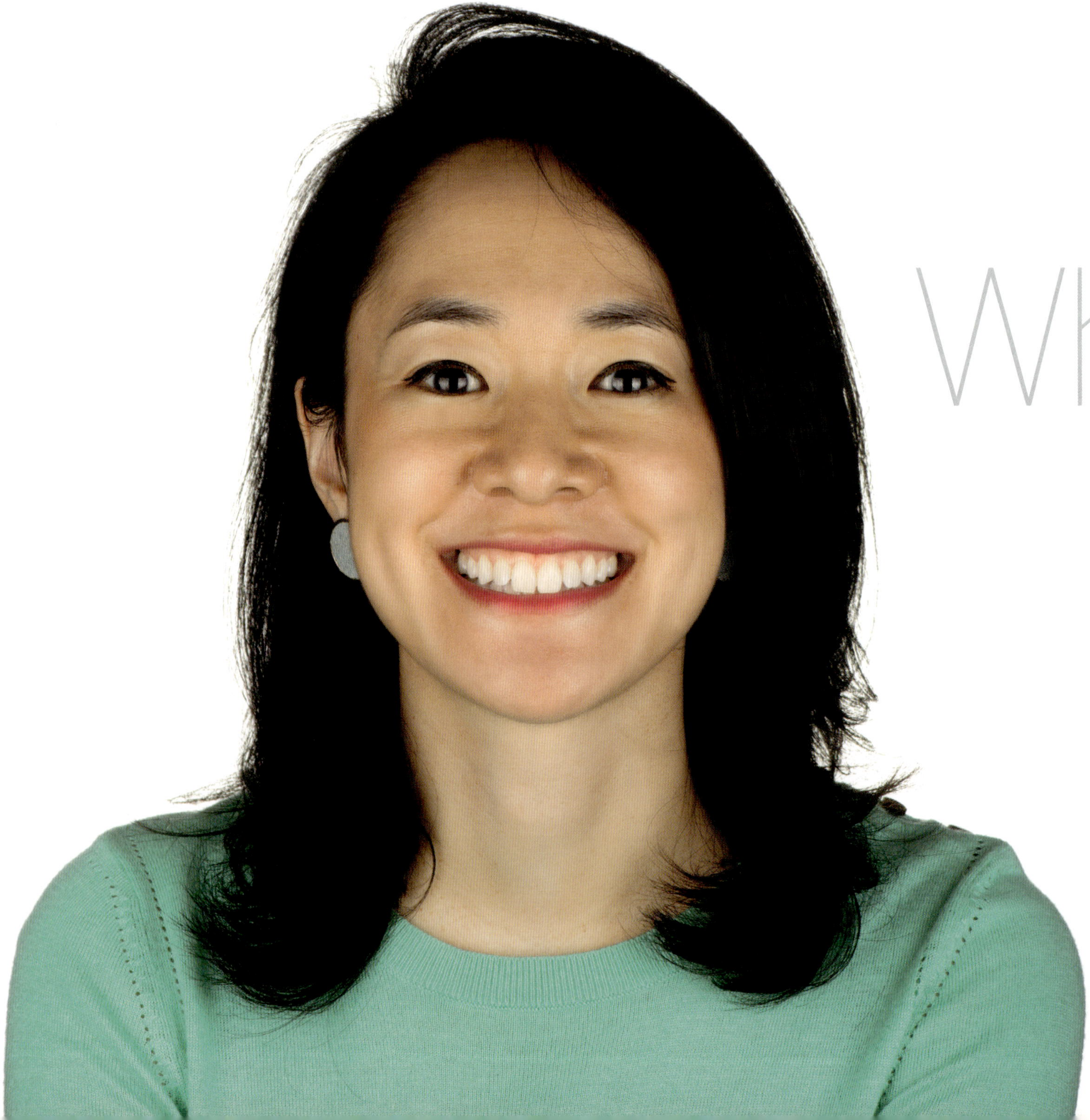

White

Background

Your background can be a white wall, or a white cloth. Anything that you can point a flash at. When using white backgrounds, it is not as common to have the subject and the background blend. However, for a maximum effect you must illuminate the background fully in order to avoid shadows. Once again, a third flash—this time pointing directly at the white background—will allow your background to appear pure white. You have to find the balance between lighting the background properly and avoiding excess or spilled light coming back around the subject. This spilled light will appear as a halo or cloudiness around your subject. If this is present, you need to reduce the power on the background flash, place the background flash farther away from the subject, and/or separate the subject from the flash and background a bit more.

Another thing to consider is the angle and distance of this flash to the background. The closer it is to the background, the smaller the white circle of light that you will create. This will result in a background that might be white in some areas but gray in others.

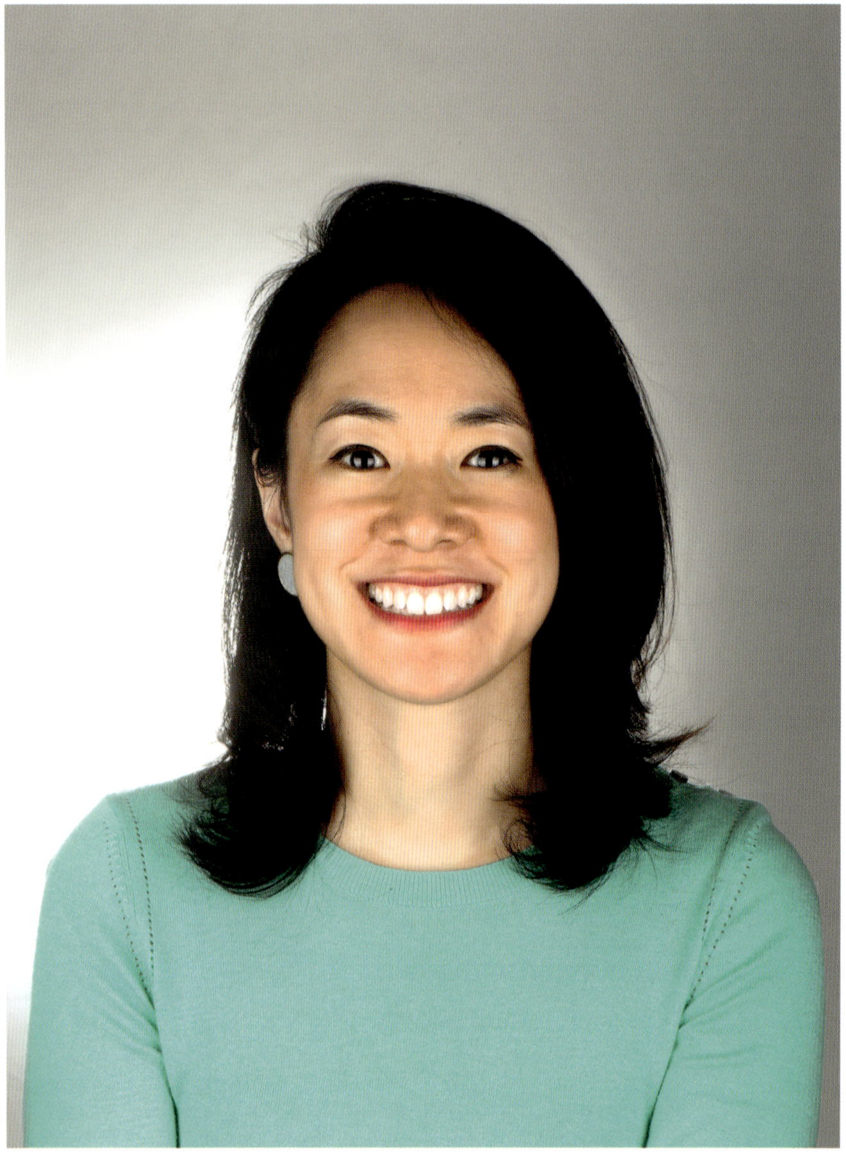

Background flash too low or too close

When the background flash is positioned too low, off center, or too close to the white background, the result will be a gray gradient background with a white overexposed area. Things you can do:

- Elevate the flash
- Tilt the flash upward
- Increase the distance between the background and the flash

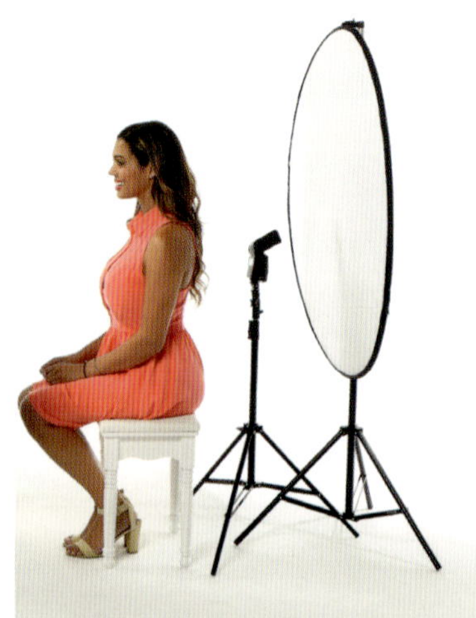

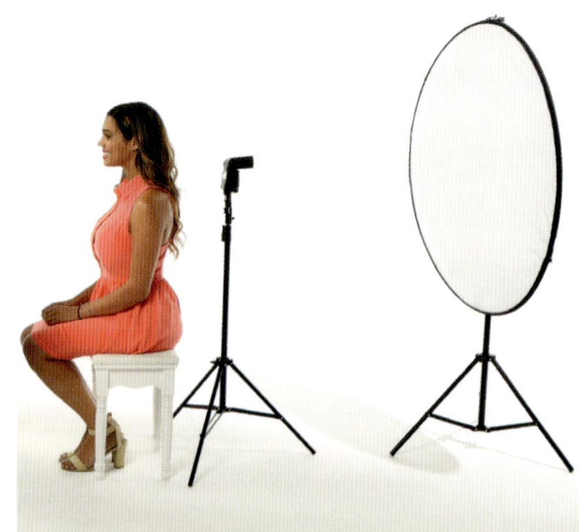

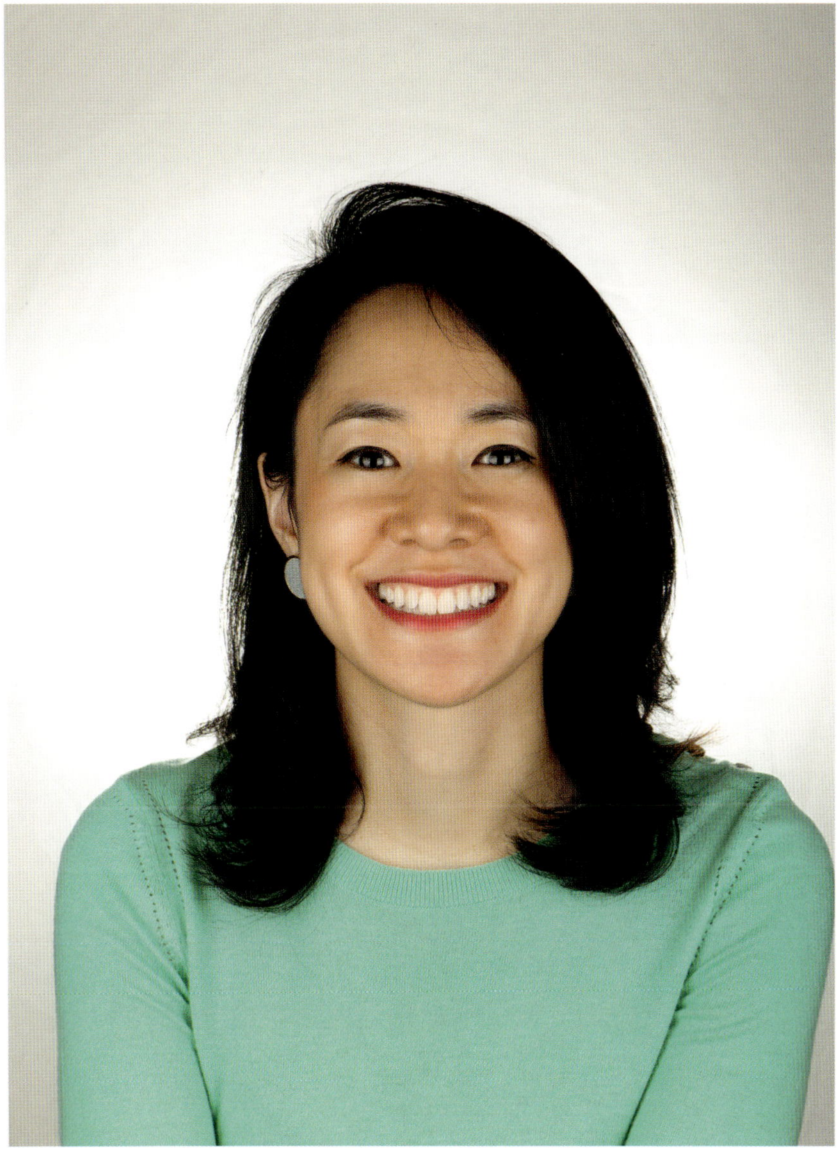

Background flash needs more power

When the power of the background flash is not high enough, the white background appears gray. Things you can do:

- Increase background flash power
- Decrease the f-stop

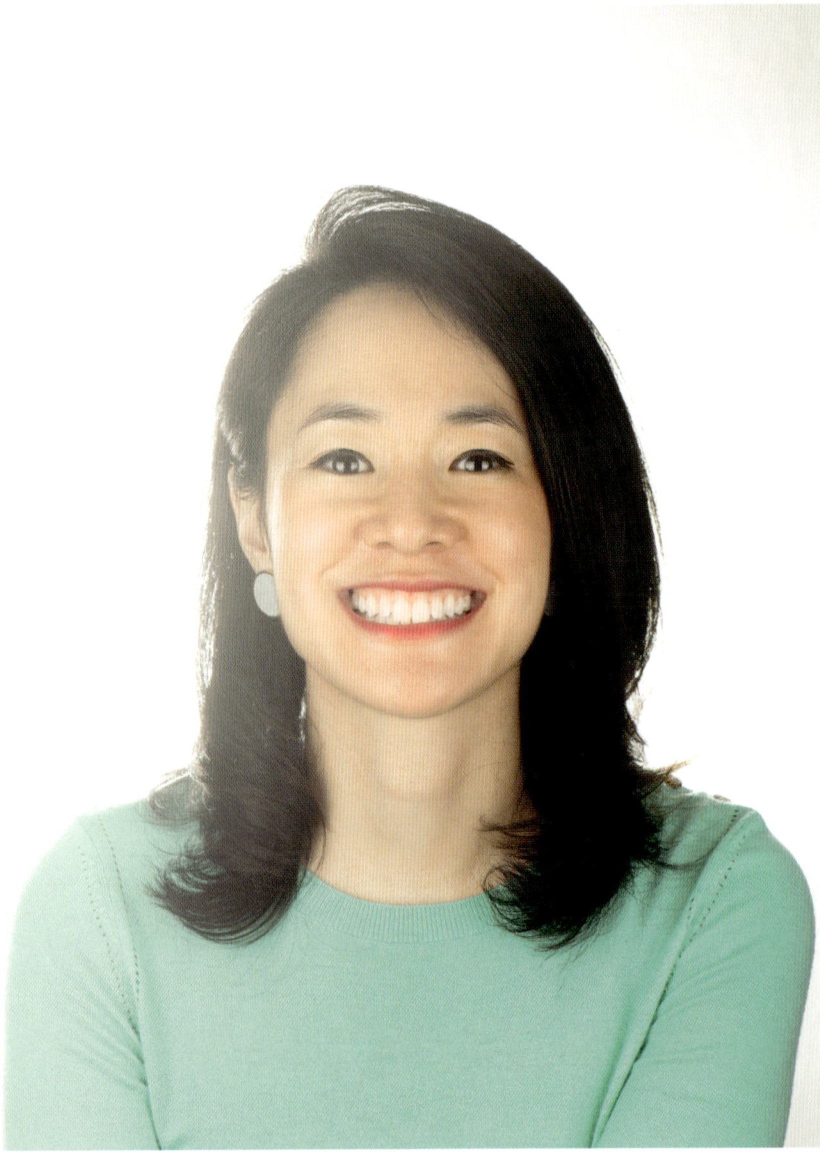

Background flash too powerful

When the background flash power is too intense, you will notice that cloudiness will overtake your subject. The edges of the subject's hair will look overexposed and yellow, and the image will seem blurry. Things you can do to fix it:

- Reduce the power of the background flash
- Move the flash and the background away from the subject

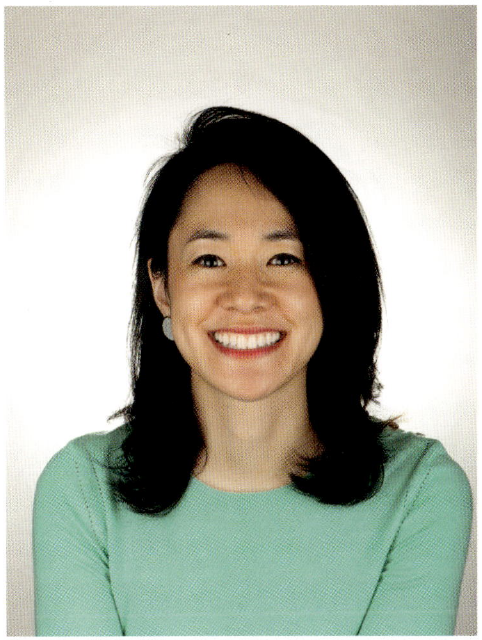

Too weak

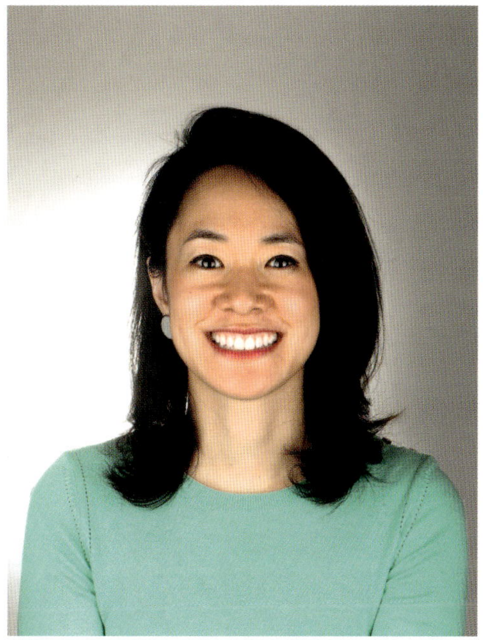

Too low

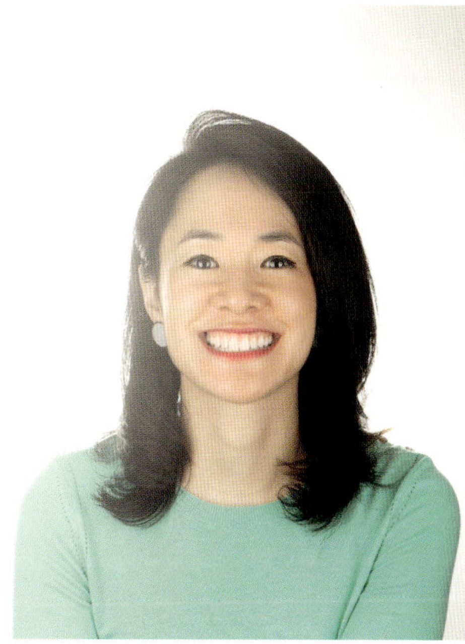

Too strong

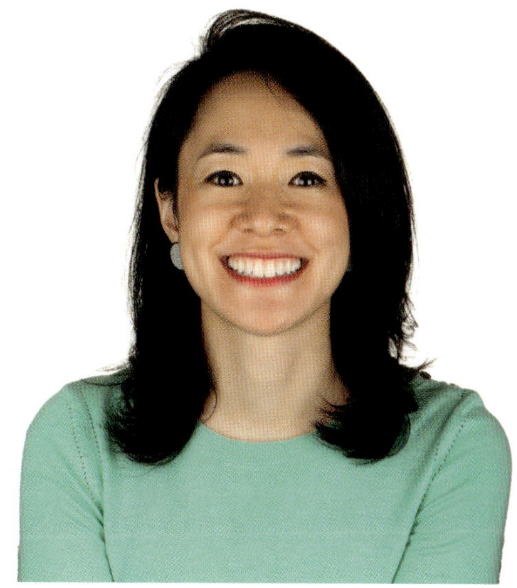

Perfect

Intraoral Photography

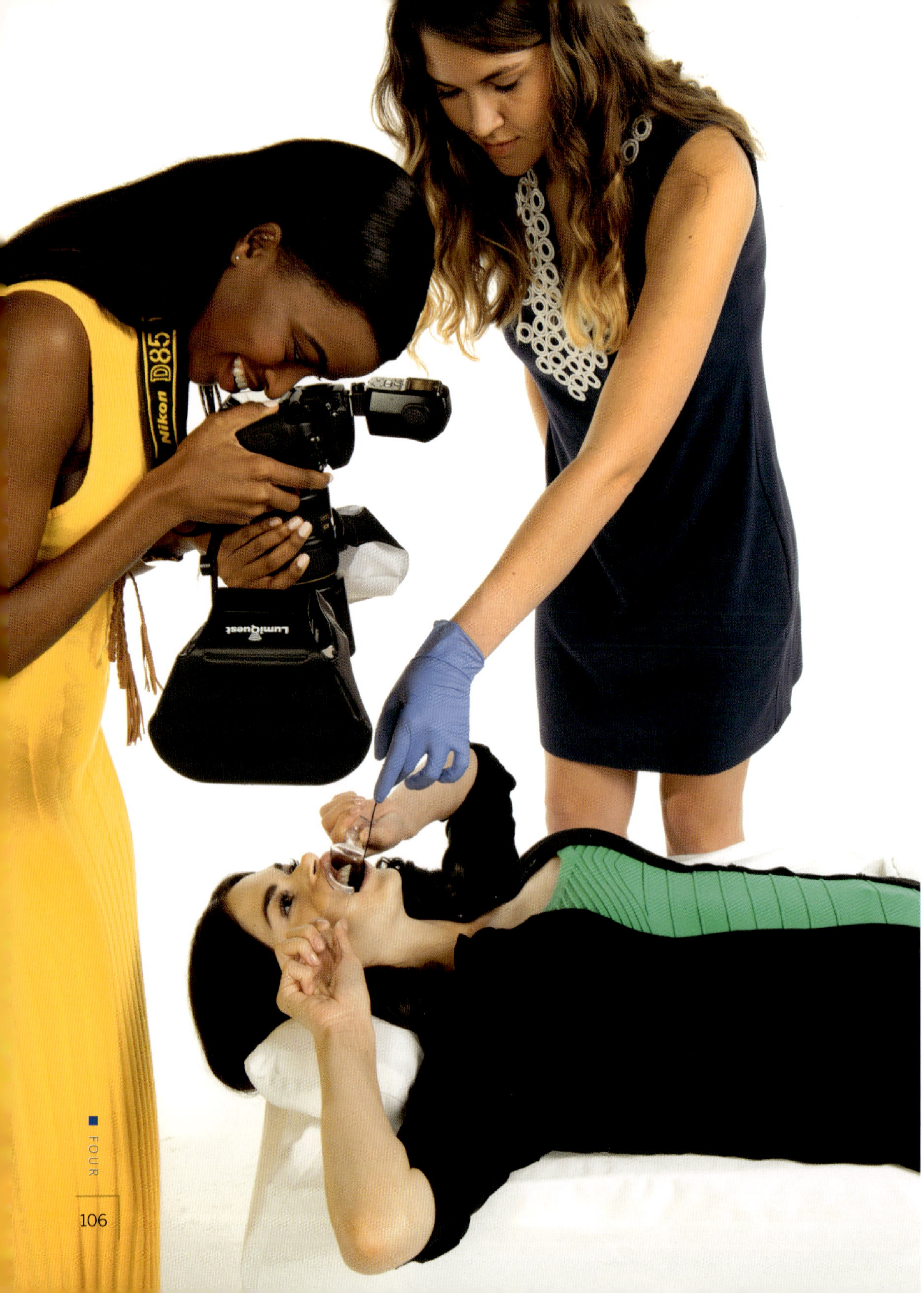

The intraoral protocols are the most important part of what we do in dental photography. Undoubtedly, digital photography and the penetration of dentistry into social media have created a wave of artistic dental photography that has inspired the masses. However, we cannot forget that the most important aspect of dental photography continues to be that meant for documentation and peer-to-peer communication. Most people who struggle with intraoral photography tend to think that somehow it is an easy task that they are not good at. Well let me tell you something: That is just not true.

Intraoral photography is not a simple task. We face many challenges in intraoral photography: confined and dark spaces, less-than-ideal physical surroundings, a moving and sometimes uncooperative subject, and equipment that many do not know how to properly use. I will simplify the intraoral protocol by showing you how I do it. I am sure there are other ways of doing it as well, but this is one way that I know works.

Flash settings

As previously discussed, most of us will be taking intraoral photographs either with a ring flash or a dual-flash system. The dual-flash system might be mounted on a circular base around the lens or it might be placed on a bracket that allows for expanded, independent movement of the flashes.

Whether you are using a ring flash or dual flashes, you should use them on manual mode, not on TTL mode. TTL or "through-the-lens" mode will allow the camera to decide the "correct" exposure for the photo you are about to take. If the photo is not properly exposed and you decide to modify any parameter, such as aperture, shutter speed, or ISO, the camera will read the environment once again and readjust to counter-balance what you just did. You do not want that. You want full control of your parameters.

Place the ring flash in manual mode. My preference is full power or 1/1 as it appears on the flash setting. Some people might argue that you can place the flash at ½ power and increase your ISO to compensate for it. They do this to increase battery life and shorten the recycle time. I like my ISO at 100 to keep the image noise down as much as possible.

Patient positioning

I take 95% of my intraoral photographs with the patient in a fully supine position. That is, I place the dental chair as low as it can go and fully flat. With the patient laying parallel to the floor, I position myself behind the patient's head. Using a ring flash, my lighting and flash settings will not change. Using a dual-flash system with brackets, my flashes will have to be adjusted at various points during my full intraoral protocol to avoid creating unwanted shadows. All my photos are going to be upside down from this position, which is something I will correct quickly on my computer after transferring the files. Because I find this position to be the best for a fast and efficient intraoral protocol, I am a big advocate of an 85 mm macro lens on a cropped-sensor camera. From this position, most people who have a cropped-sensor camera (ie, most of you) and a 100 mm or 105 mm lens will struggle to take a properly framed photo. The reason is that you will find yourself too zoomed in. You will do the little tippy-toe dance trying to get yourself higher in order to fit the smile in your frame, especially those of you who are shorter that 5'10". With an 85 mm lens, this problem is practically solved, depending on how low your chair can go.

How far are you willing to go to get the best photo?

Your photos will only be as good as your light source.

Ring flash

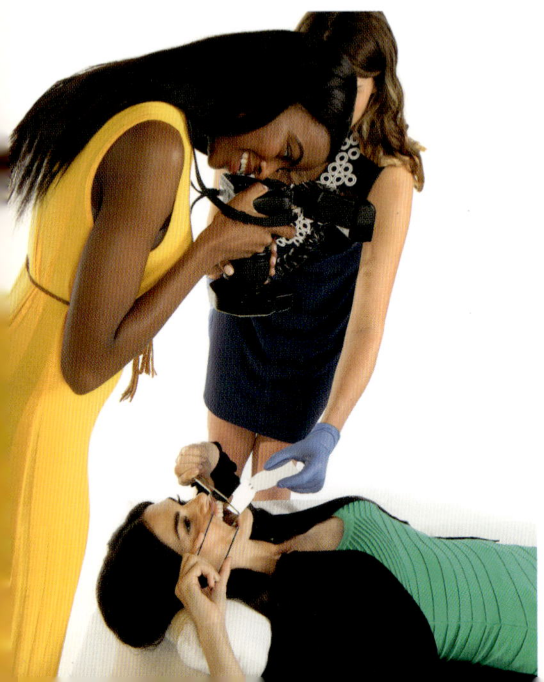

Dual flashes

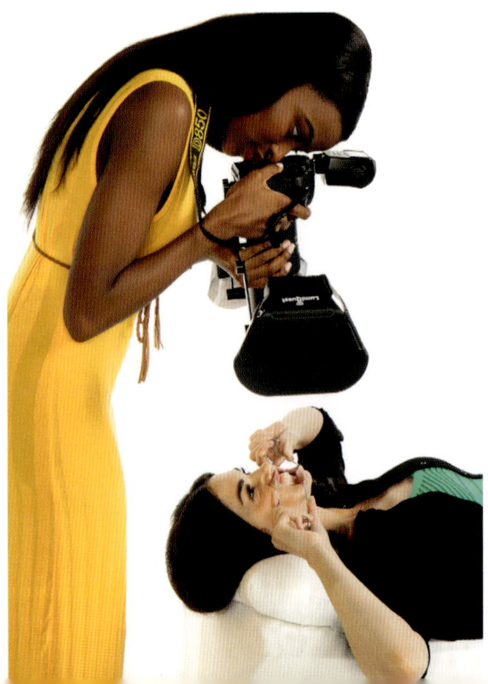

Speedlights

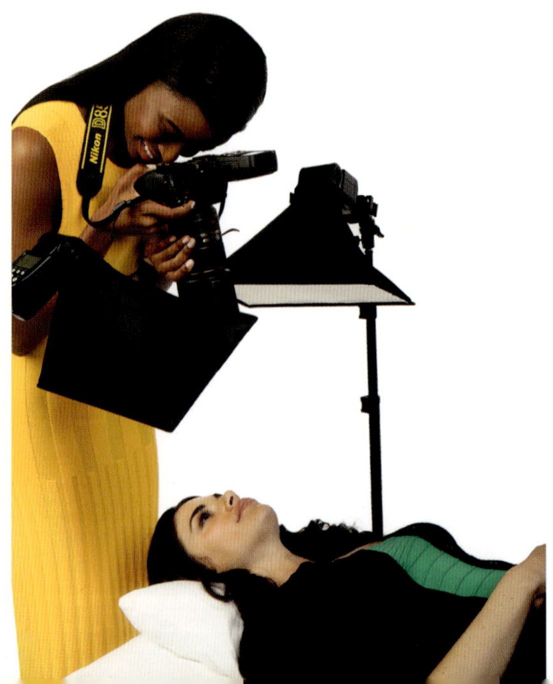

Strobes

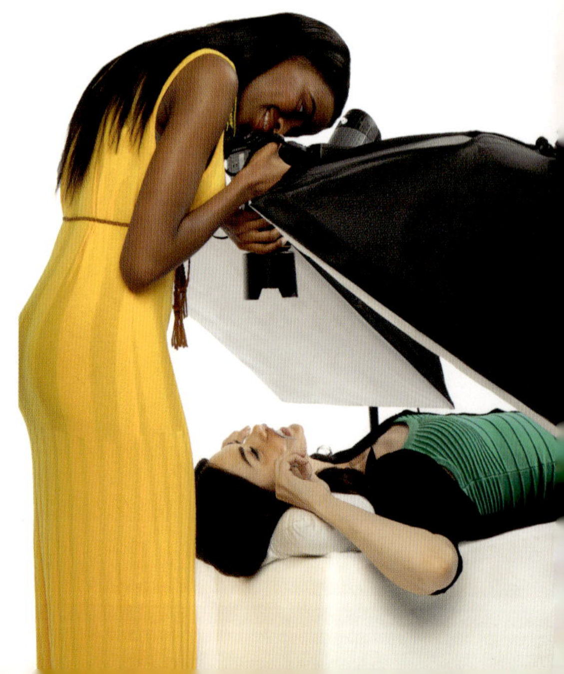

The Simple Protocol:

This chapter is about a simple intraoral protocol that works every day, without disrupting your clinic flow. I want you to be able to take great intraoral photos every day without having to spend an extra session to do so. However, photography is all about lighting. For this reason, you will see a variety of lighting setups throughout this chapter. But one thing will remain constant: the protocol. It does not change that much, even when you change the lighting systems.

If you want to know what I use every day in clinical practice, I use the speedlight setup. As explained earlier, it is simple, inexpensive, and easy to store. But the main reason I choose it over the other setups is because the speedlights with a diffuser are independent of my camera. Once I set the exposure, I am free to move and my lighting conditions do not change. With the ring flash or dual flashes, the lights move with you, which alters your exposure every time you move, and strobes are just not practical for most offices due to their size.

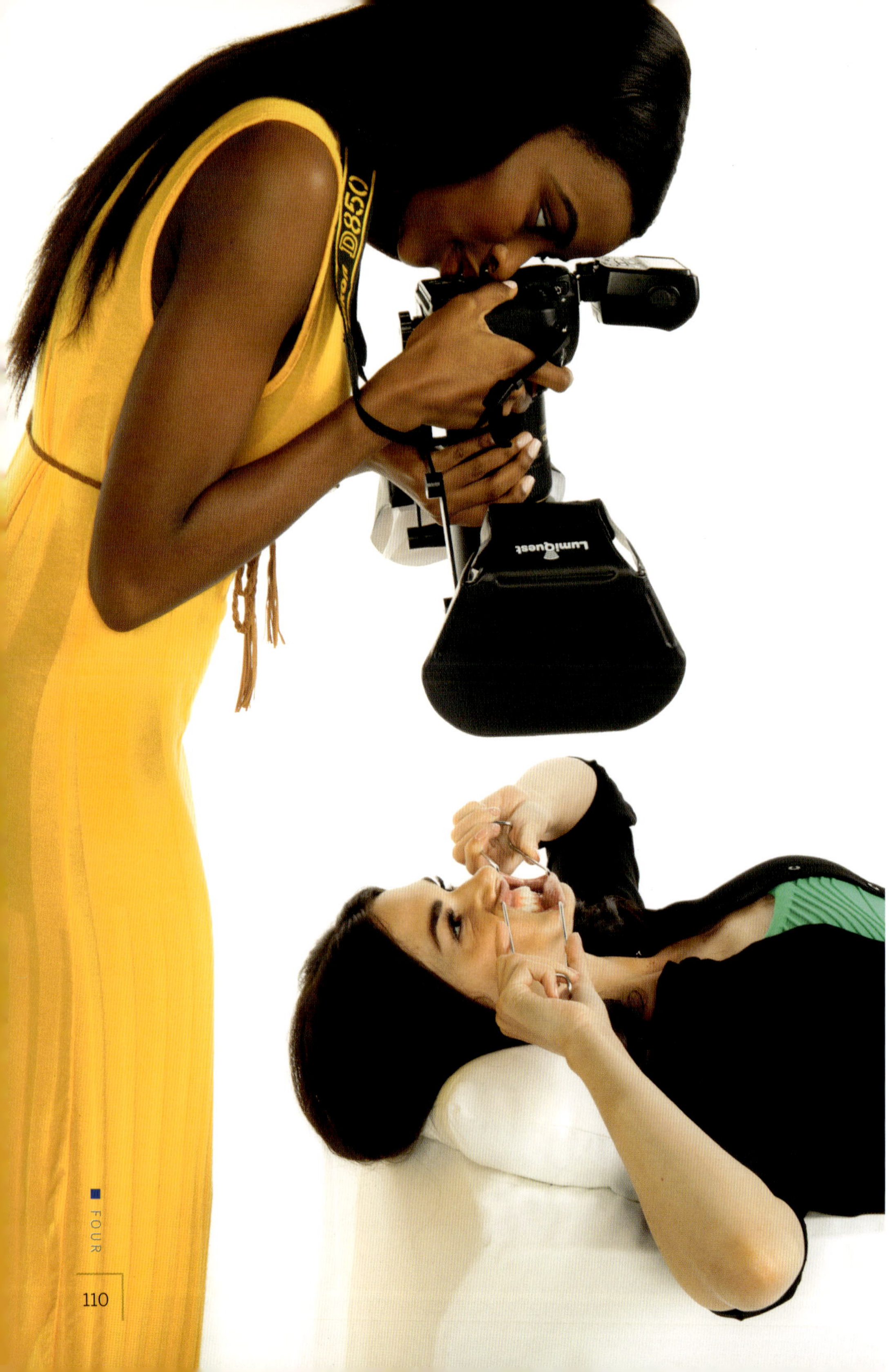

The Simple Protocol: Frontal Views

The first photo I take is a reposed smile. I use the first few photos to adjust my exposure, using all the tools we covered earlier: aperture, shutter speed, ISO, etc. I take full advantage of my histogram at this time as well. My dual flashes are open as wide as they can be on the brackets with the bouncer/diffuser on them. However, you must be careful not to have them on each side of the patient's face (180 degrees) or you will create a place of underexposure running vertically in the middle of the patient's face. The bracket wings should be wide open as long as the flashes are at 45-degree angle to the patient's face. Flashes are on manual mode and full power, no TTL.

From this position and with this setup, I will take all the following photos:

- Gray card, for white balance correction
- Lips in repose
- Relaxed smile
- Full smile
- Closer shots of all the above, but you must be careful and understand that as you move in closer, so do your flashes: Exposure will increase, and DOF will decrease
- Full dentition with retractors
- Maxillary anterior 6 to 8 teeth
- Maxillary anterior 6 to 8 teeth with contraster
- Shade-evaluation photos

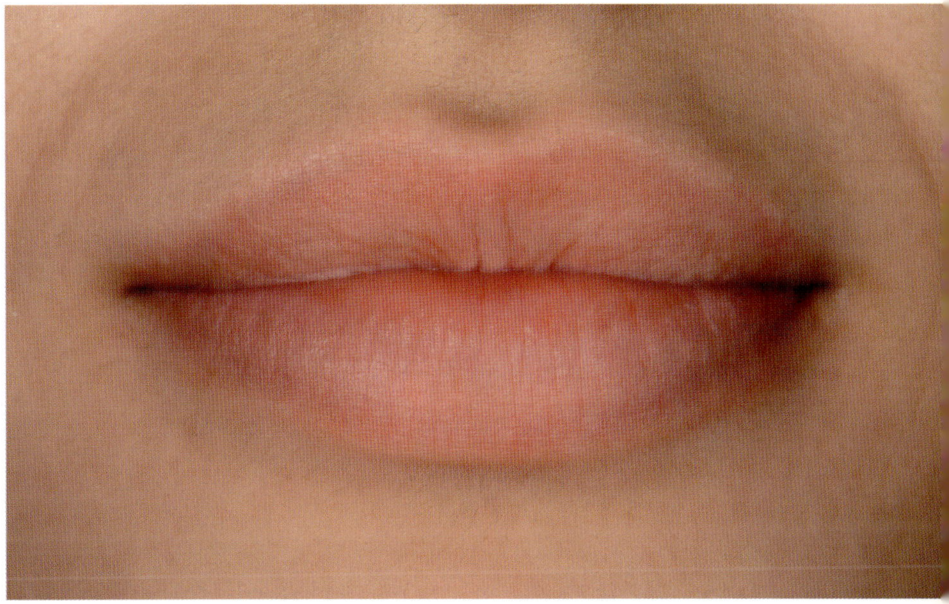

Advanced Tip

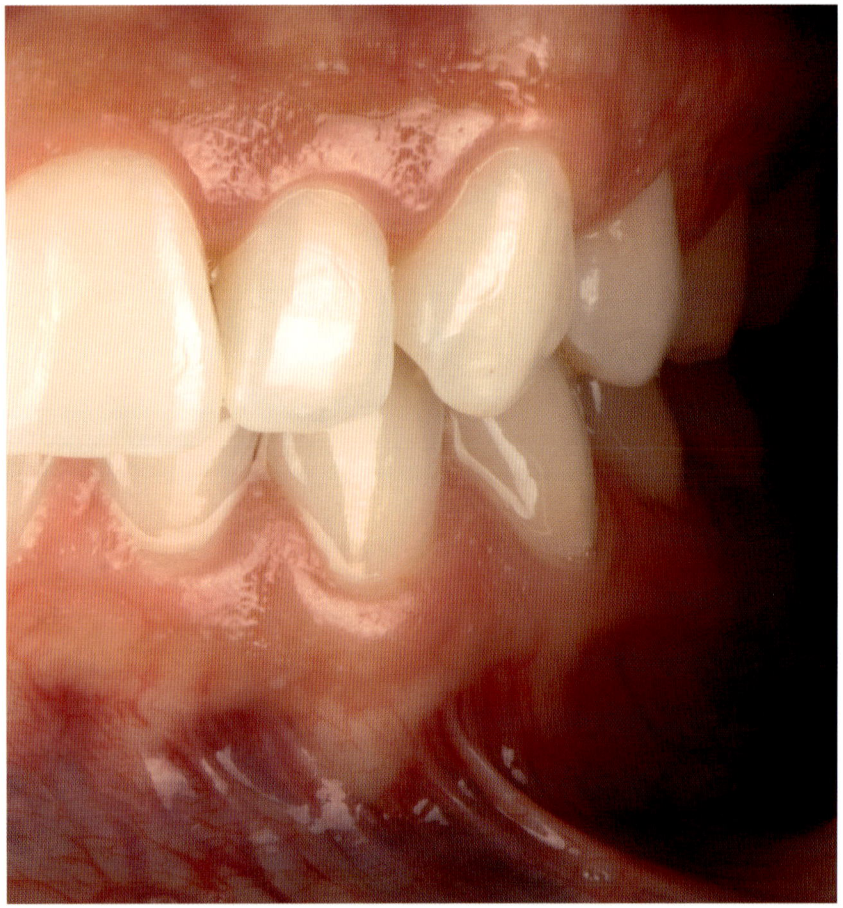

Underexposed buccal corridors

BUCCAL CORRIDORS

If you continue to have your bracket arms wide open while attempting to take the intraoral shots, you will have significant shadows on the buccal corridor areas. The ways to overcome underexposed buccal corridors:

- Close the wings and place the flash units in a ring position*
- Elevate yourself farther from the patient: This will straighten the angle of light reaching farther back into the posterior area
- Have the patient/assistant not only pull the retractors sideways but also forward; stretching the lips anteriorly will open up the buccal corridors

**Owners of ring flashes should not rejoice as if you had just won a small battle. Ring flashes are not better than dual flashes, even if at some point you need to use your dual flashes in a similar configuration to that of a ring flash. Dual flashes achieve nicer and more pleasing photos, as long as the light from the flashes is bounced and diffused.*

Note on contrasters

Positioning the contrasters to achieve a pure black background is a tricky thing. Ask the patient to position the retractors at 10 o'clock and 2 o'clock, the "smiley face position," as I call it. I place the contrasters as close to parallel to the occlusal surface as possible, trying to avoid a 90-degree angle between the contraster and the axis of my lens. This position of the contraster will diminish any light bouncing back from it and create a pure black background.

These anterior shots can be taken with the flashes at an open-wing position or at a more closed position. It depends on the effect you are trying to give to the photo. The more open the wings are, the more texture and shadows will result on the teeth. The line angles will be especially more prominent. However, you might want to close the wings a bit if you also want to include the premolars in the shot while properly exposing them.

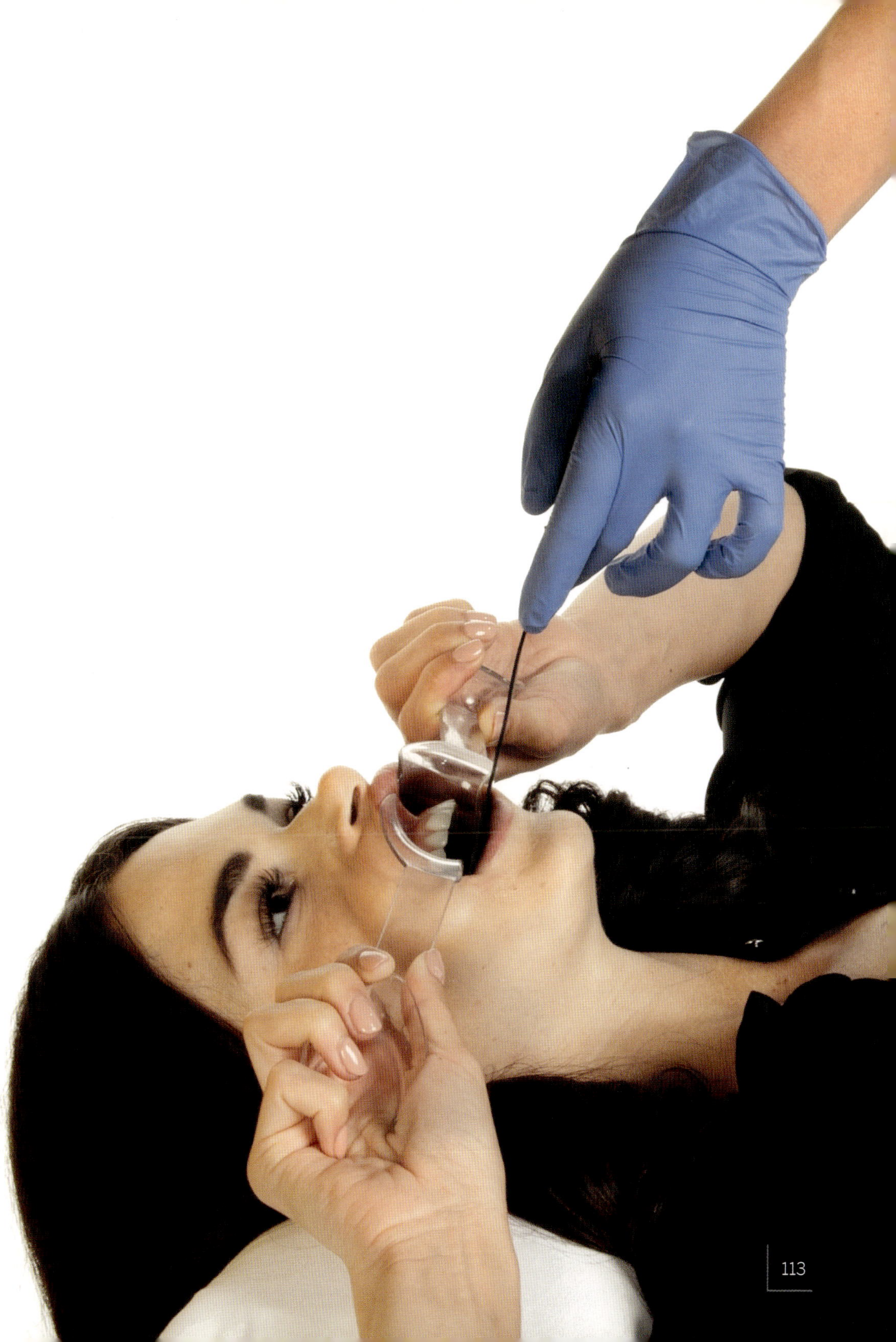

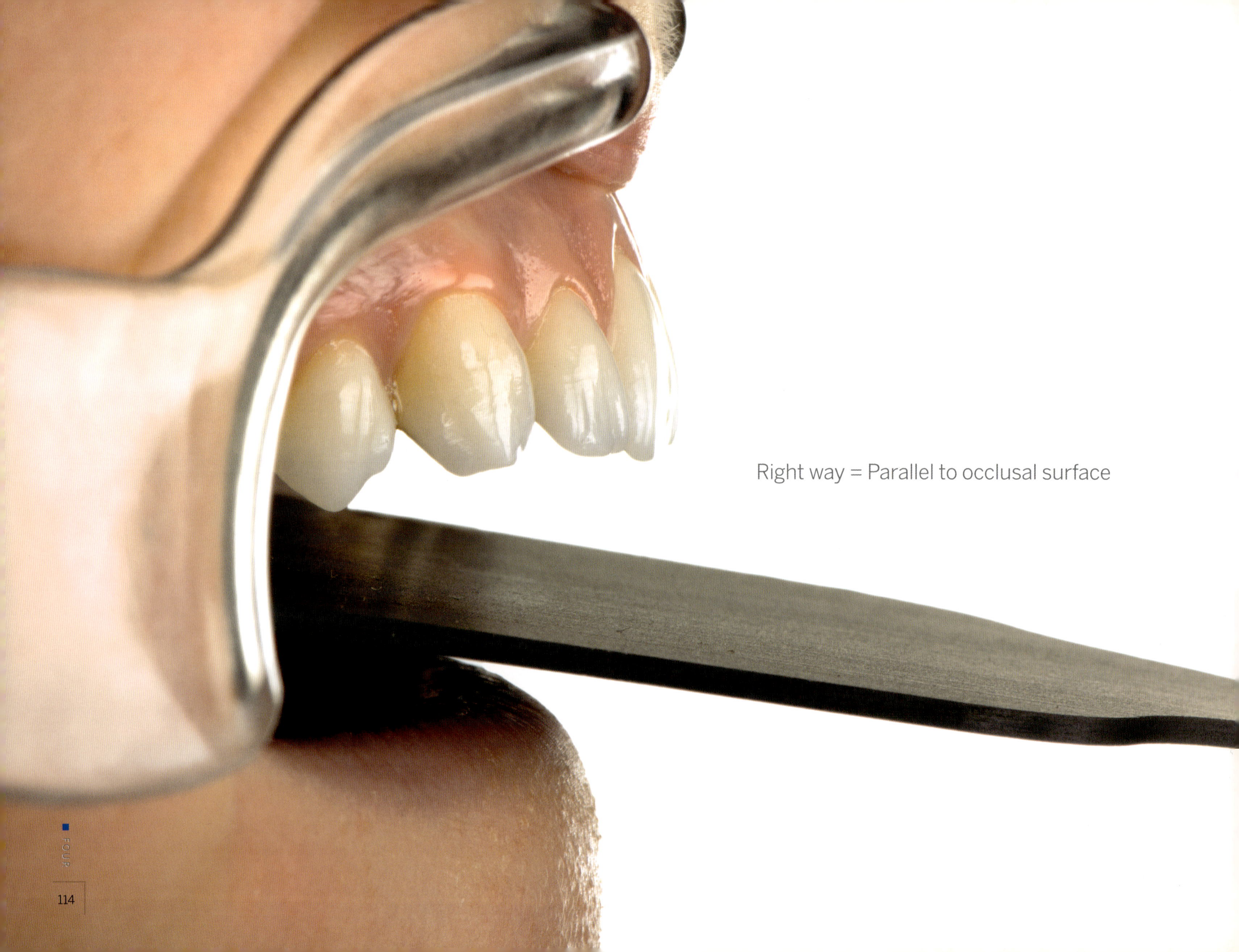

Right way = Parallel to occlusal surface

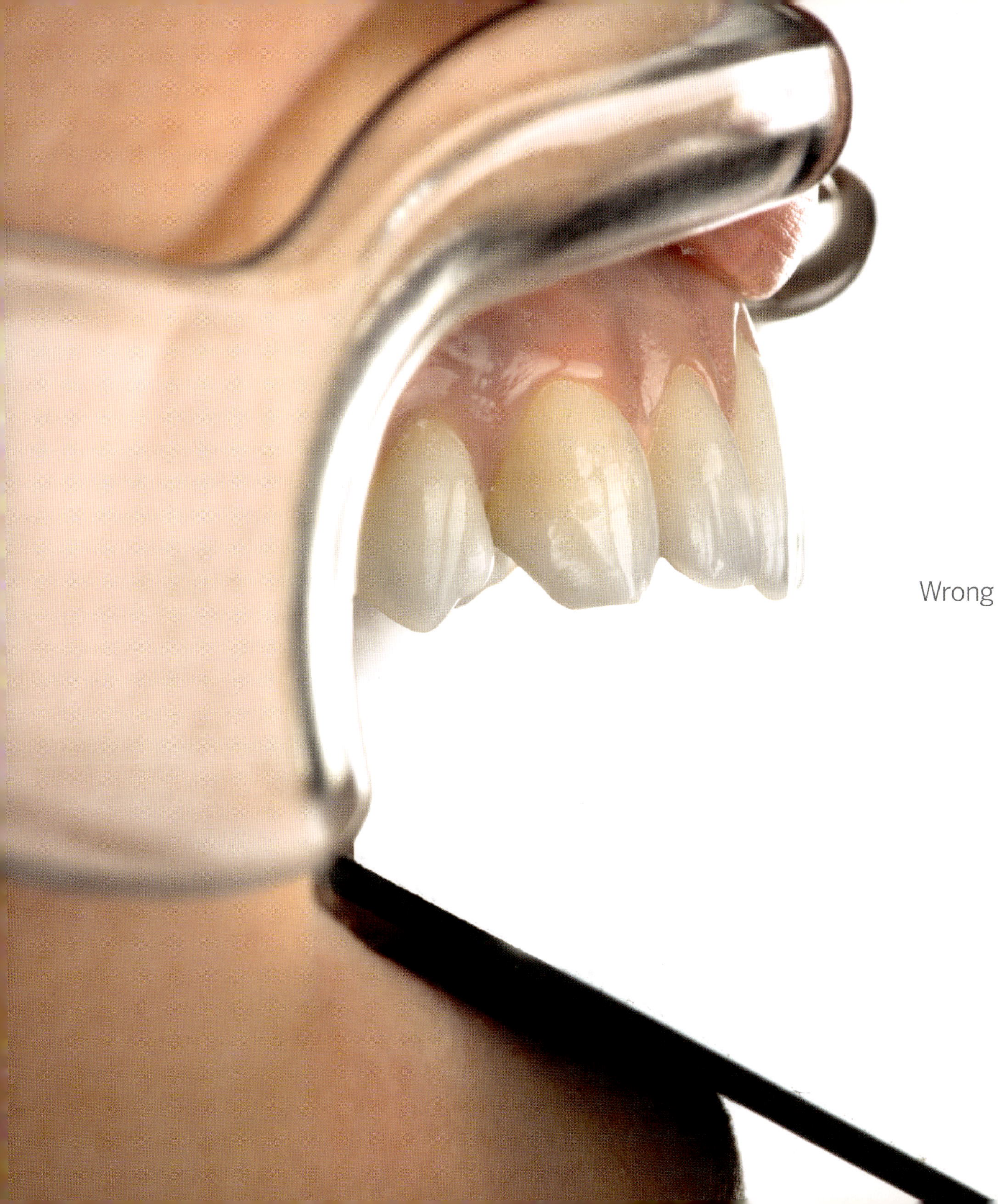

Wrong way = Angled to occlusal surface

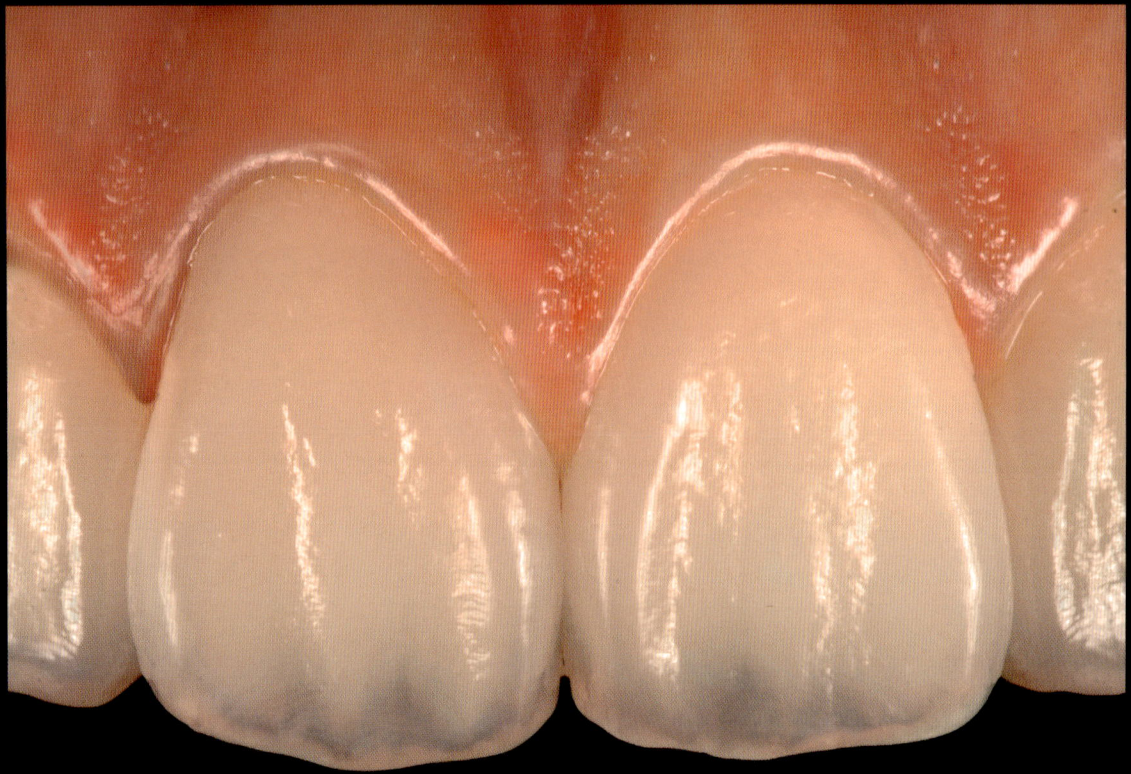

Advanced Tip

TRANSLUCENCY

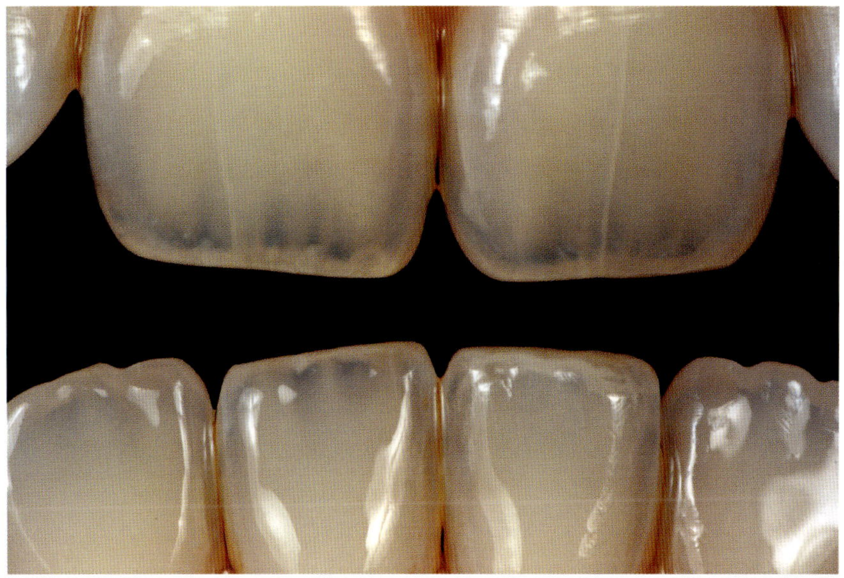

If you want to show translucency, underexpose your photo and then increase the exposure in post-processing.

Diminishing distance

As you move closer to the anterior teeth, you need to start worrying a bit more about the consequences that arise from the diminished distance. If your flashes are attached to your camera, exposure will increase dramatically. You will have to reduce your shutter speed (higher number) and/or increase your f-stop. You could reduce the power of the flashes as well. And if your ISO was for some reason higher than 100, you will need to lower that as well.

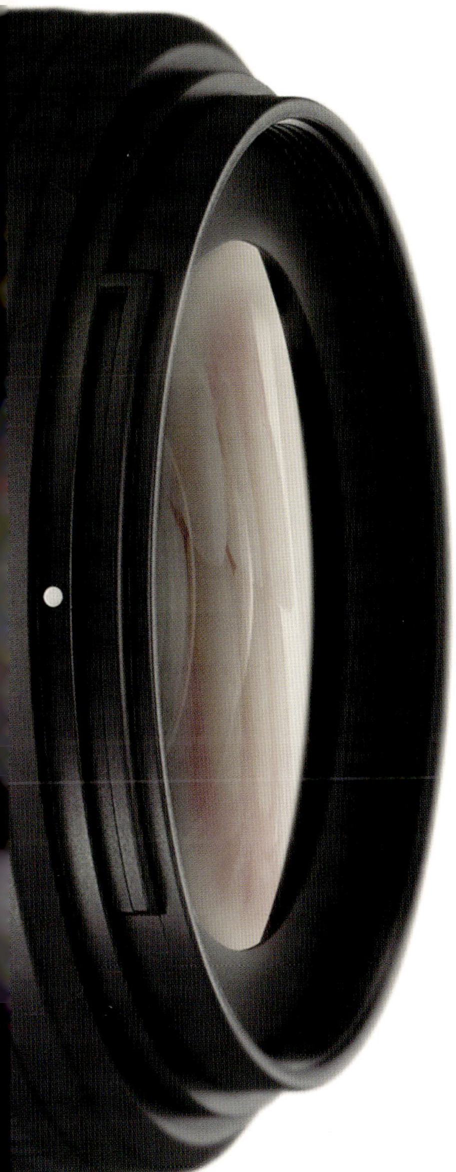

Remember the "1/3, 2/3 rule"

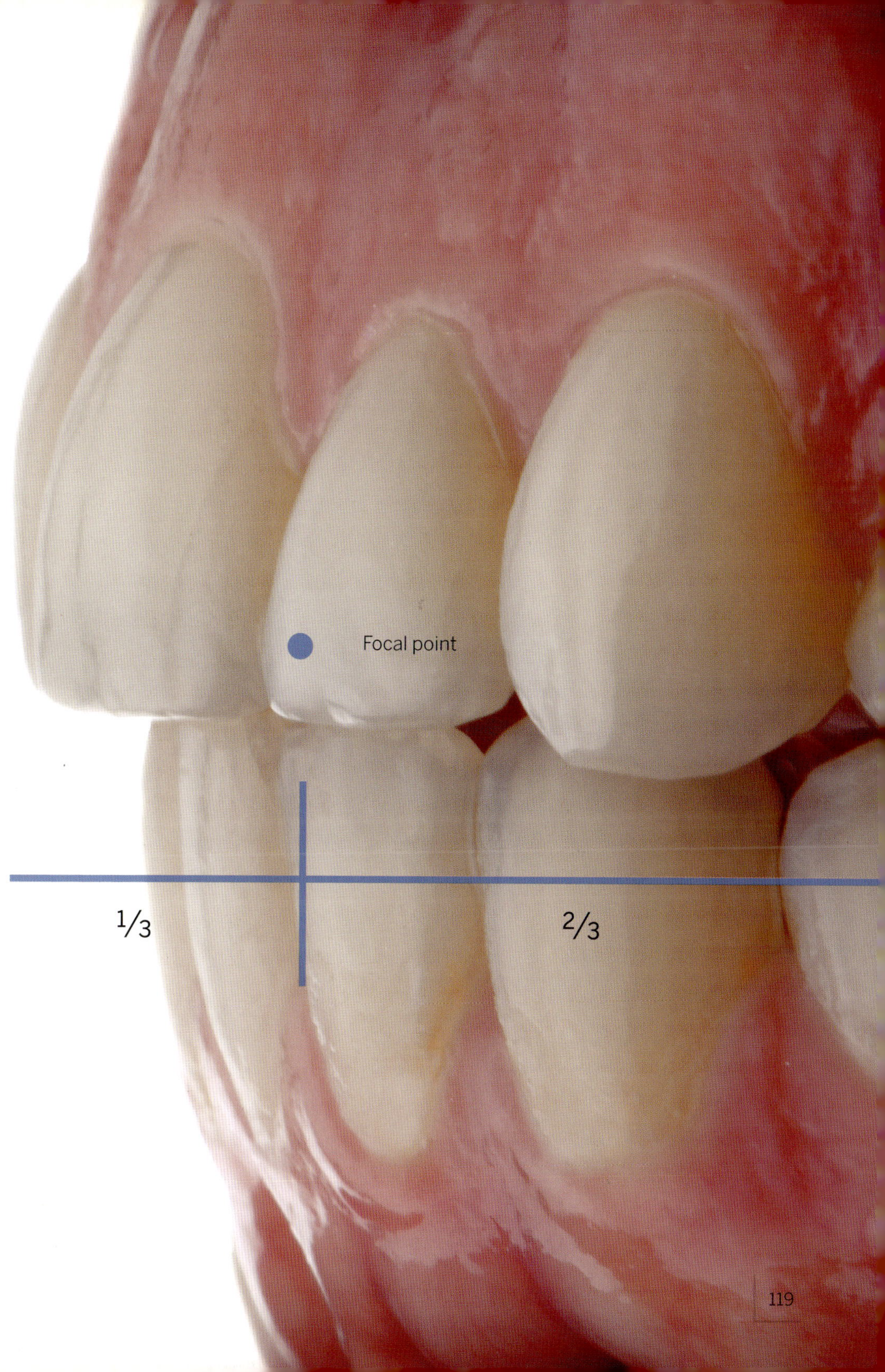

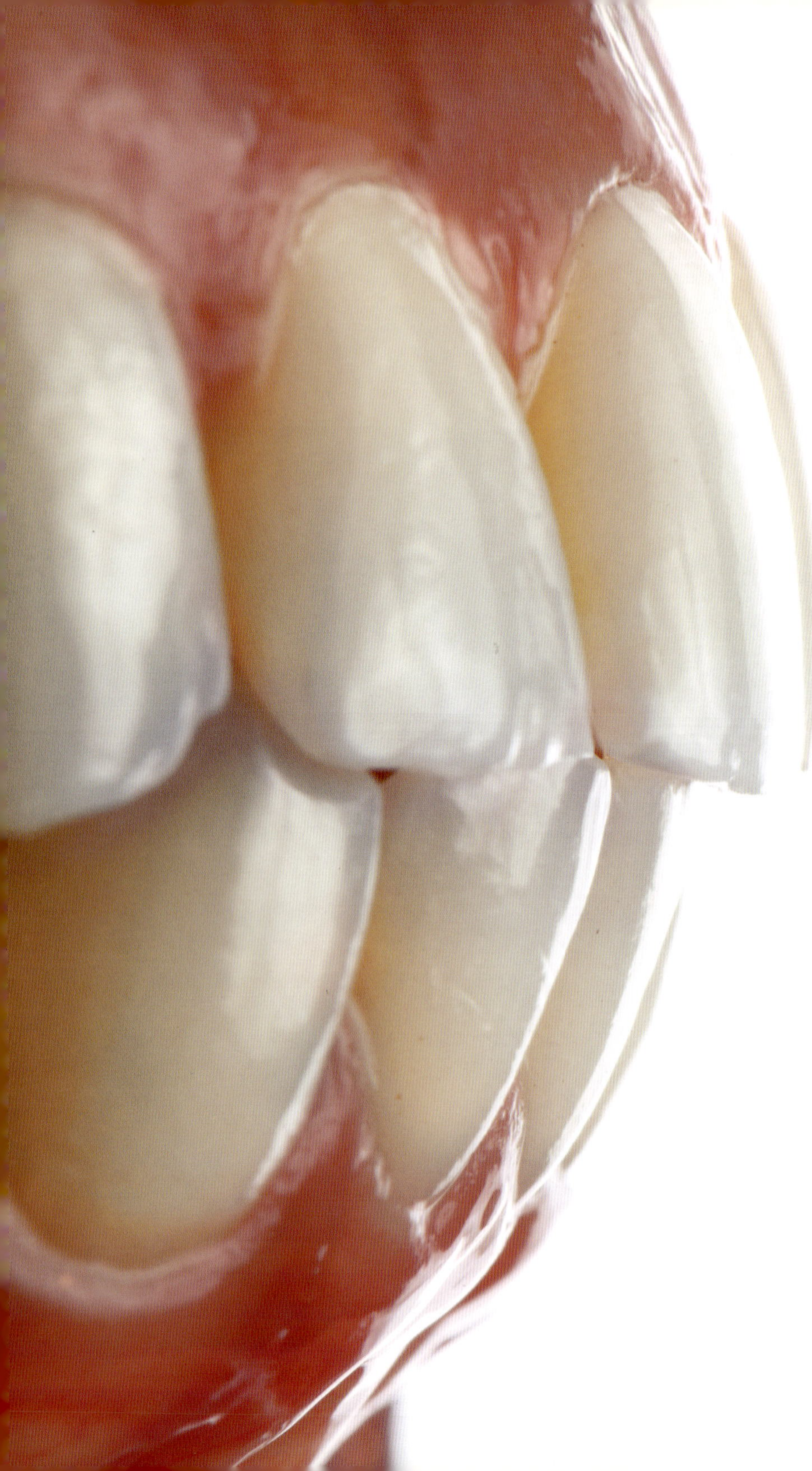

Narrow depth of field

Notice how the central incisors are sharp but the canines are blurry. As I got closer and closer to take this shot, the DOF decreased. The f-stop should have been increased to compensate for the shorter distance.

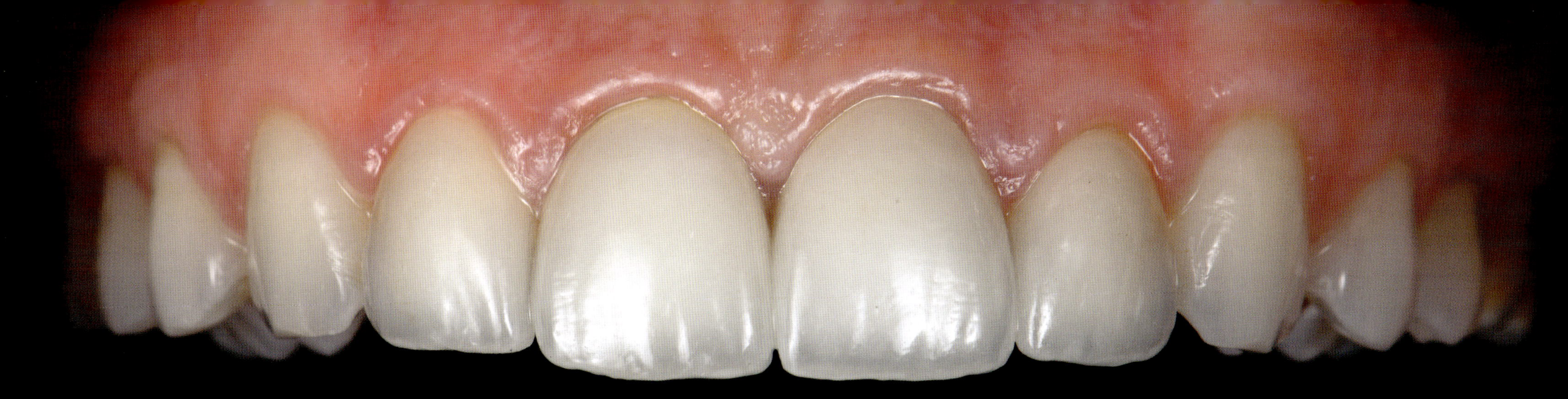

Underexposed buccal borridors

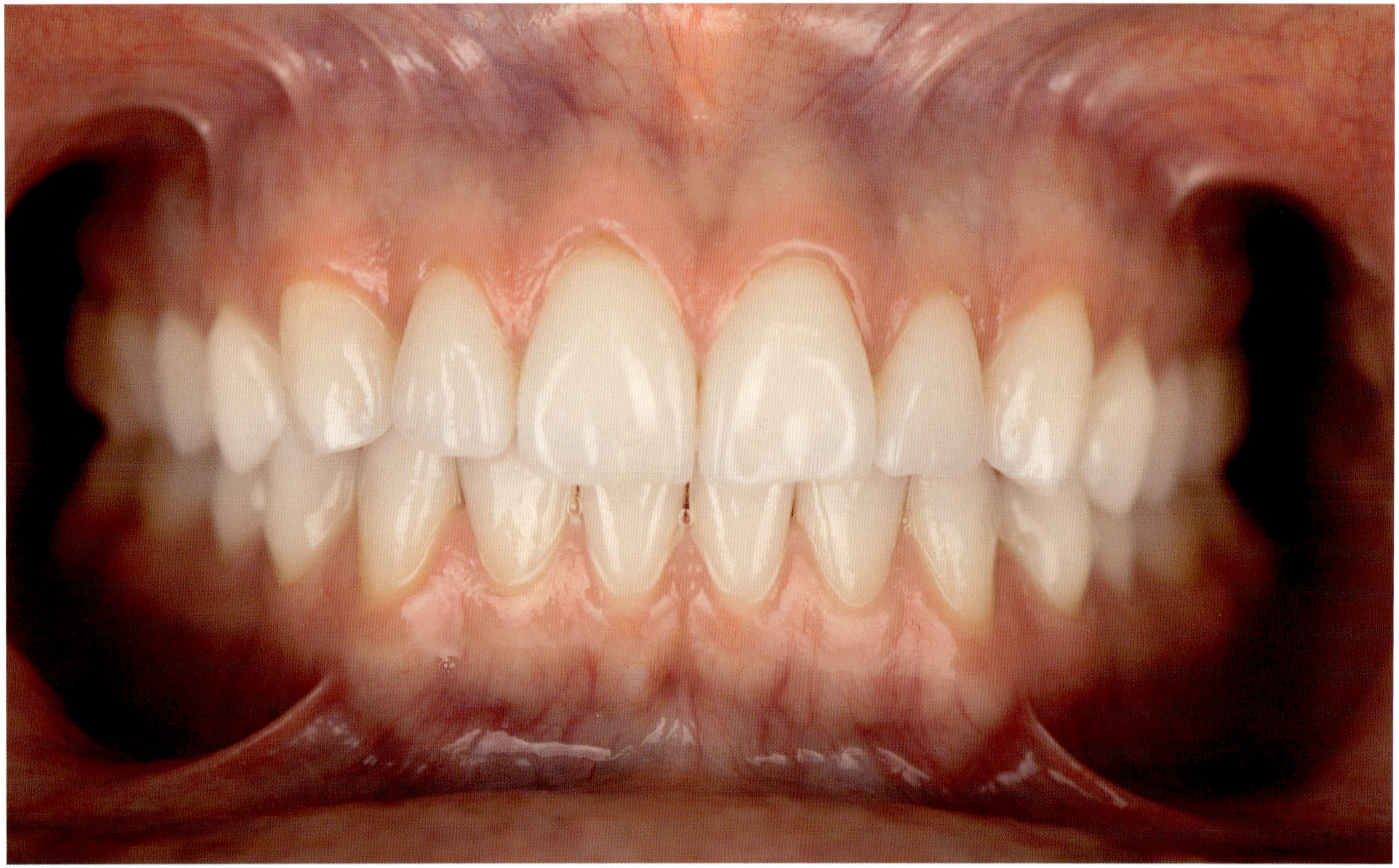

DOF too narrow = Posterior area out of focus

Need to increase f-stop to 32 or higher

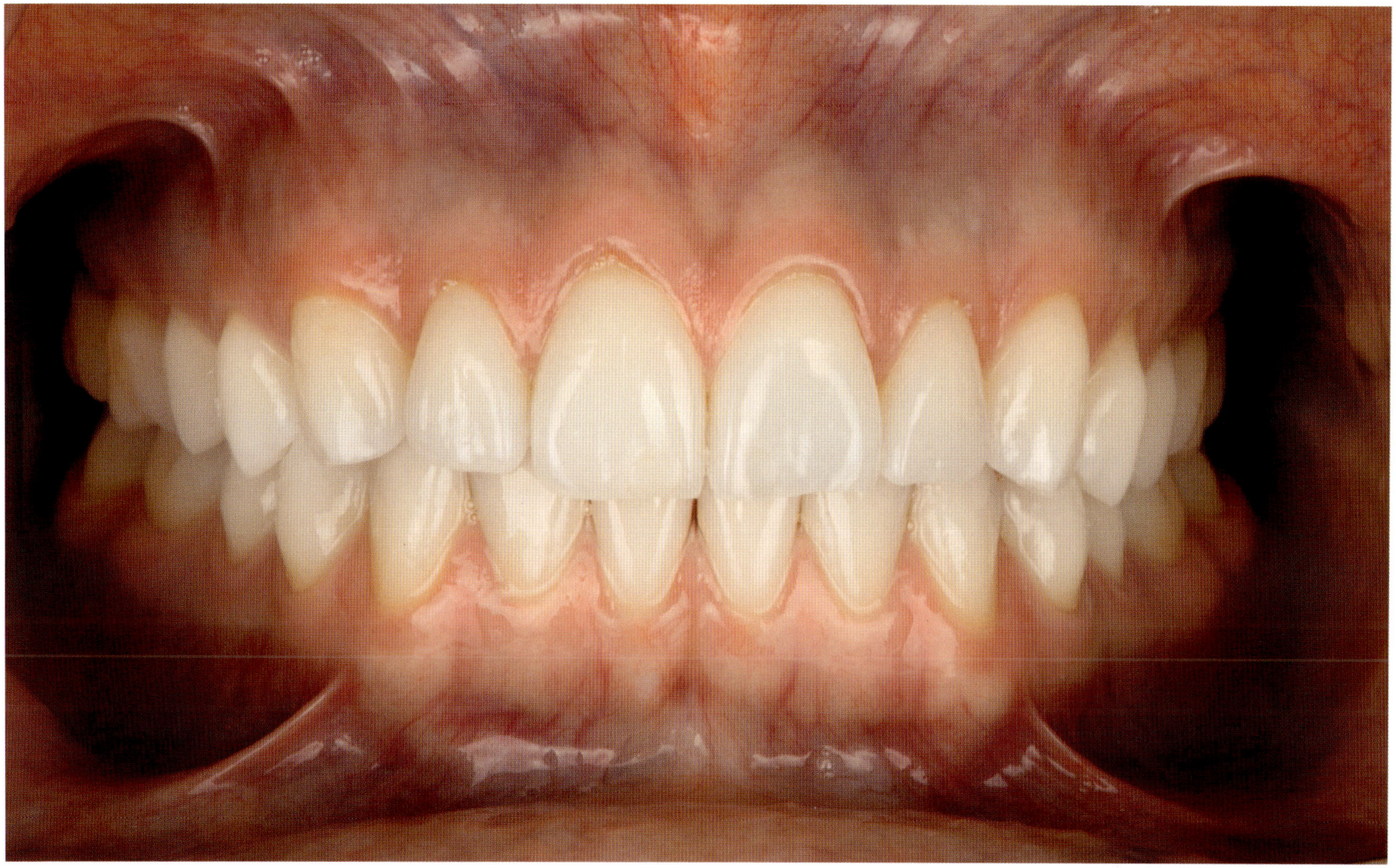

DOF appropriate = Posterior area in focus

F-stop = 32

The Simple Protocol: Maxillary Occlusal Plane

After I place the metal retractors or the cut-off C-shaped retractors, I then ask the patient to put their chin up and hold their breath. I place the double-sided stainless steel occlusal mirrors. The posterior part of the mirror *should not* be placed against the occlusal surface of the teeth; it should be as far back as possible but without touching the maxillary teeth.

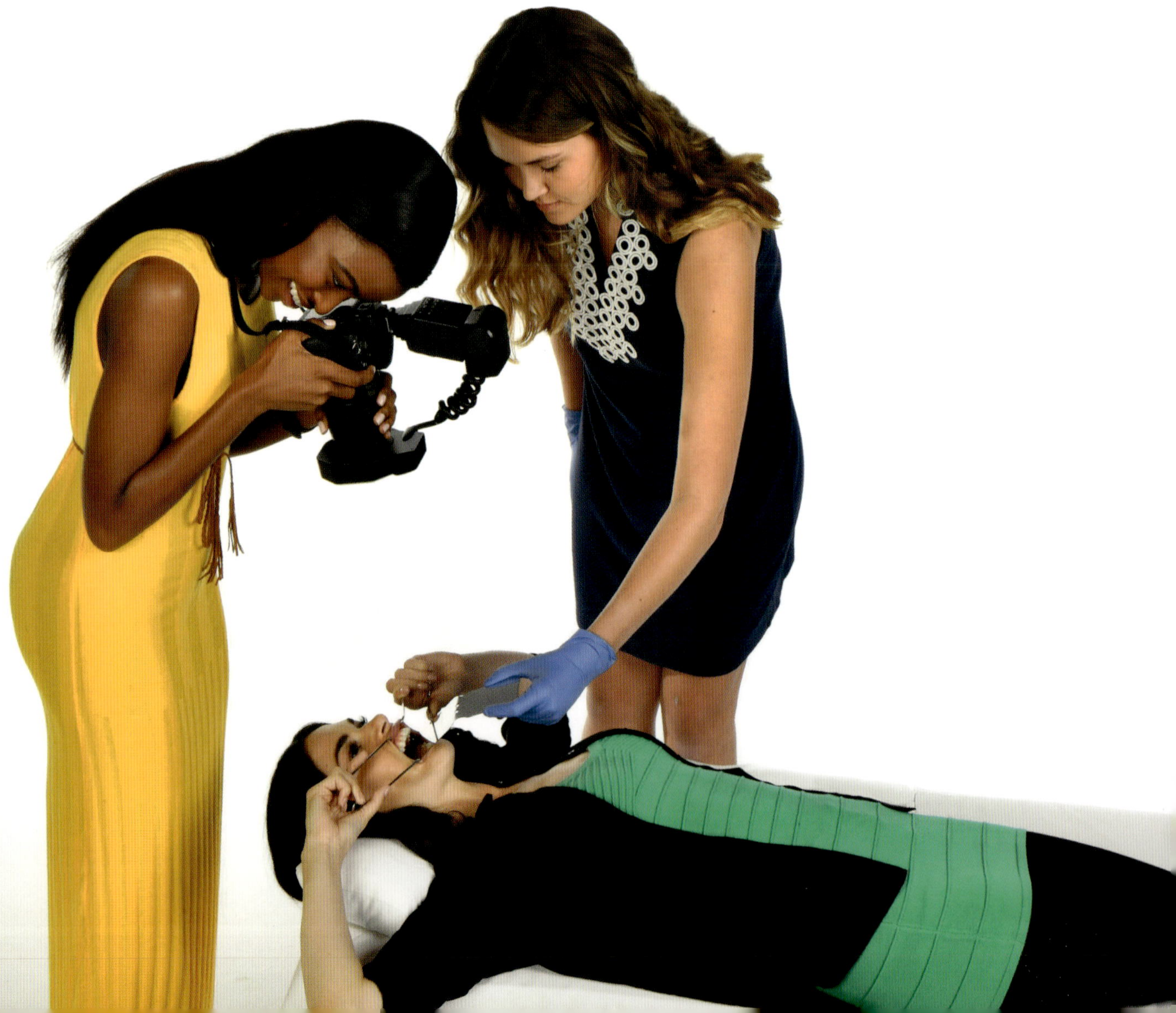

Diffused speedlights

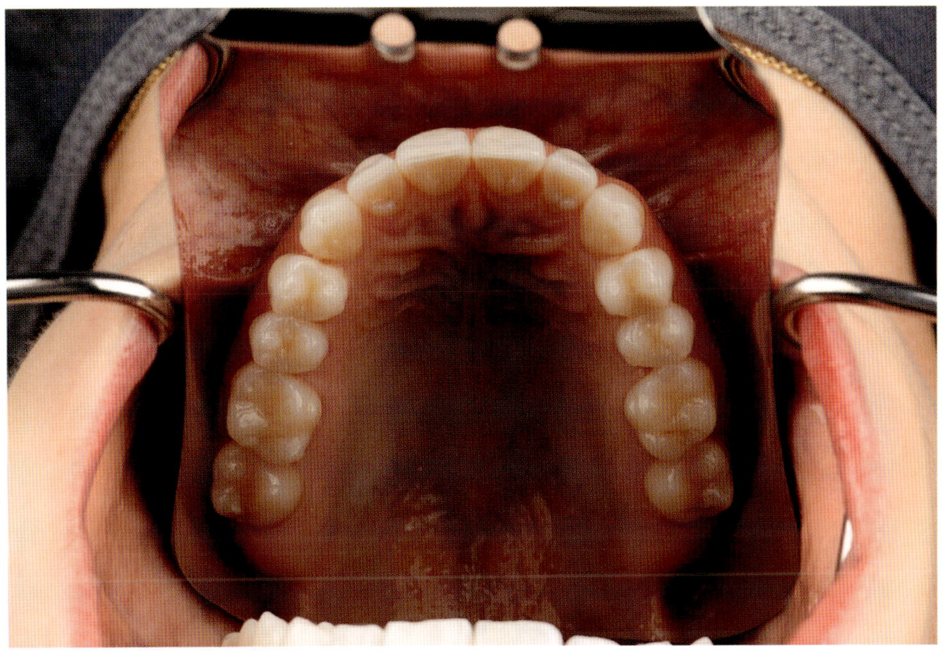

Complete field of view

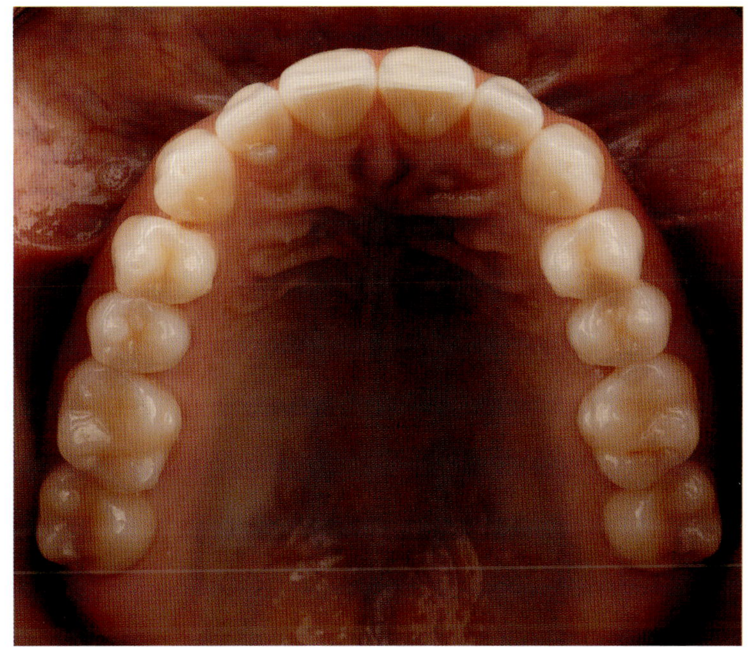

Final cropped photo

Three-quarters of all shots are done without changing position.

As of now, I have achieved 75% of my intraoral shots from the same position. I had no need to move the patient or myself. And that is not all. I take the shade measurements from this position as well. So how is that for simplifying the intraoral protocol? What if I tell you that 90% or more of the intraoral photos you have seen from me are taken in this position? Prep shots, temps shots, surgical shots, before and after shots, etc, all with the patient in a supine position and me standing at 12 o'clock.

MIRRORS

Stainless steel mirrors have several advantages that I love. They will not break. They are light, thin, and front-surface. They are less expensive than most glass front-surface mirrors by a significant amount, and their shape is ideal for the job.

But there is another advantage that is important, at least for me. That is the fact that I can heat them up quickly with my butane torch that I use for modifying the occlusal rims on a denture. I grab the torch, I light it up, and I do four quick side-by-side passes. Swighhh, swighhh, swighhh, swighhh, and done. (That was the sound of the torch moving side to side, by the way.) In less than 3 seconds, the mirror is at body temperature and no fogging occurs.

Trust me, it works beautifully. No need for water or any little motor fan. No need to blow air or anything like that. Just swighhh, swighhh, swighhh, swighhh.

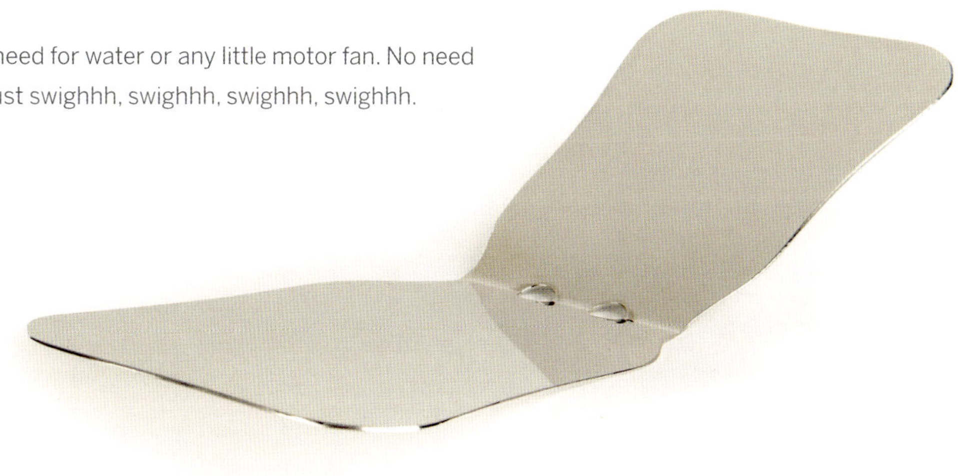

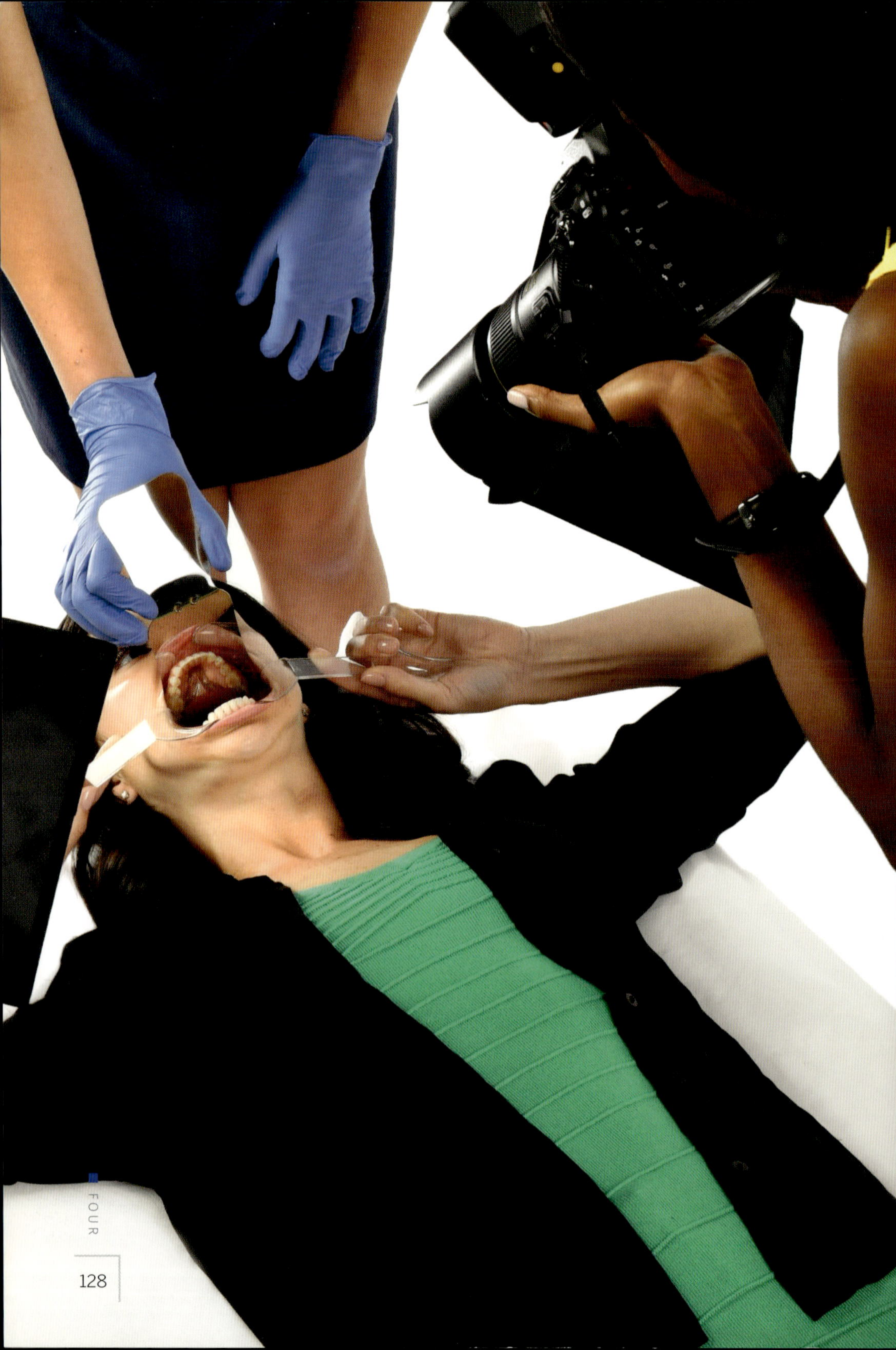

The patient stays in the same position, but I move toward the 5 o'clock position. I ask the patient to use the retractors on the 4 o'clock and 8 o'clock positions to separate the lower lip from the mandibular anterior teeth. Then I ask the patient to place their tongue on the roof of their mouth. As I introduce the mirror underneath their tongue, I ask them to now relax their tongue. I push the ventral part of the tongue posteriorly with my warmed-up mirror. I place the mirror at 90 degrees to my field of view and take the photo.

The Simple Protoco Mandibular Occlusal Pla

Diffused speedlights

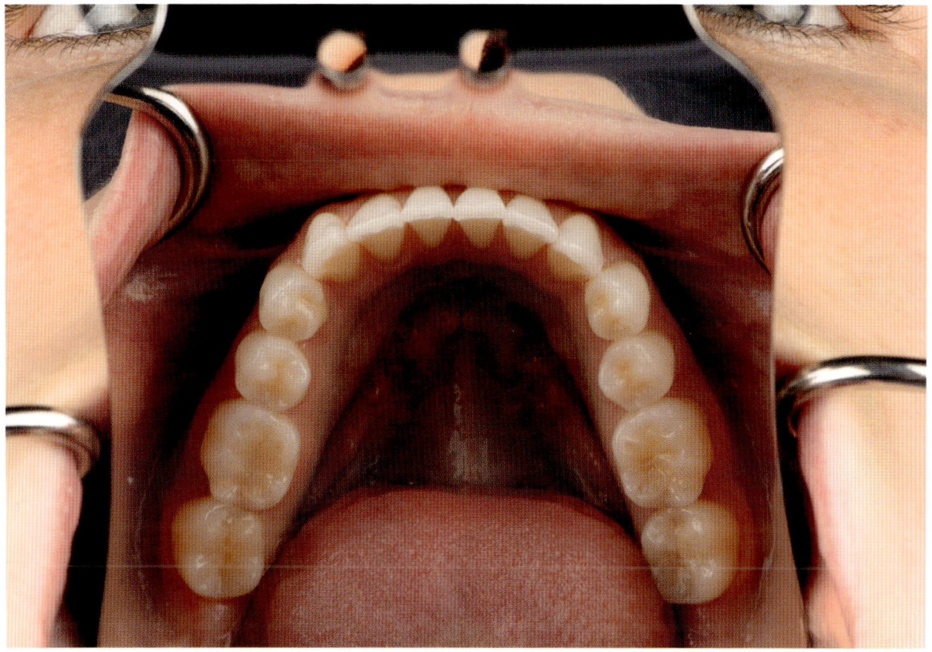

Complete field of view

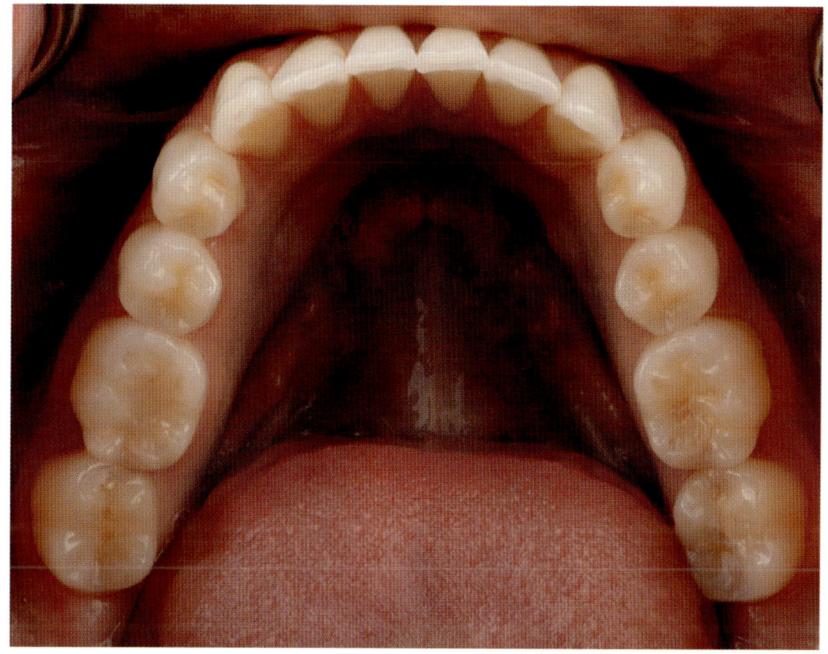

Final cropped photo

The Simple Protocol:

Posterior Lateral Photos

For the first time, I place the patient's chair at a 45-degree angle. For the left side lateral shot with mirrors, I place myself on the right side of the patient. I place the dual flashes at 3 o'clock and 12 o'clock, or most likely I will use a ring flash. A retractor is placed on the right side, and the patient is asked not to pull too hard on it. With the mouth open and using the stainless steel lateral shot mirrors, I ask the patient to bite down into maximum intercuspation. The mirrors are moved as posteriorly as possible. Once there, the most posterior part of the mirror has to be pulled outward, away from the buccal surfaces of the posterior teeth. This is the only way to fully photograph the posterior buccal surfaces properly.

The most common mistake made at this stage is to lean the posterior part of the mirror on the buccal surface of the second molar and pull outward on the anterior region. This creates a 30- to 40- degree angle between the buccal surfaces of the teeth and the mirror, which must be avoided. The mirror and the teeth have to be separated and parallel with each other.

- Place chair at 45-degree angle.
- Use one retractor to pull the contralateral side gently.
- Warm the mirror with the torch.
- Adjust your dual flashes to 12 o'clock and 3 o'clock, or use a ring flash.
- Separate the posterior teeth from the mirror.

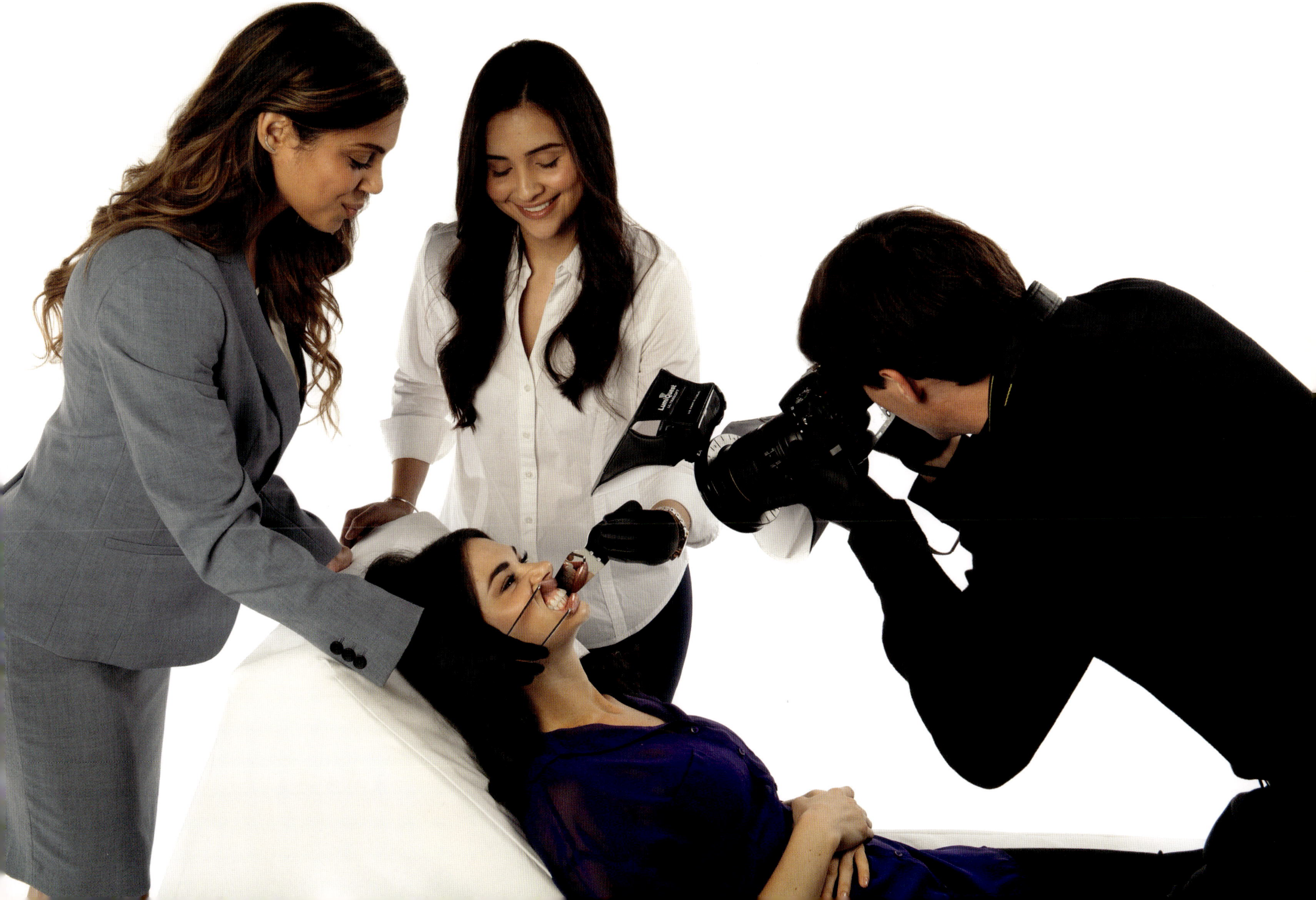

Ring flash

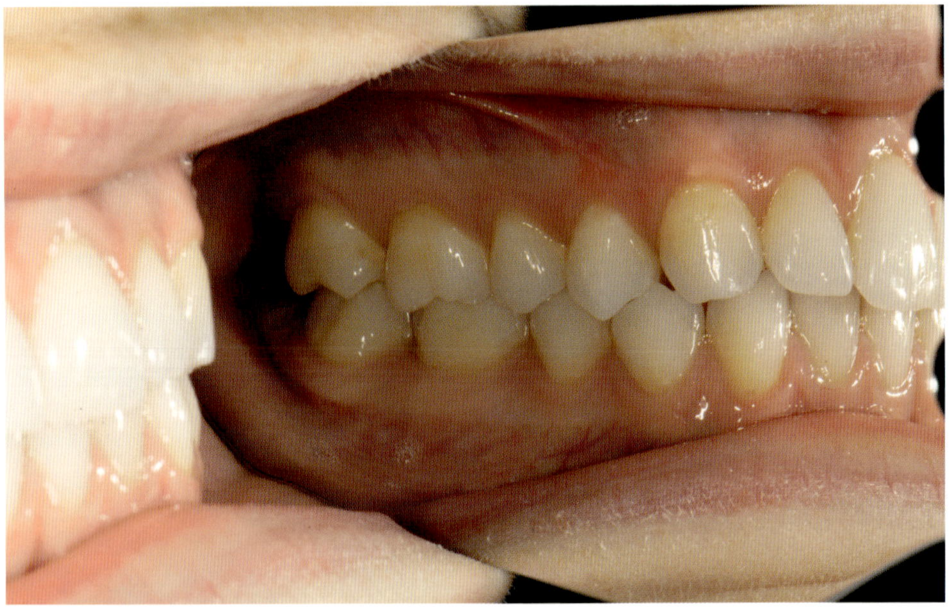

Posterior lateral photo of left side with complete field of view

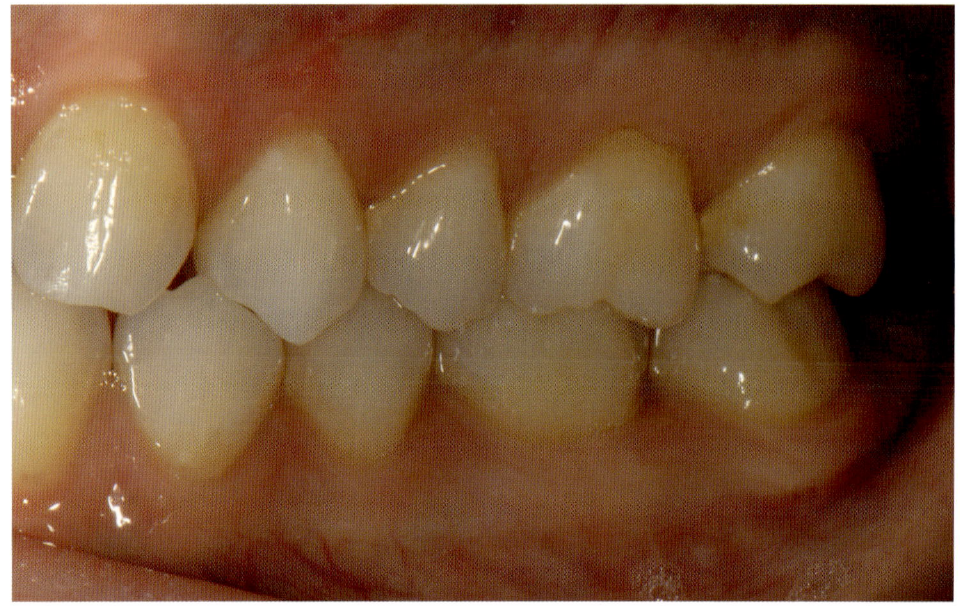

Posterior lateral photo of left side, cropped and mirrored

On Quick Guides

If you are flipping through this book trying to find a set of pages where I give you what camera settings you should have for every type of shot, then you are wasting your time. I am a fervent believer that such "quick guides" are not only unhelpful but misleading.

The only way that a quick guide with a set of f-stop, shutter speed, ISO, and flash power parameters can work is if the camera, the lights, and the patient are always in exactly the same position for every photo. When using a ring flash or dual flashes, you will move back and forth and so will your light distance and intensity, resulting in over- and underexposed photos every time, if parameters are not actively adjusted.

If you are using speedlights or strobes, your light might be more consistent, but your distance with the subject will change. As you try to compensate for DOF, you will change your aperture and thus your exposure will differ from shot to shot.

We will not even mention that those quick guides are never to be found in the operatories, neither can you go around reading them while taking photos. The best way to learn photography is by understanding three little things: aperture, shutter speed, and light source.

Know Your Limits

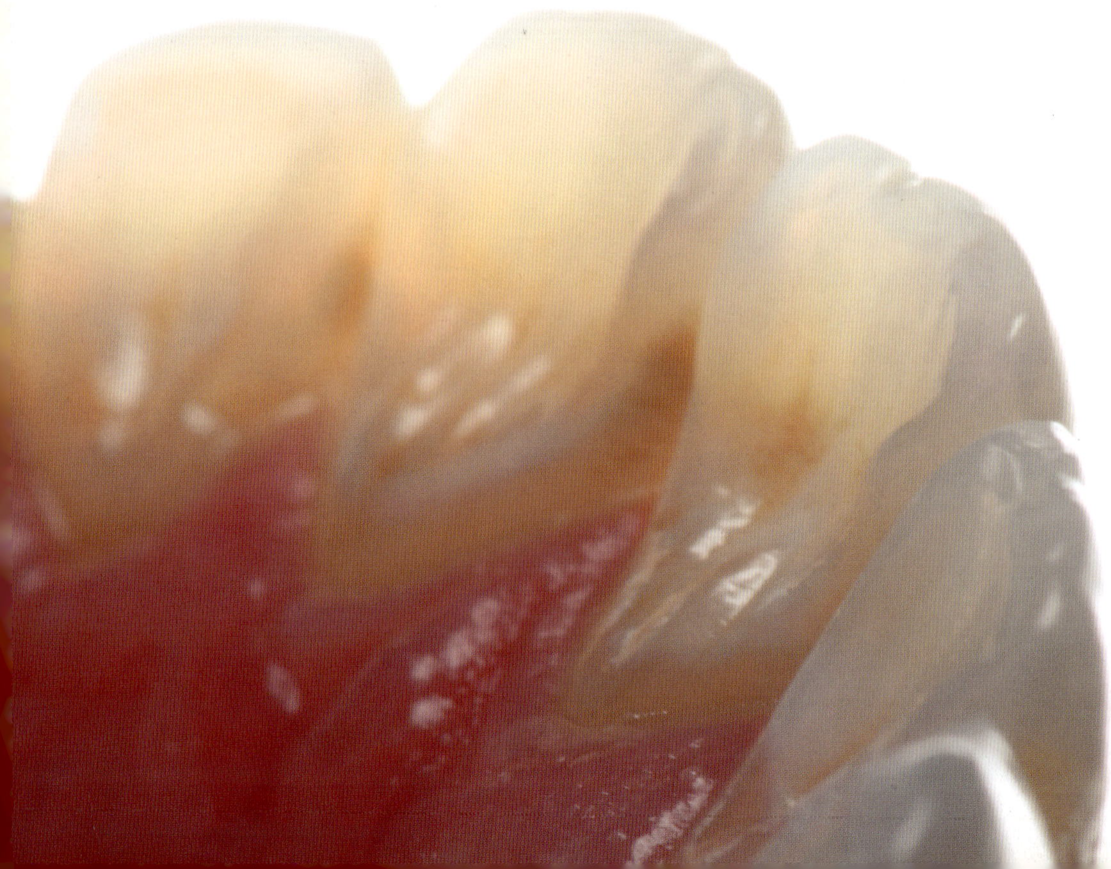

Aperture

f/22 to f/36 for intraoral or f/16 to f/36 for portraits

Shutter speed

1/100 s to 1/250 s

ISO

100, if possible

Flash

Full power and manual mode

Knowing those limits and understanding how to correct for exposure is all you need.

The Simple Protocol: Summary

This concludes the basic day-to-day intraoral protocol for any new or existing patients. There are always more shots that could be discussed, such as lateral movements, but I find them all to be variations of the previously discussed photos.

- Start with the patient laying flat. Position yourself behind the patient.
- Camera settings: f-stop = 32, shutter speed = $1/125$, ISO = 100, flash = full power
- Find the right exposure using the histogram as a tool.
- Take the frontal and occlusal shots:
  - Gray card, for white balance correction
  - Lips in repose
  - Relaxed smile
  - Full smile
  - Full dentition with retractors
  - Maxillary anterior teeth, with and without contrasters
  - Maxillary occlusal plane
  - Shade-evaluation photos
- Move to the 5 o'clock position.
  - Take the mandibular occlusal plane shot.
- Place the patient at 45 degrees.
  - Take the lateral shots.

You are done.

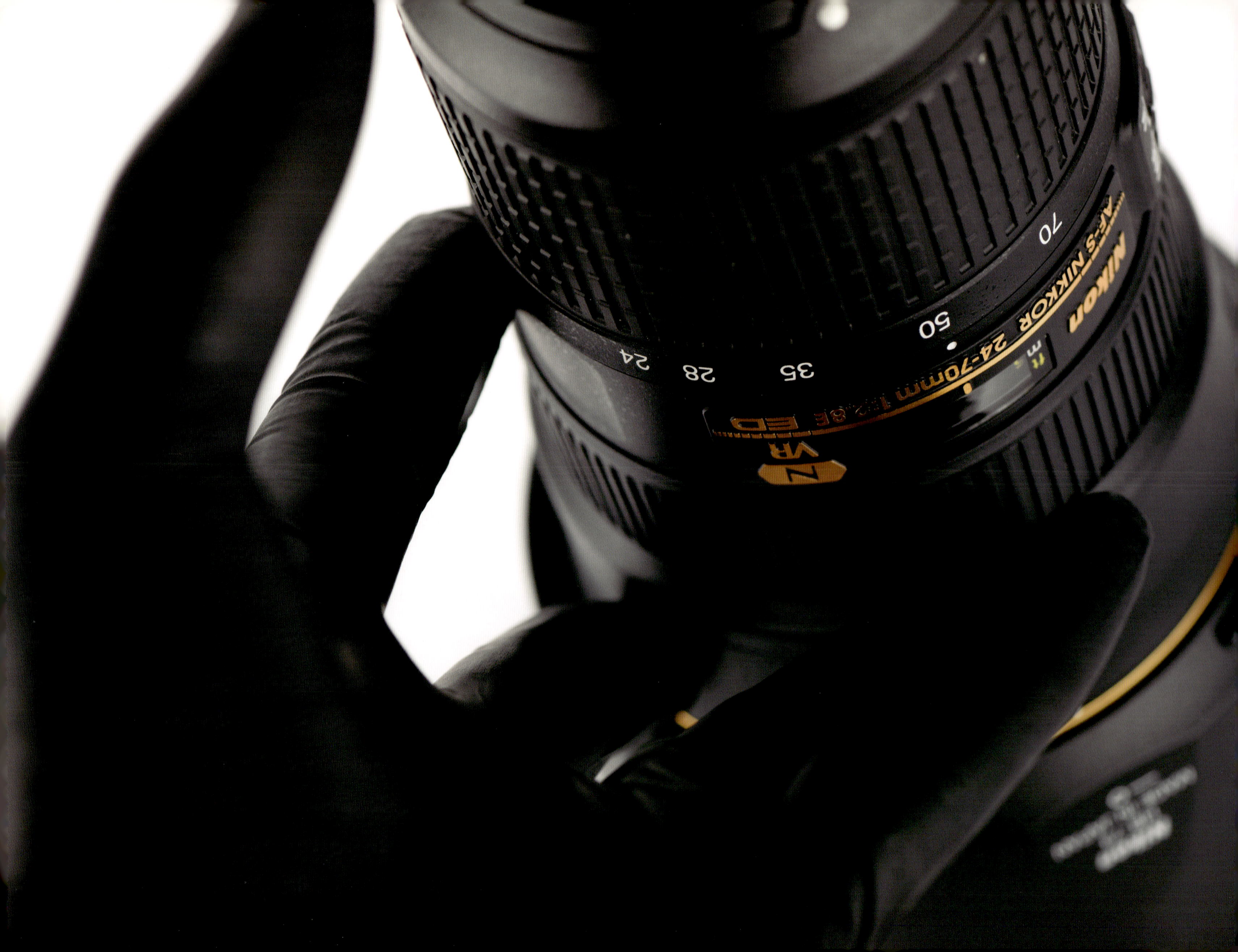
Nikon
AF-S NIKKOR 24-70mm 1:2.8E ED
VR
N
24
28
35
50
70

Encore:

Black Gloves

It is important for me to mention that in order to be a great dental photographer, you must have certain things. They include the desire to be better, the understanding that some gear is necesssary, and the will to practice your techniques. However, it seems that the number one requirement for true success is . . . black gloves.

It is for this reason that I made sure that as I created this book for you, I had on my black gloves. Without them, you and I could never reach excellence.

Artistic Dental Photography

Let the Controversy Begin

Artistic dental photography has arrived and it has brought with it some controversy and rejection. Social media has modified the notion that all dental photography must be for the purposes of documentation and presentations only. We have challenged the idea that we must show perfectly centered photos with no character or visual appeal. We have confronted the notion that dental photos must use the lighting, DOF, and composition to depict exactly what the treatment plan is. Some find such artistic photography absurd, a thing that has no place in the dental profession. I have a theory, however. I believe most haters of artistic dental photography are part of a group who, deep inside, wish they could do it themselves but feel frustrated when they try to do it and fail. To those I say, "Do not worry. Here is your chapter. Here is how it's done." Artistic dental photography is for everyone and it is here to stay—to evolve, to evoke, to inspire.

This chapter covers the following concepts and more:

THE GLOSSY EFFECT

CHIAROSCURO

CHROMATICITY

MAKEUP

light

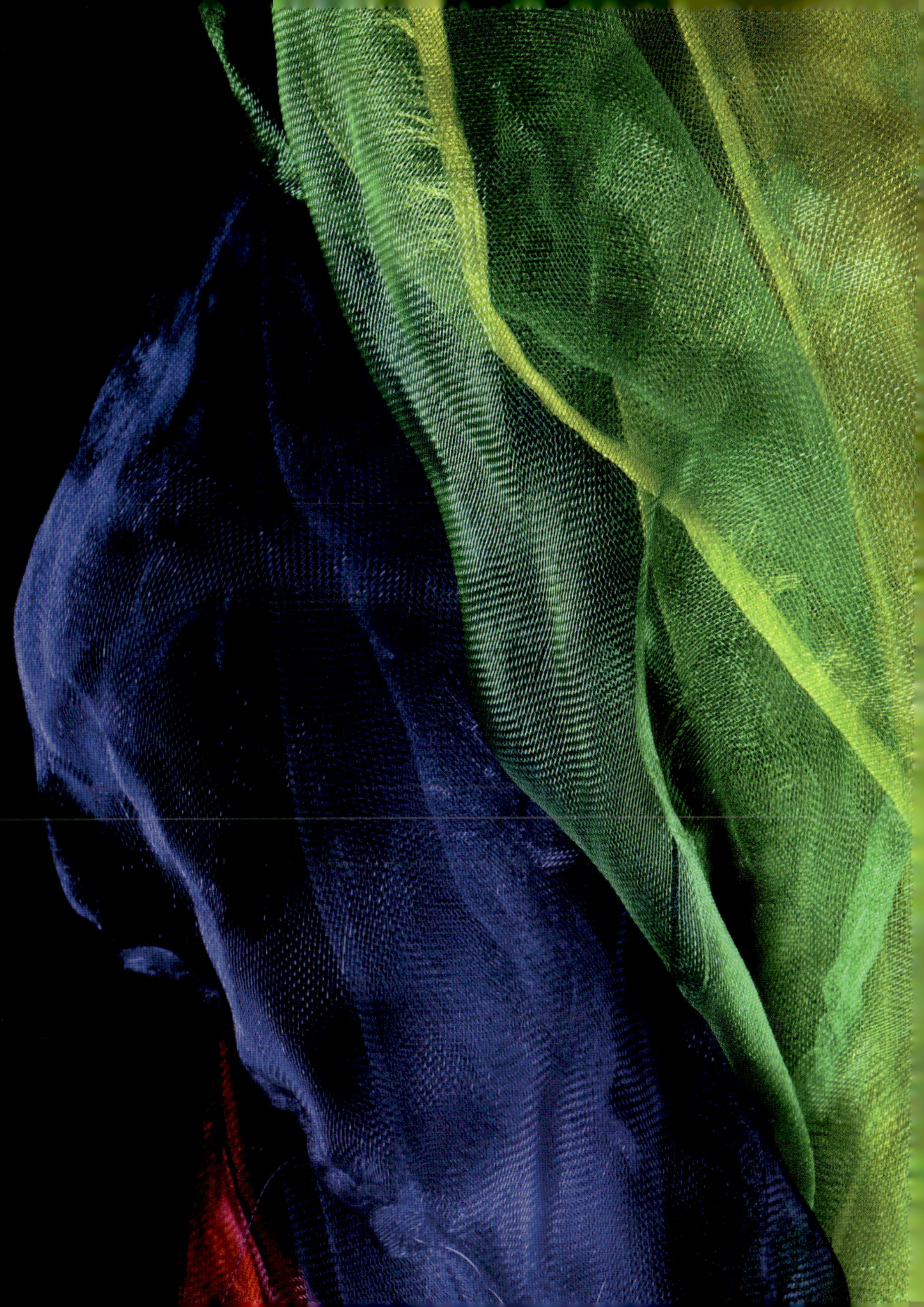

The Glossy Effect

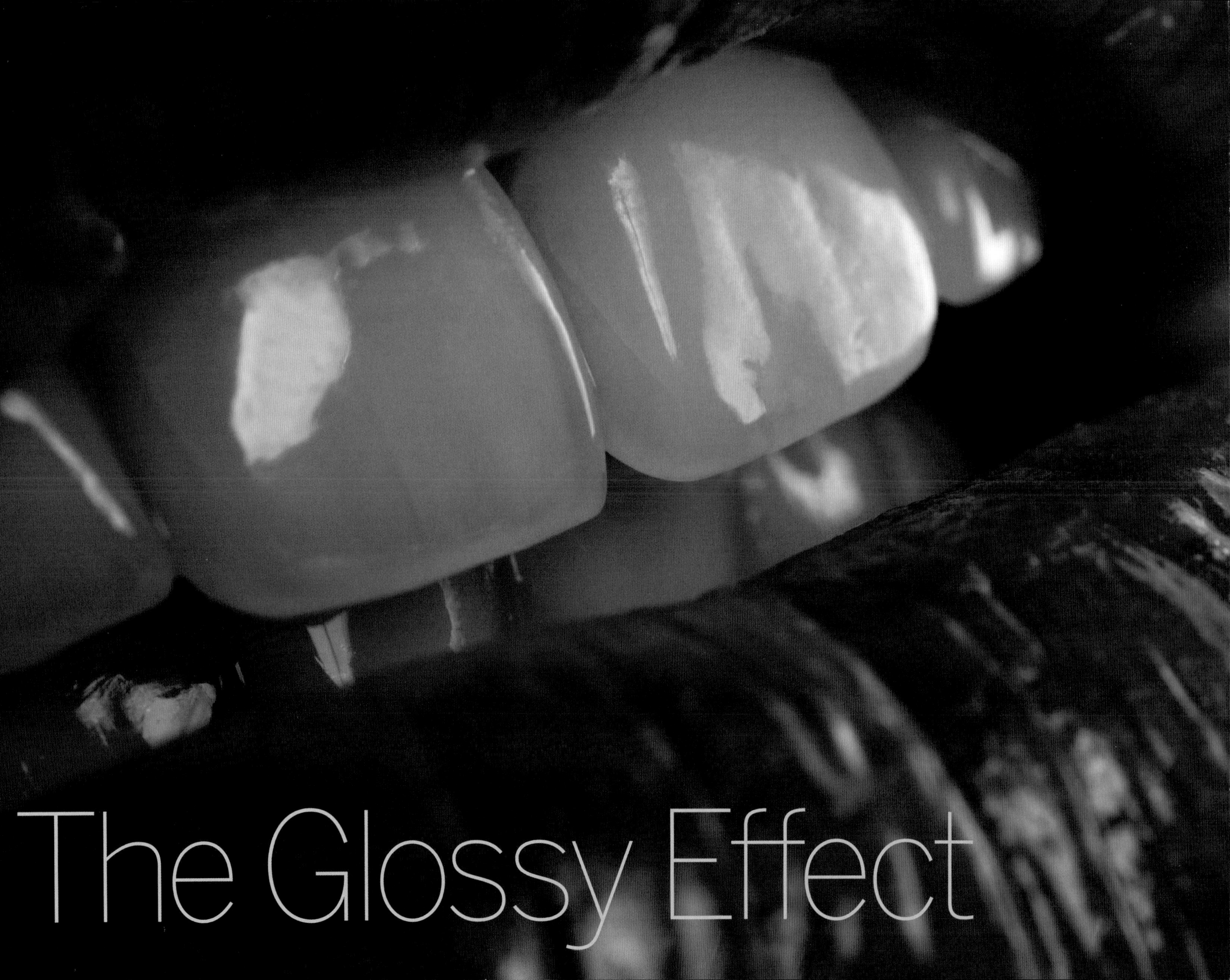

This technique will allow you to achieve glossy textures on teeth and gums. Although I have been using this technique for a long time, I always had trouble explaining it. One day, Dr Carlos de Carvalho simplified it for me. He said:

"In order for teeth and gums to look soft and glossy, you must increase the size ratio of the light source with respect to the subject. At the same time, you need to have highly diffused light. The way we achieve such large ratio of source to subject size is by bringing the diffused light source as close to the subject as possible."

HOW IS IT DONE? DISTANCE.

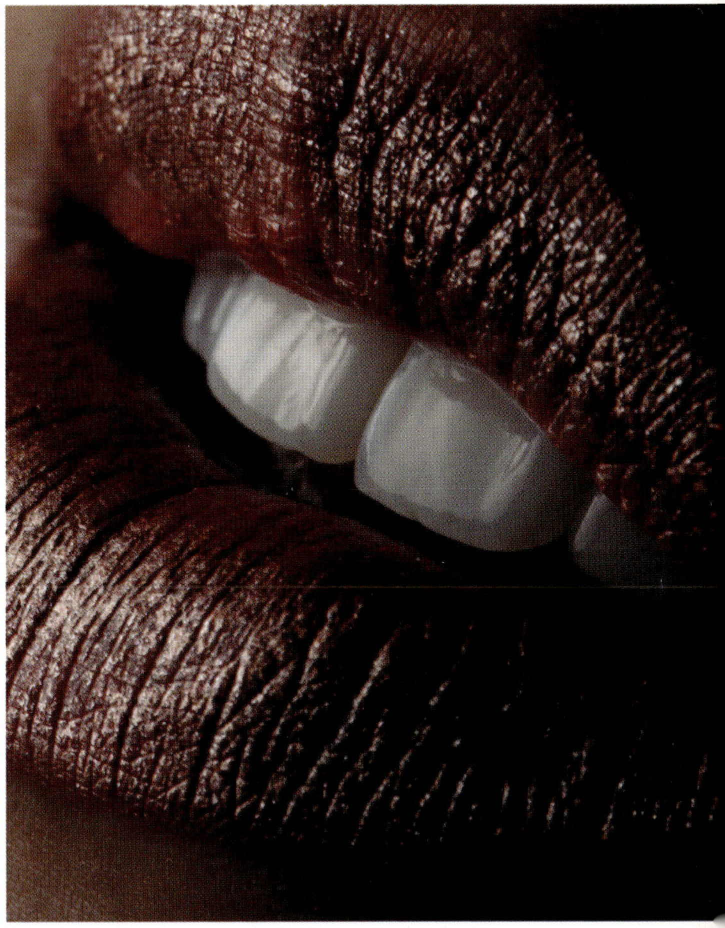

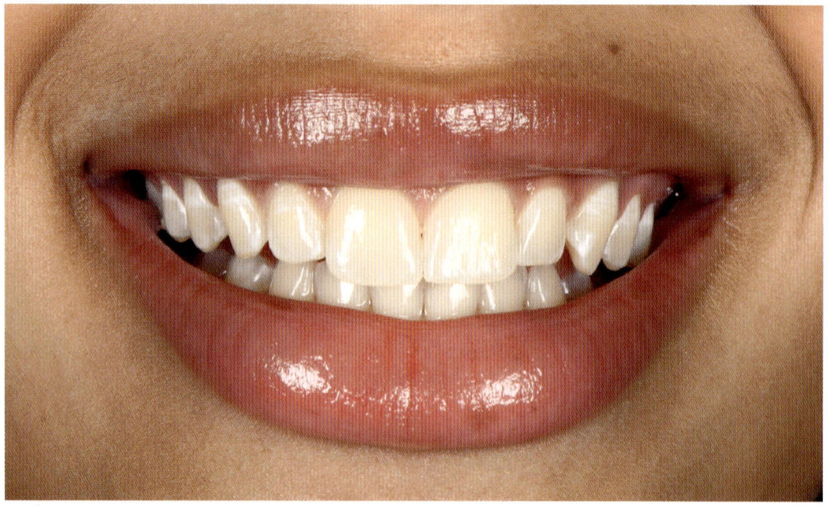

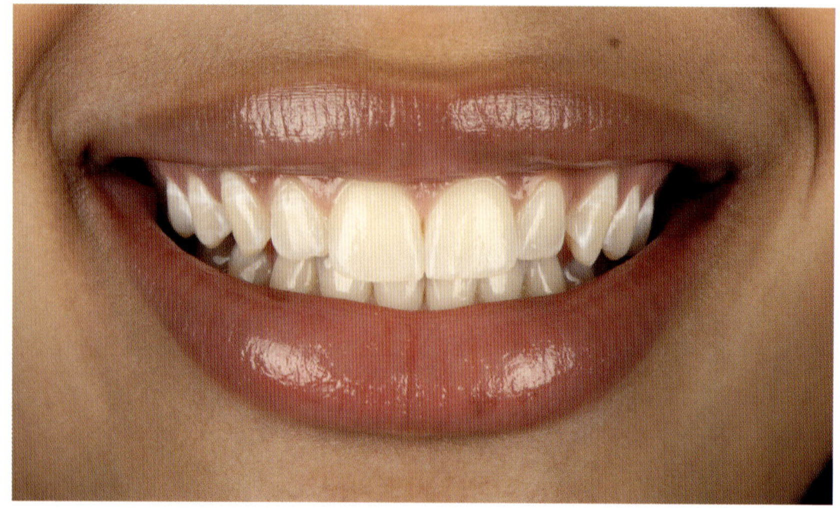

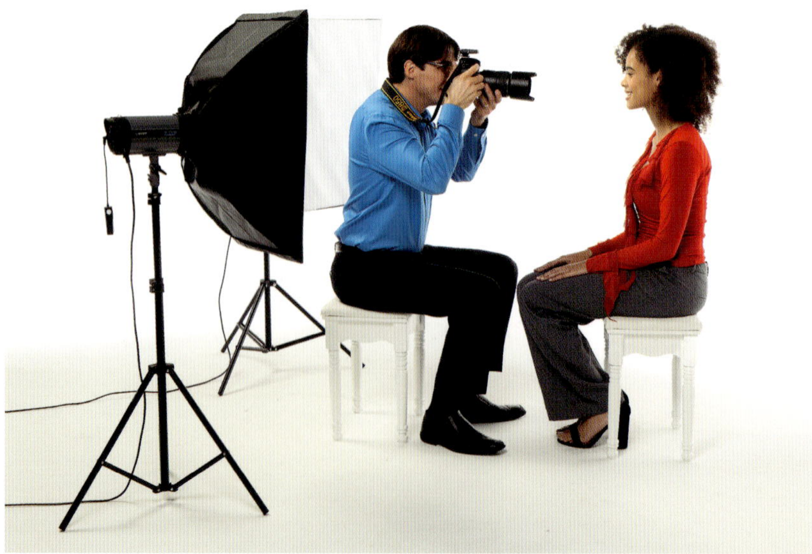

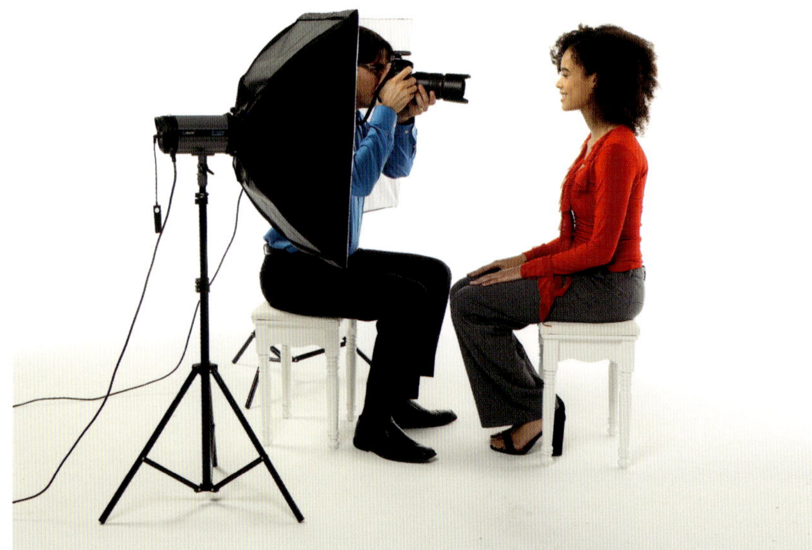

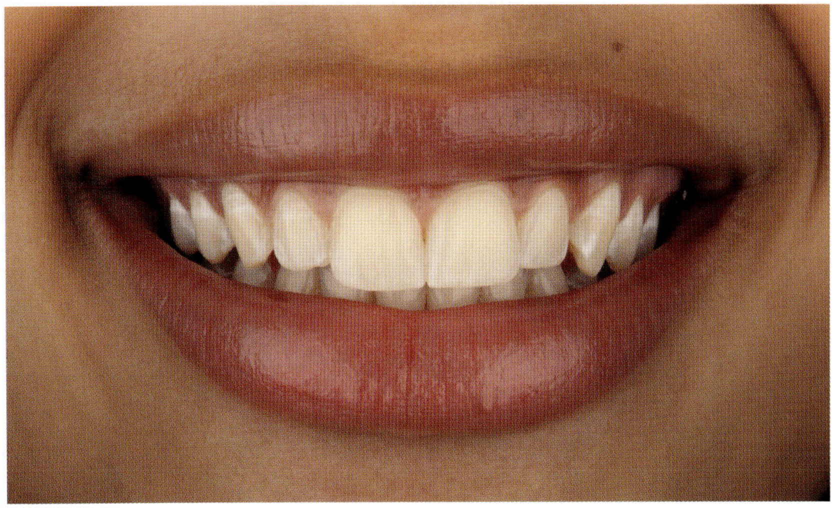

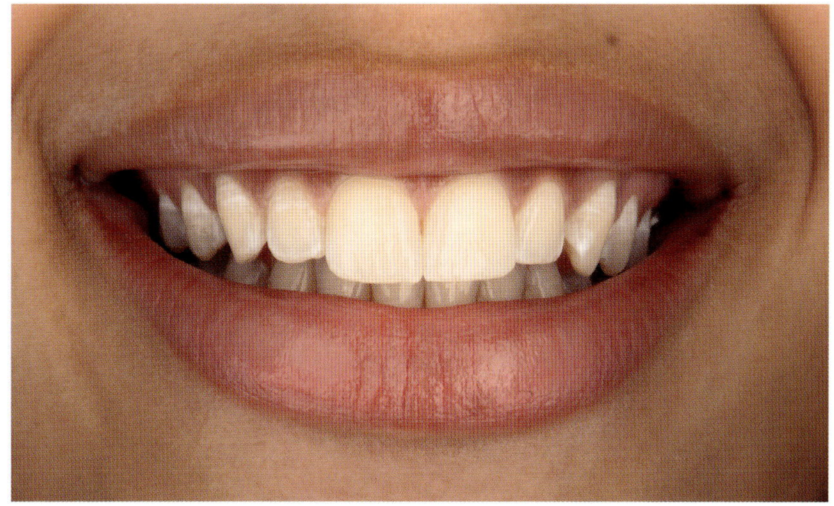

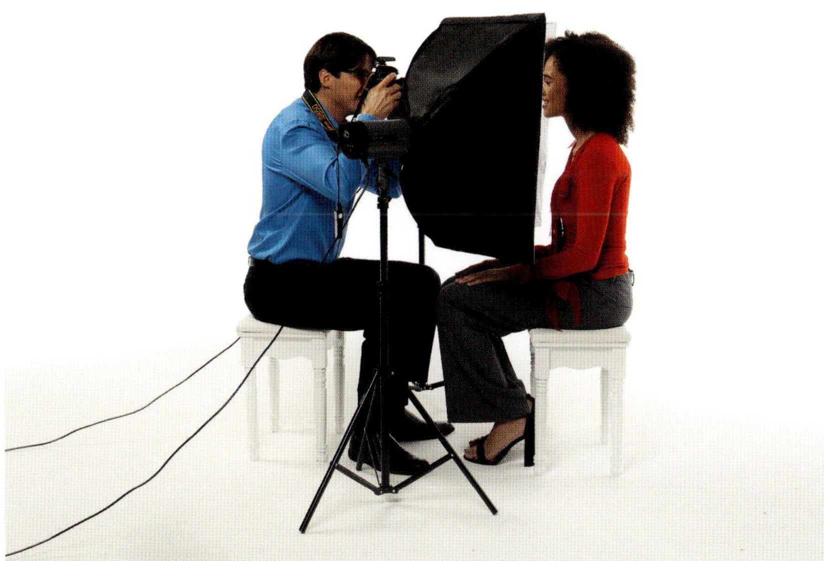

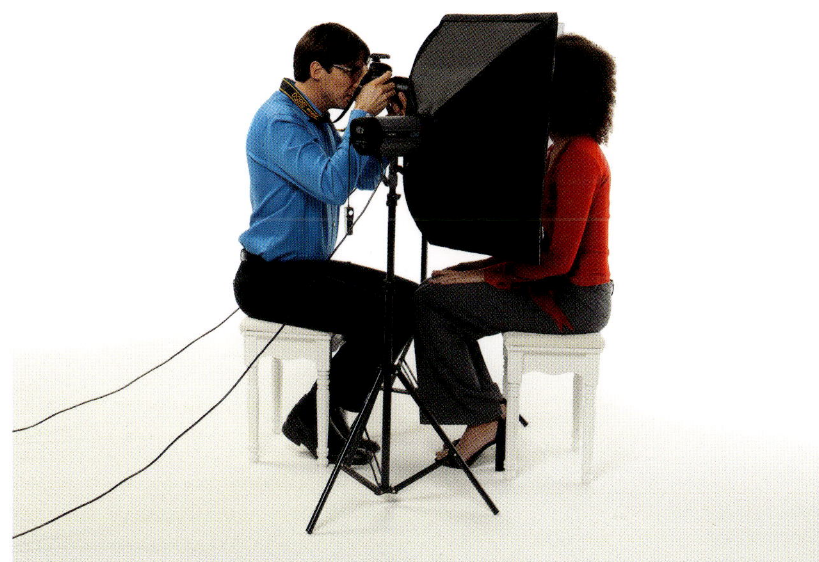

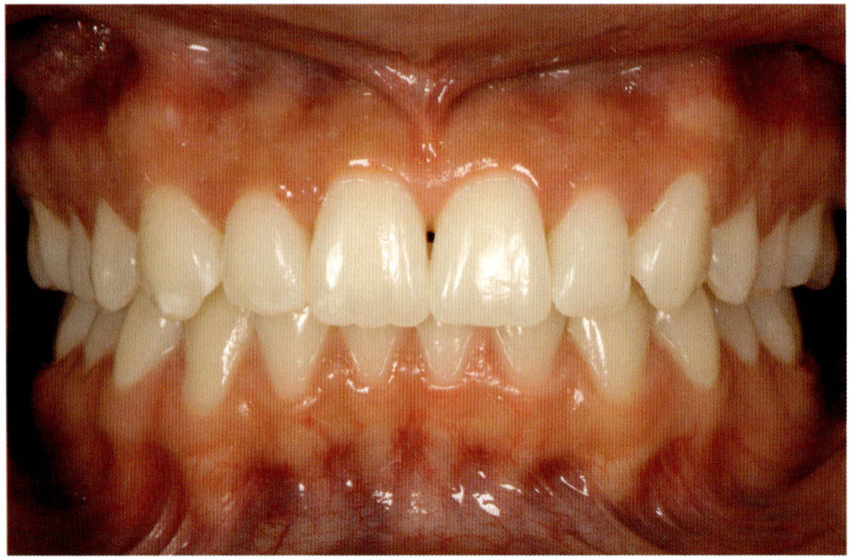

Far

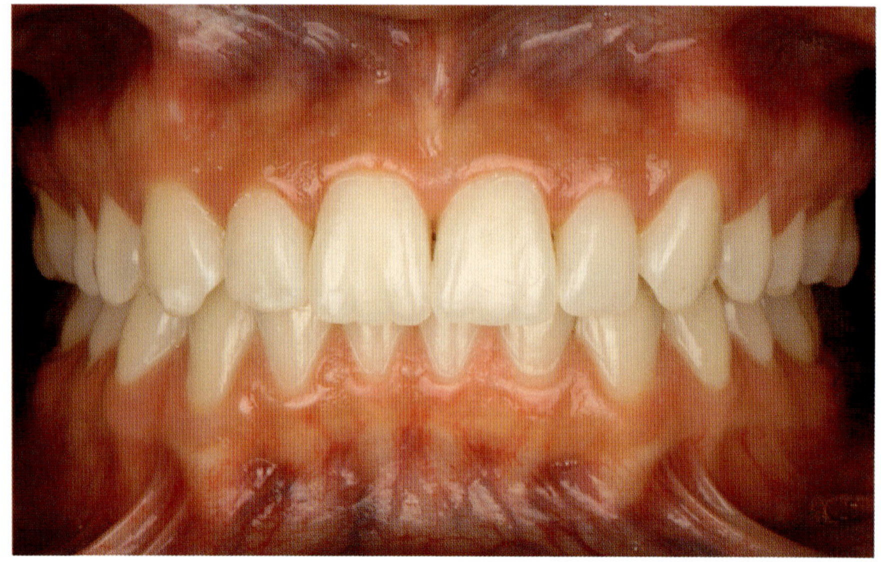

Close

As you can see, just by changing the distance of a bounced/diffused light source, we can achieve two totally different images. In this case, to correct for exposure as I moved the strobes closer, I increased the shutter speed and decreased the ISO.

A few things are worth noticing:

- Disappearance of high-intensity white spots. All those white glare patches are gone.
- Every surface becomes smoother and softer.
- Even though the light source has not been modified, the act of moving it closer creates a situation where the apparent color temperature of the light has changed. The value seems to go down, and the chroma seems to have increased.

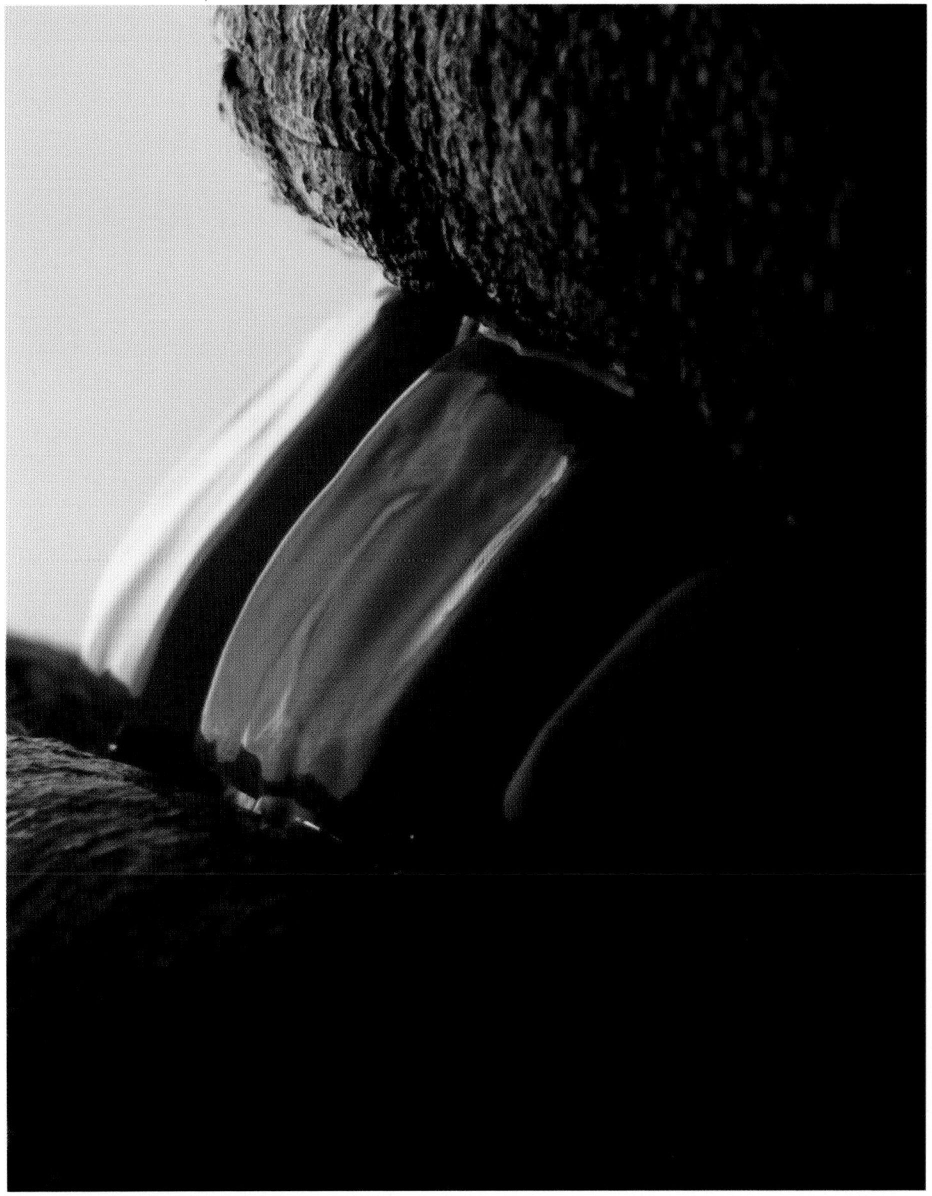

Advanced Tip

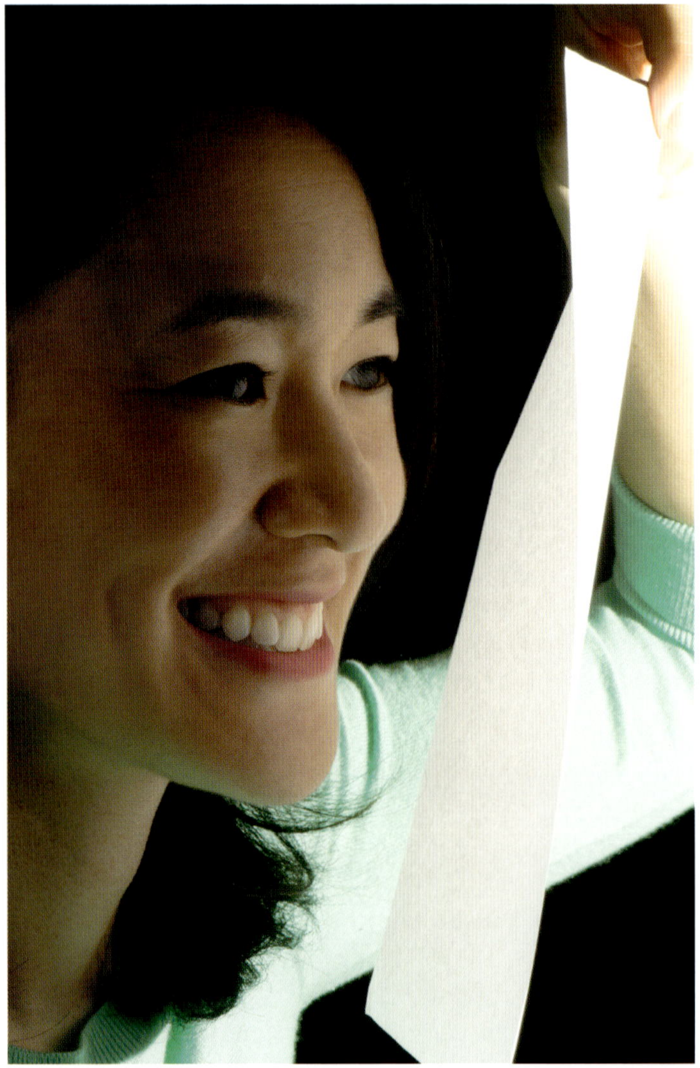

WHITE PAPER

If you think you have to invest in speedlights, strobes, or softboxes as the only way to achieve these kind of results, you are wrong. I am here to attempt to simplify your photographic needs, not to make them more and more complex. The cheapest and arguably greatest bouncer and/or diffuser is present in every dental office: white paper.

A simple piece of white paper placed in front of your subject can create almost the exact effect as described before. Things to consider:

- Tissue paper works best because it lets more light pass.
- The size has to be large enough to cover most of the incoming light. The usual 8.5 × 11 works well.
- The paper has to be placed as close to the subject as possible and not close to the source. Placing it in front of the source will do almost nothing, if the source is several inches away. In order to achieve the increase in ratio from source to subject, the paper has to be placed right in front of the subject (face, lips, teeth). At this point, the paper becomes a light source that is spread and diffused.

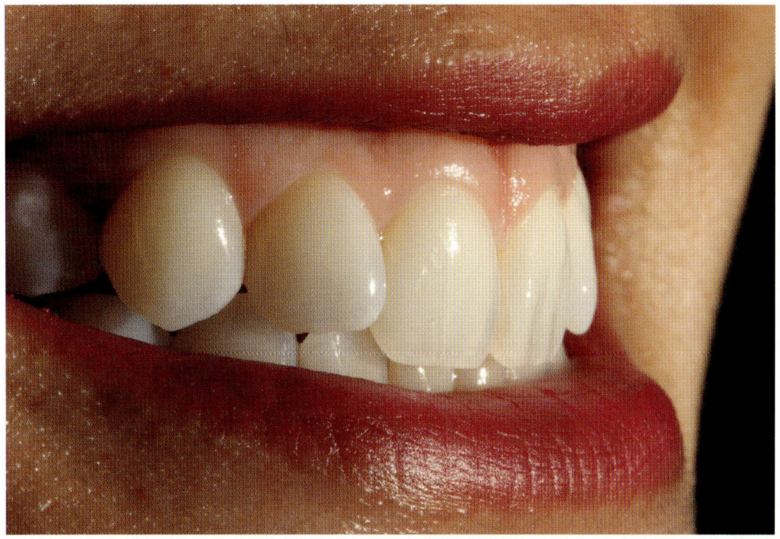

Flash

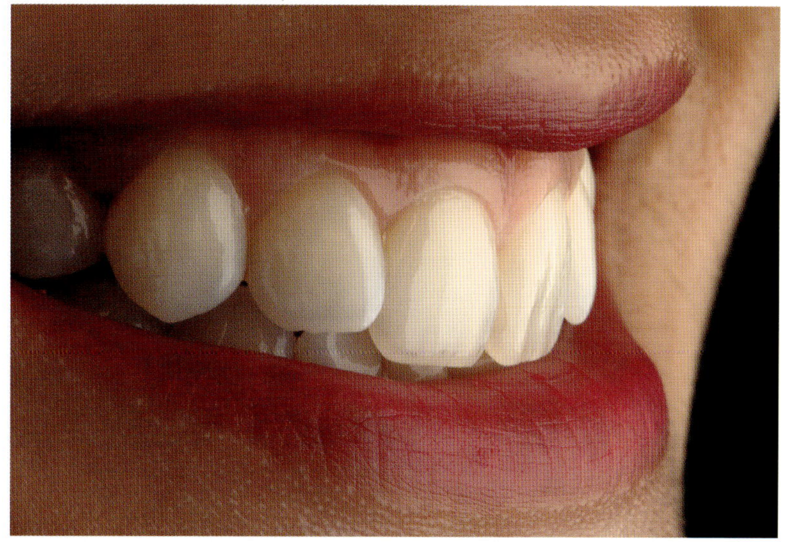

Flash with white paper

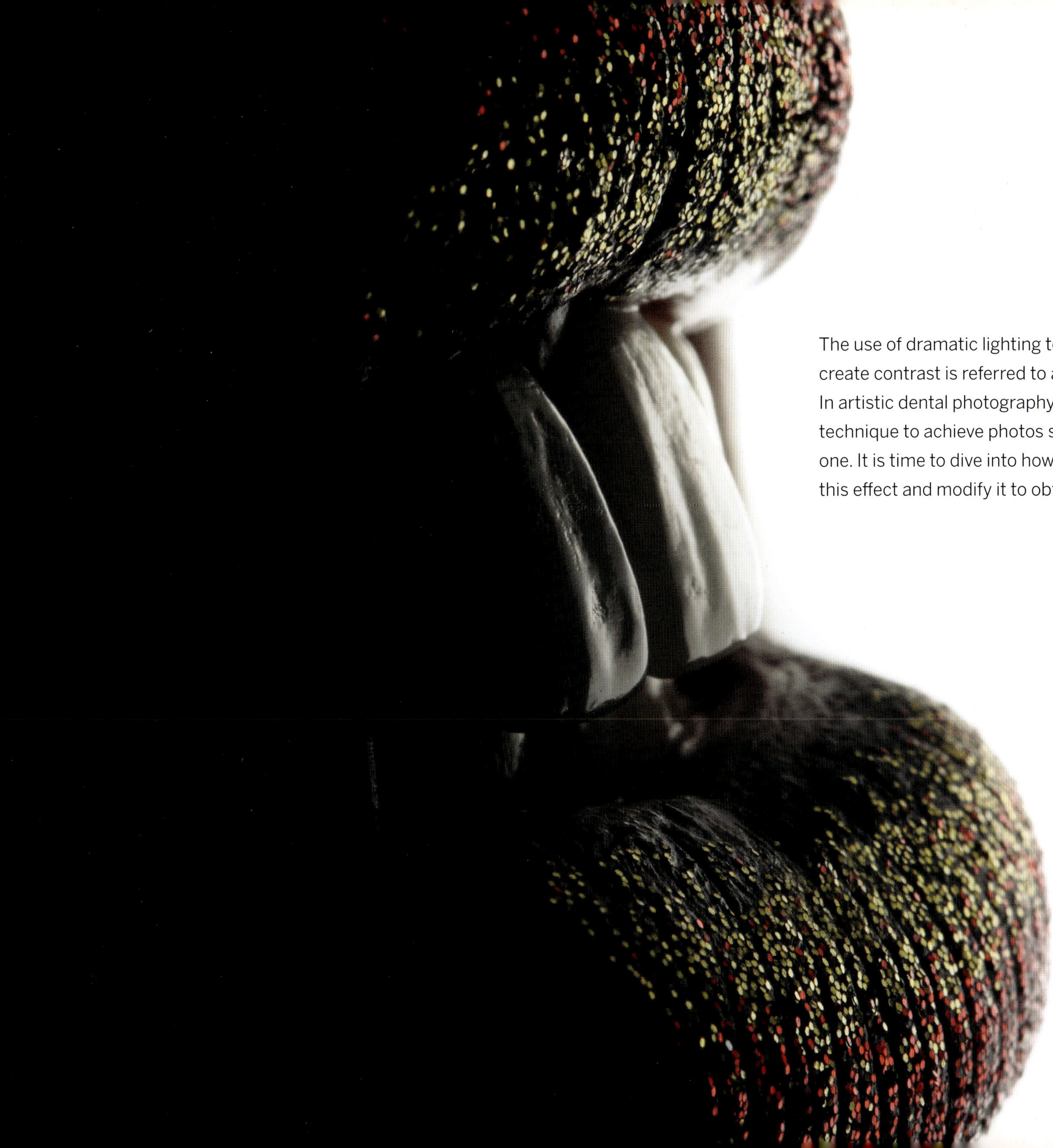

Chiaroscuro

The use of dramatic lighting techniques to create contrast is referred to as *chiaroscuro*. In artistic dental photography, I use this technique to achieve photos such as this one. It is time to dive into how you can create this effect and modify it to obtain others.

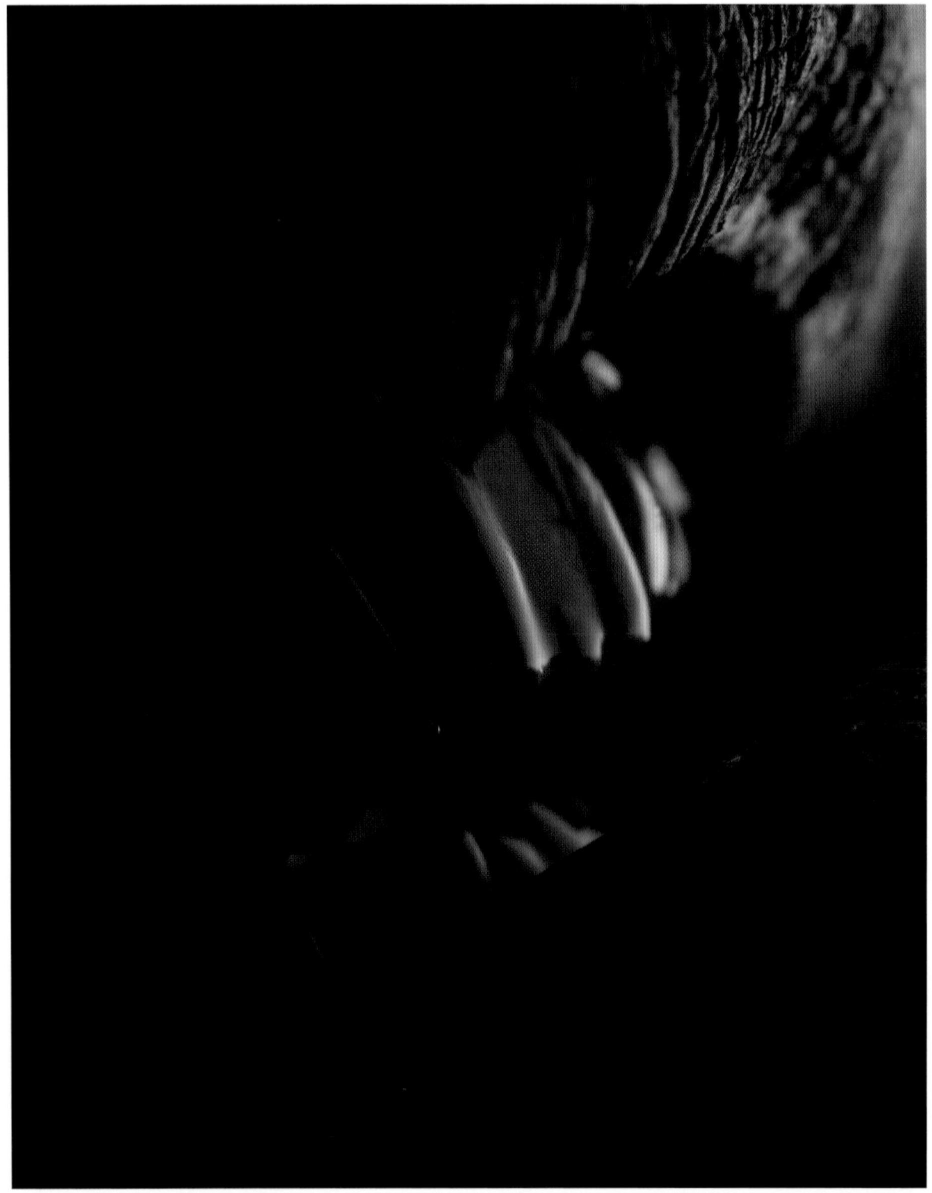

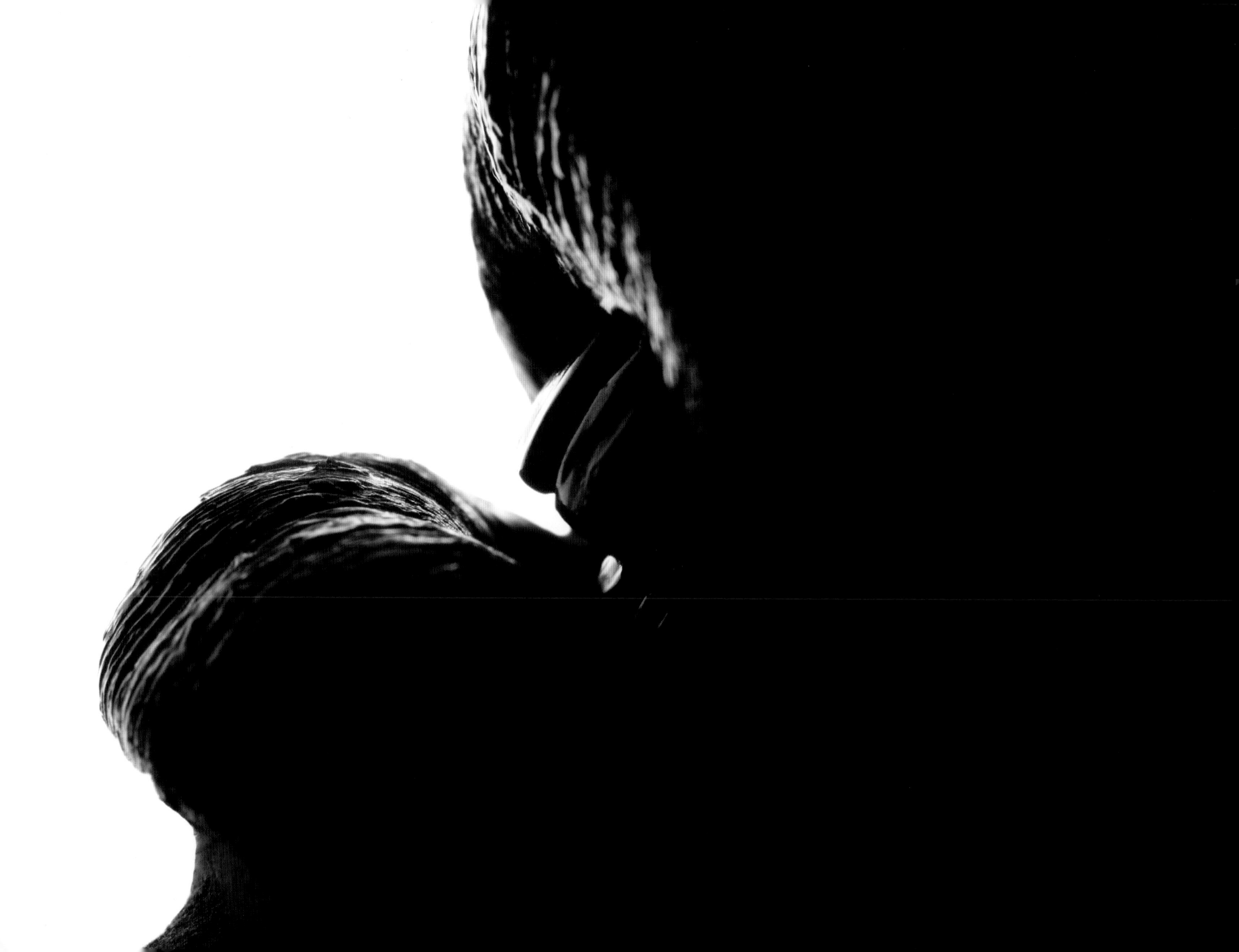

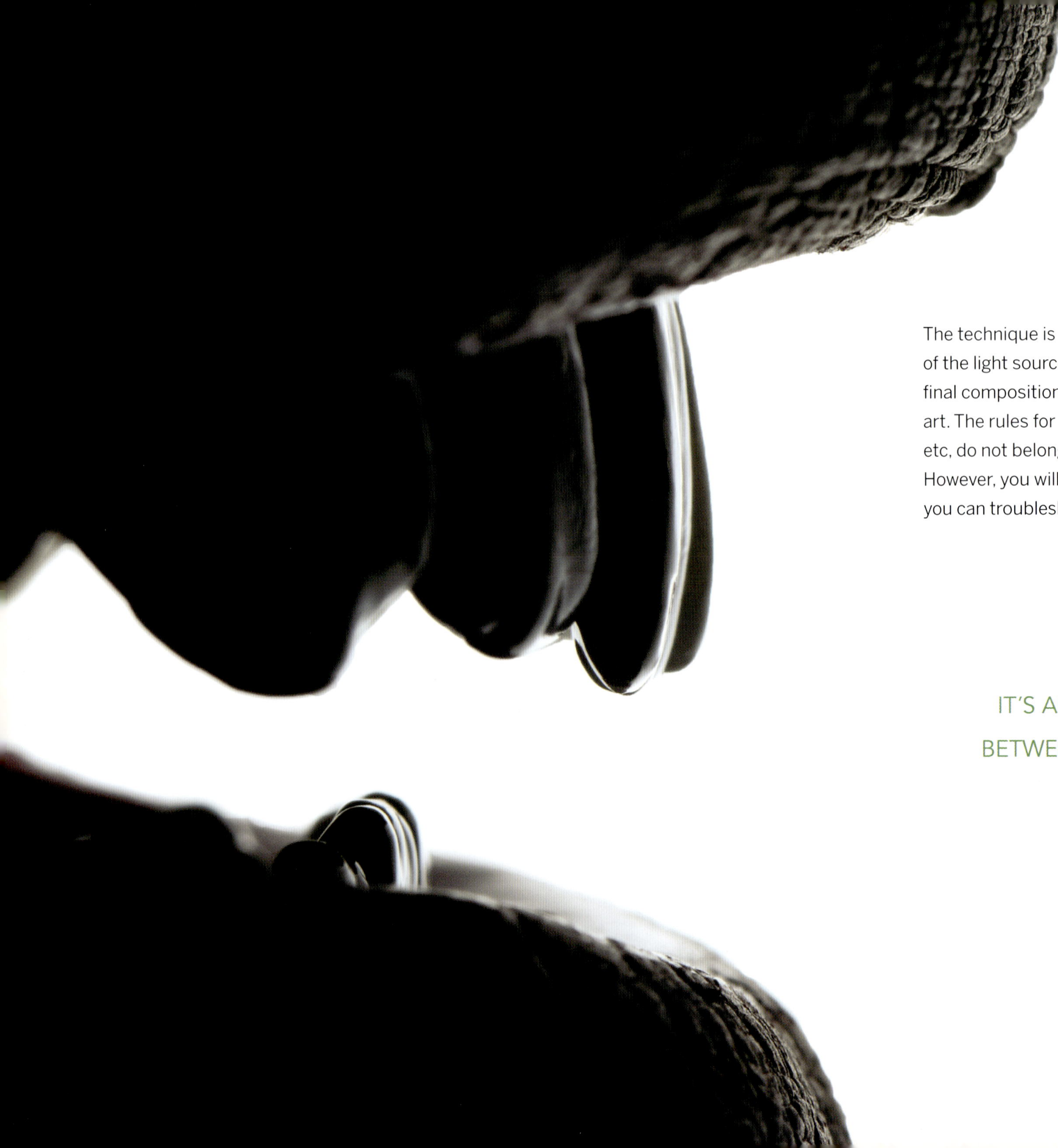

The technique is based on the direction and power of the light source. There are no set rules on what the final composition should look like. We are creating art. The rules for "perfect" exposure, DOF, angulation, etc, do not belong here. You create your own rules. However, you will need to know a few tricks so that you can troubleshoot some classic problems.

IT'S ALL ABOUT THE ANGLE BETWEEN THE CAMERA AND THE LIGHT SOURCE.

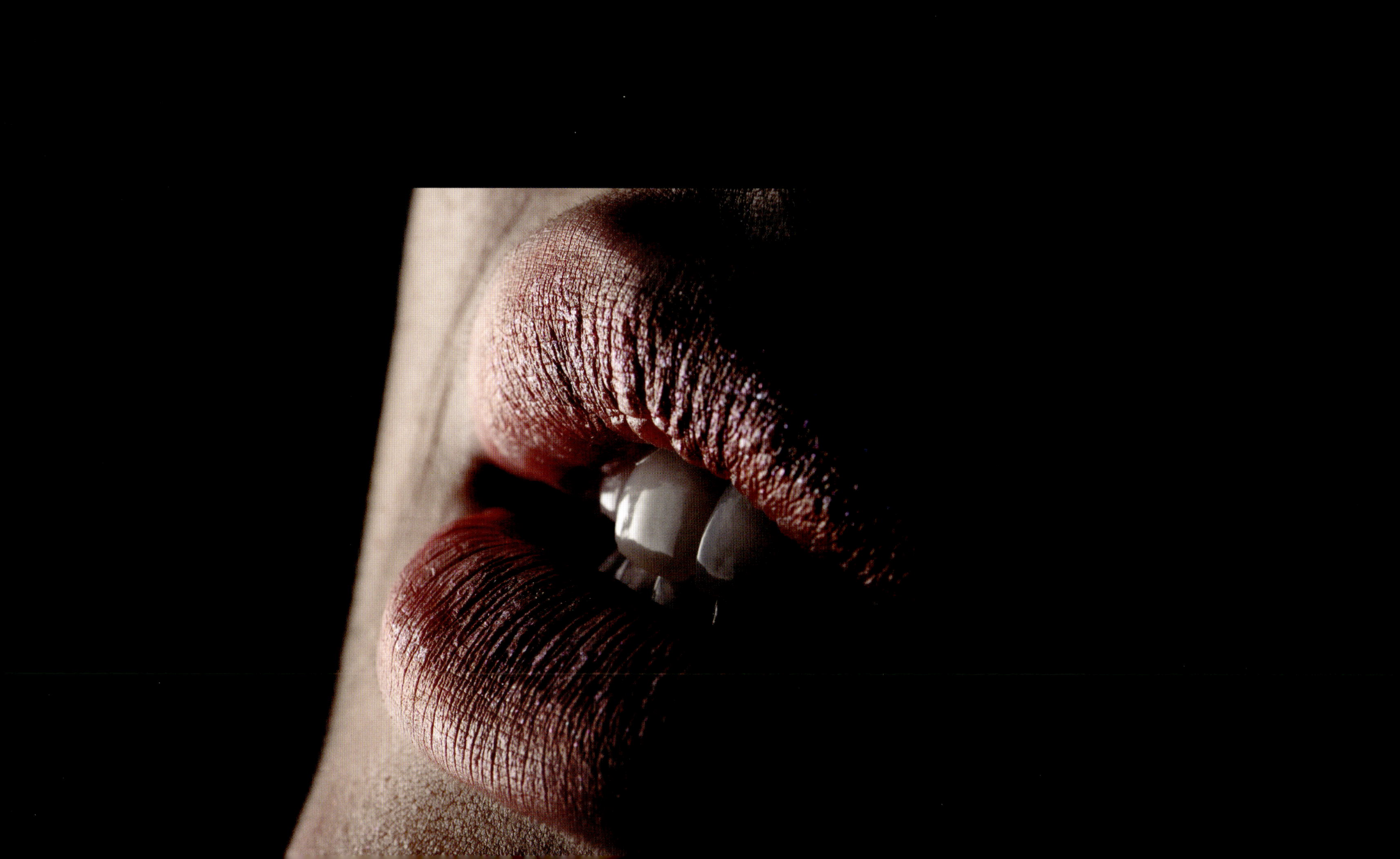

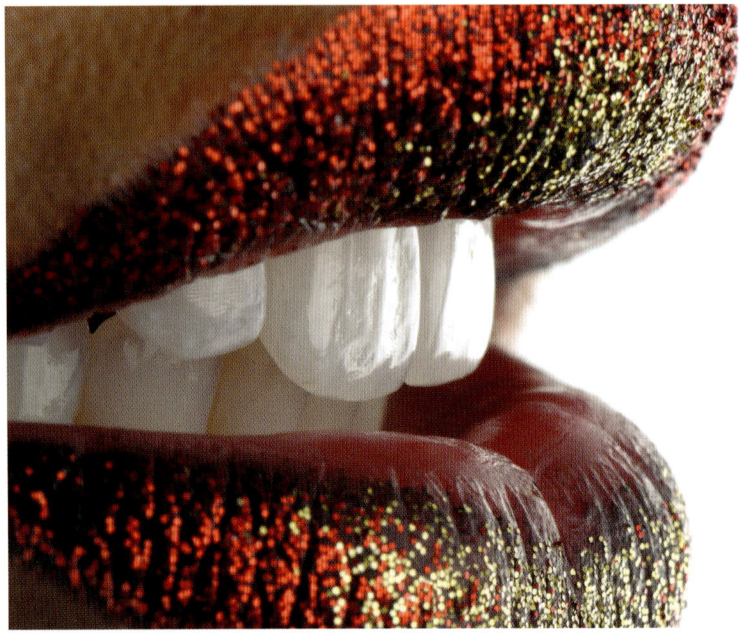

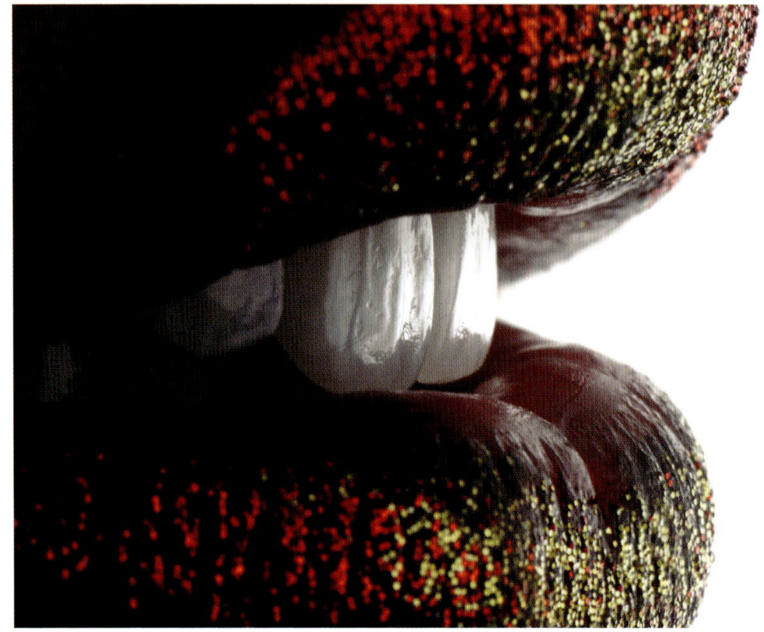

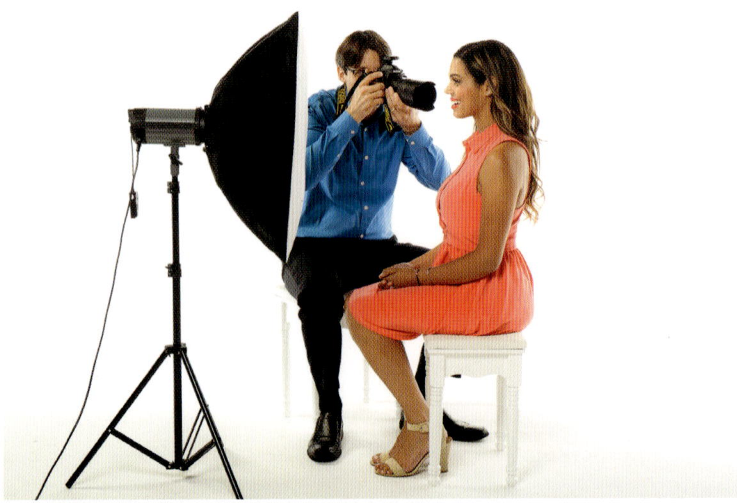

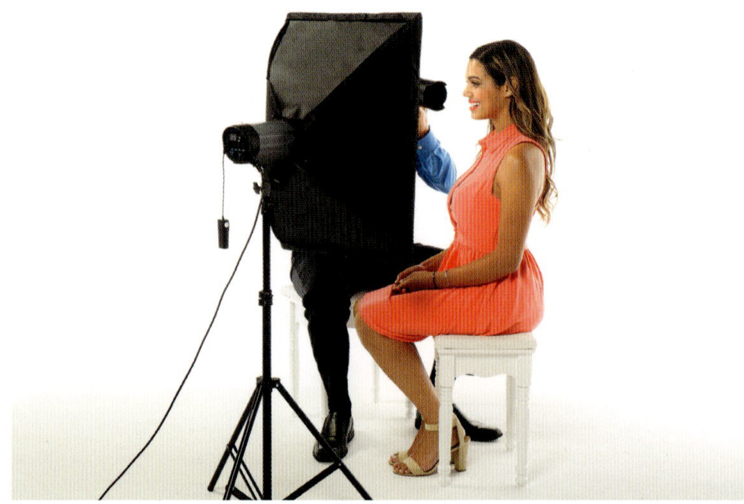

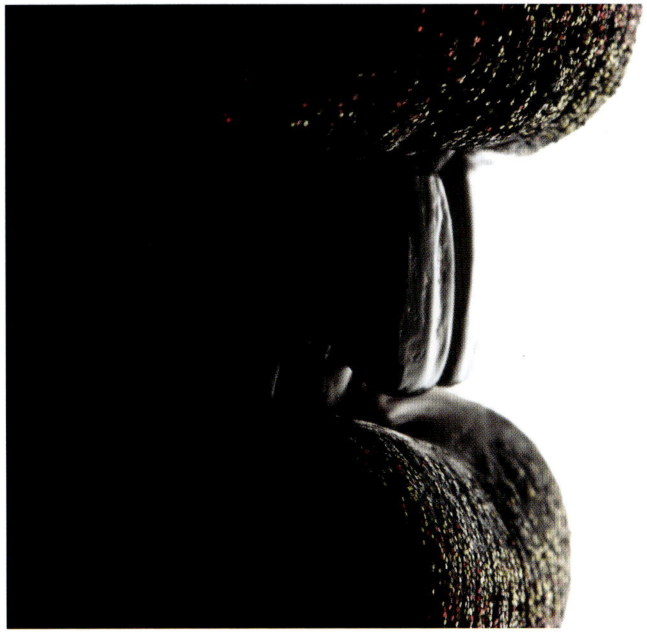

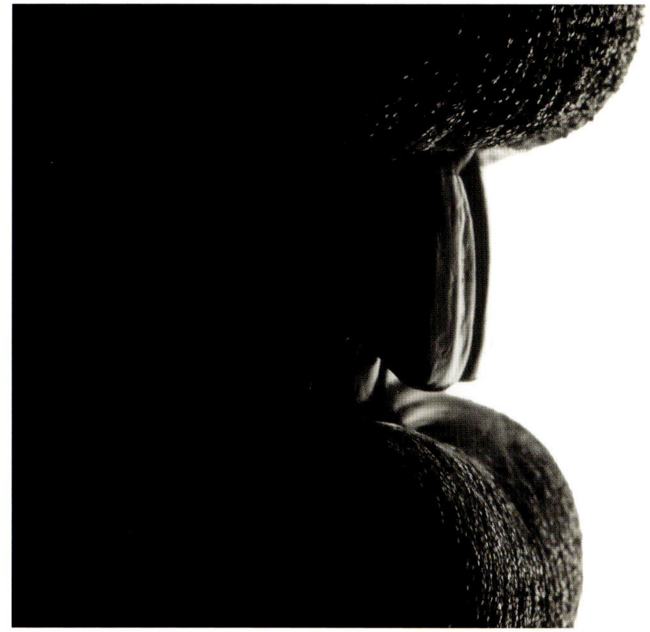

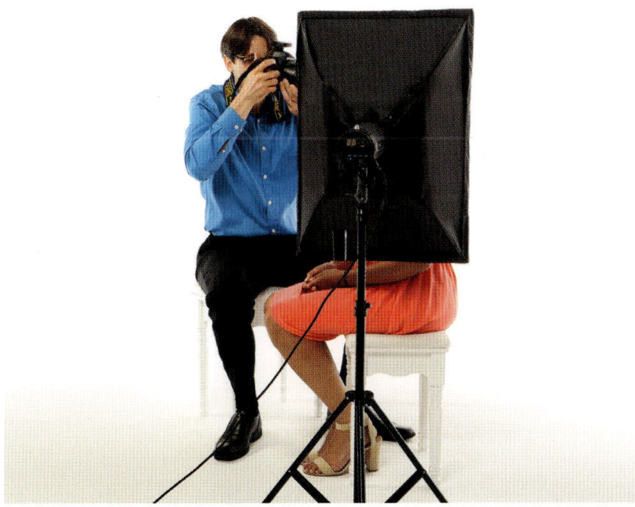

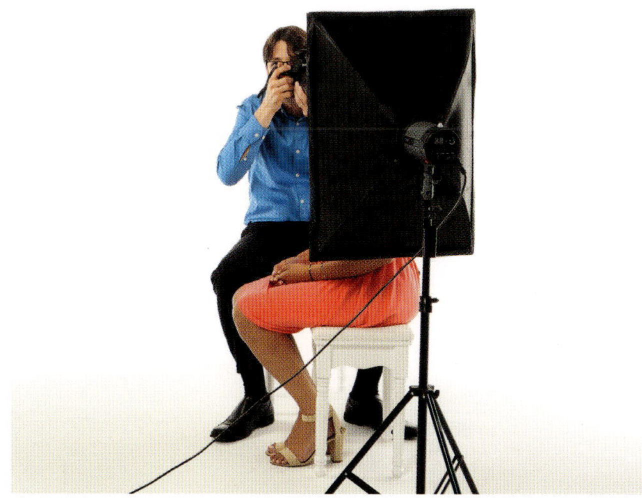

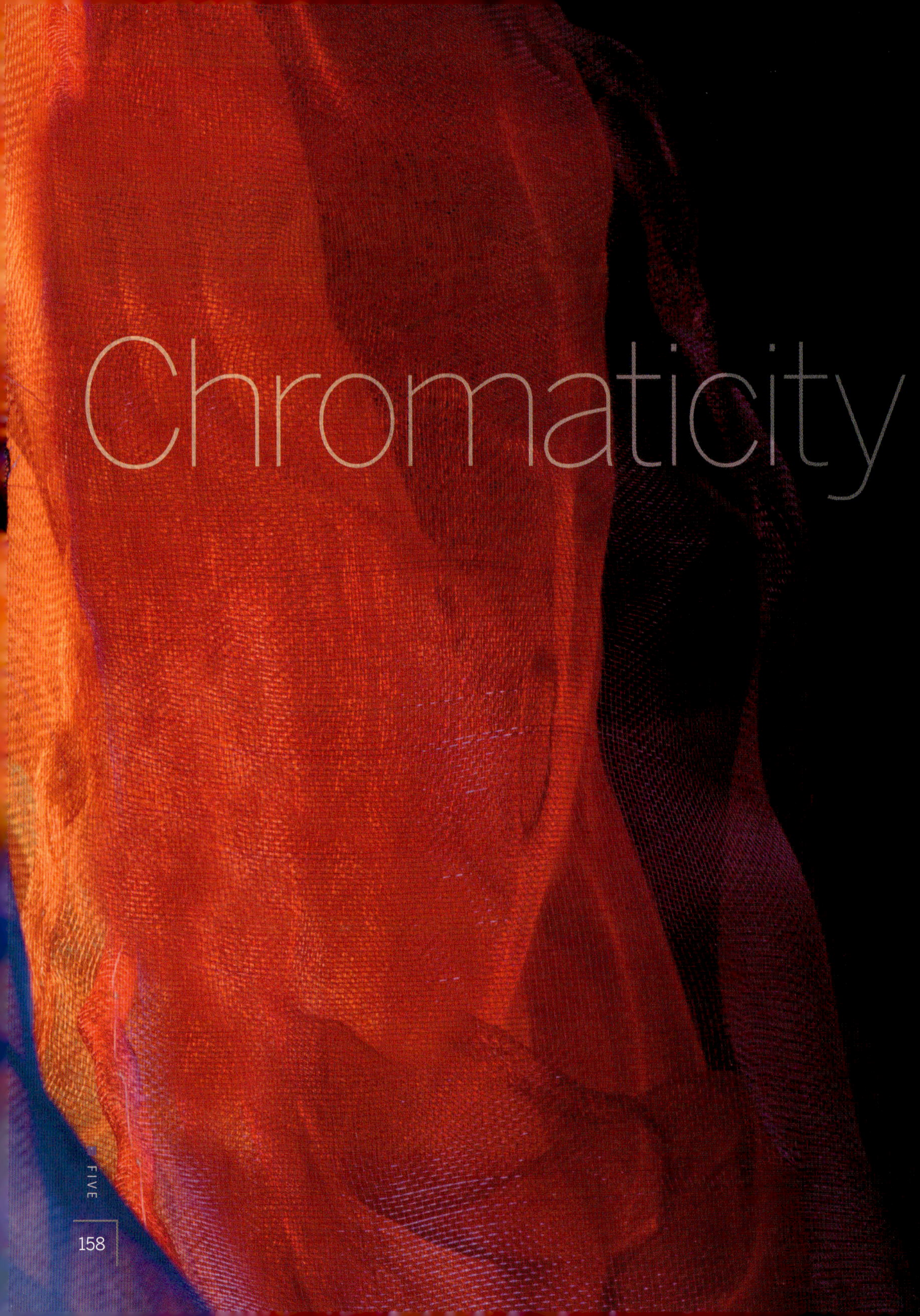

Chromaticity

FIVE

Chroma goes down as the angle increases. As we saw on the previous four images, as we increase the angle between the camera and the light source—from 90 degrees to 180 degrees—several things happen:

- Chroma decreases from colorful to almost black and white.
- Contrast increases as shadows become more prominent.
- Texture increases as microscopic peaks and valleys get filled with or deprived of light.

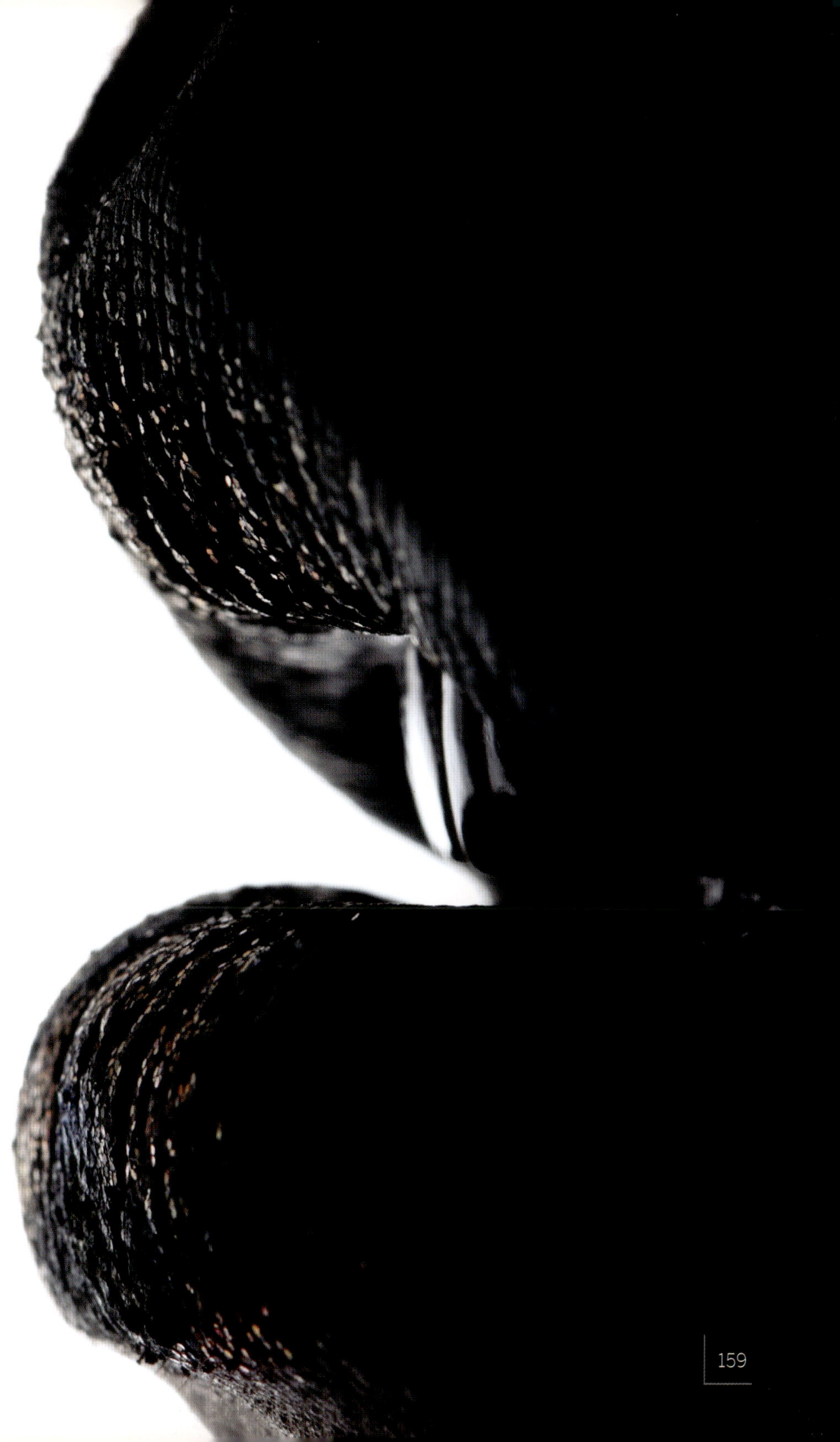

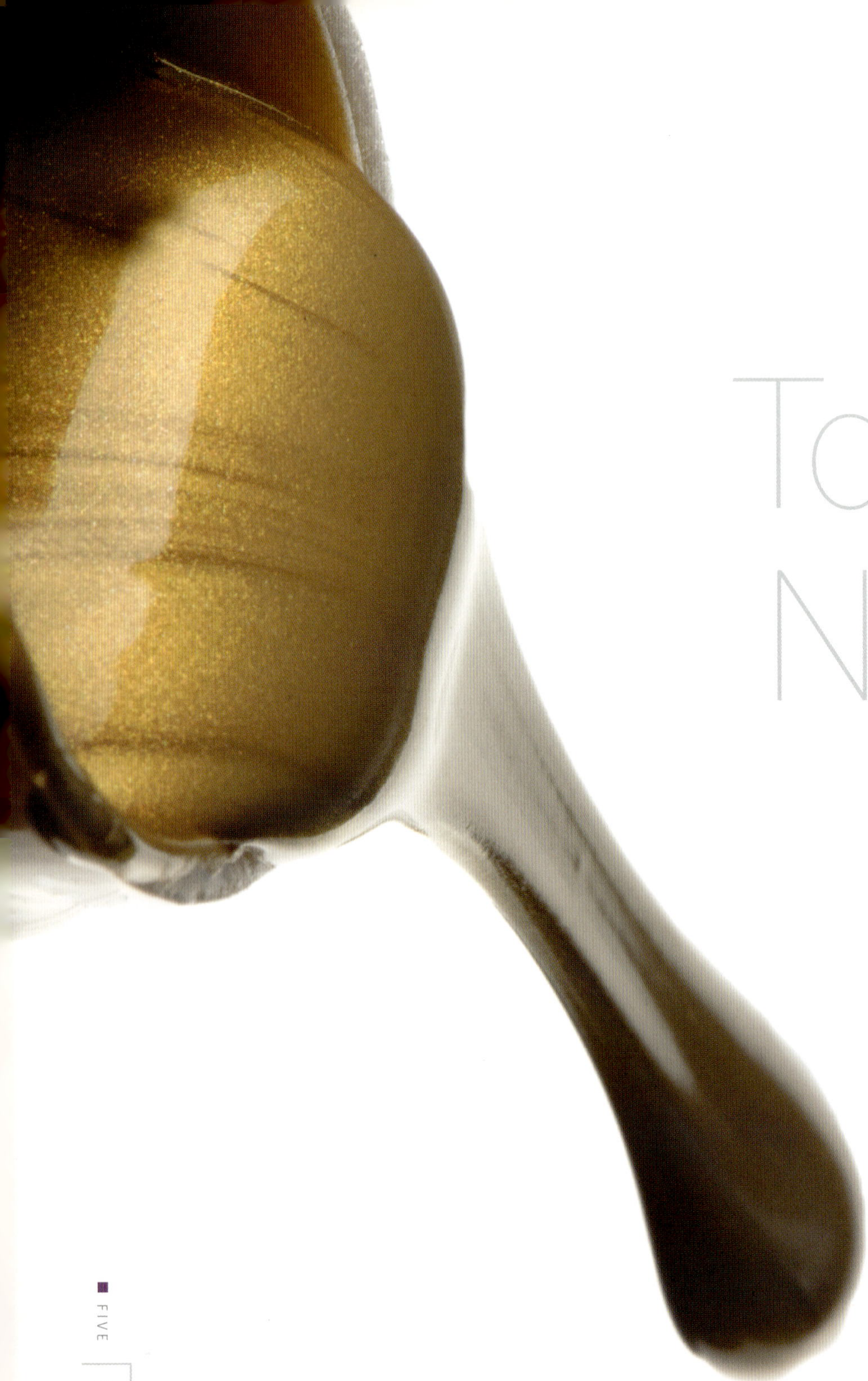

To Makeup or Not to Makeup

FIVE

Are we stepping away from dentistry in this discussion? I do not know. You tell me. And if we are, why not? If you have read until this part of the book and you are thinking of trying out all these techniques, it means you are not just a dentist. You have something inside you that resembles a photographer. You like art, images, texture, learning, improving. Good for you. As for me, I do not listen to those who criticize artistic dental photography. Neither you or I is harming anybody by taking pictures. So let's keep doing it.

One of the most satisfying ways of doing artistic dental photography is by manipulating and creating compositions that involve makeup. I do not personally do makeup on my subjects. I have had the pleasure of working with several incredibly talented makeup artists. I recommend you hire a makeup artist one day and have the satisfaction of doing your own artistic photo session. Your knowledge of photography and lighting will improve so much during that session that it will feel as if you took the ultimate dental photography course.

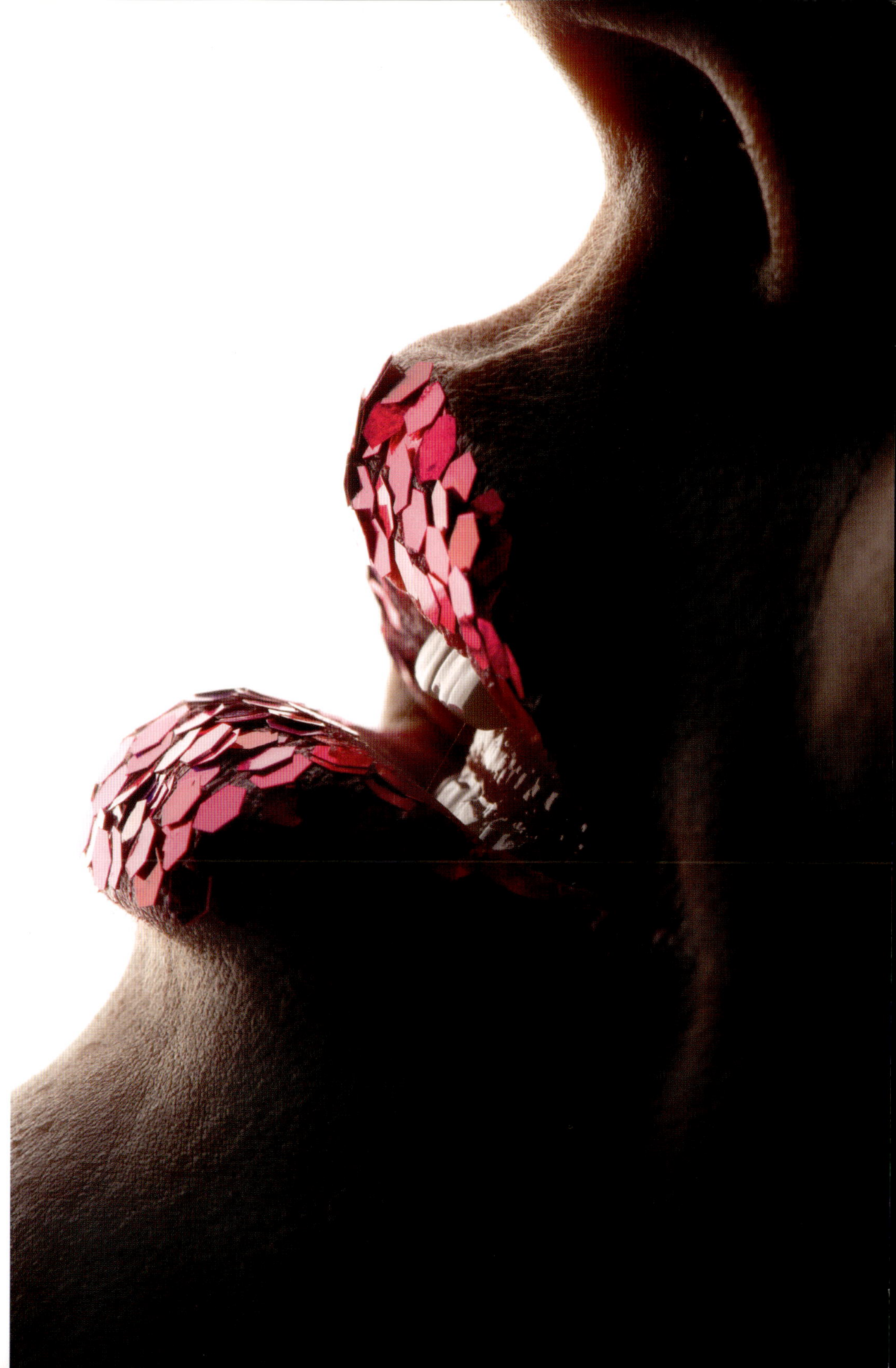

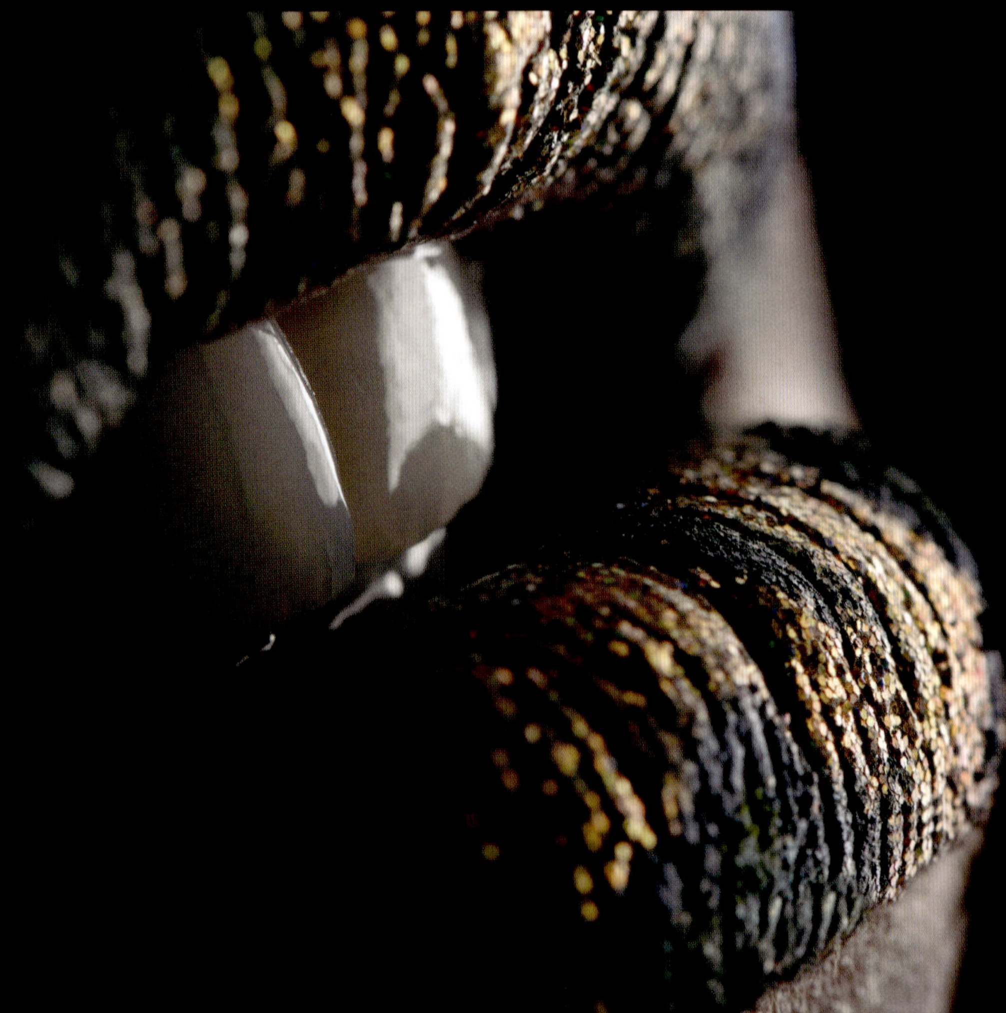

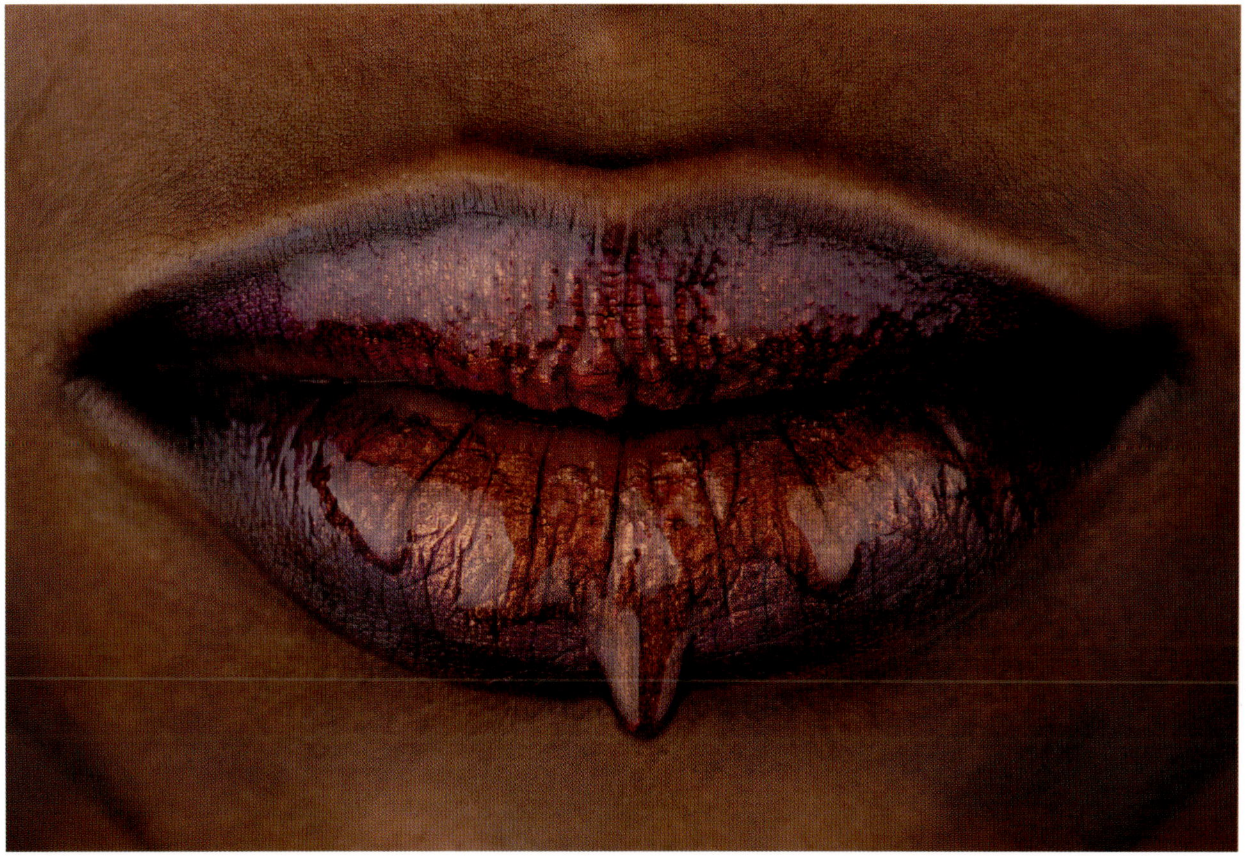

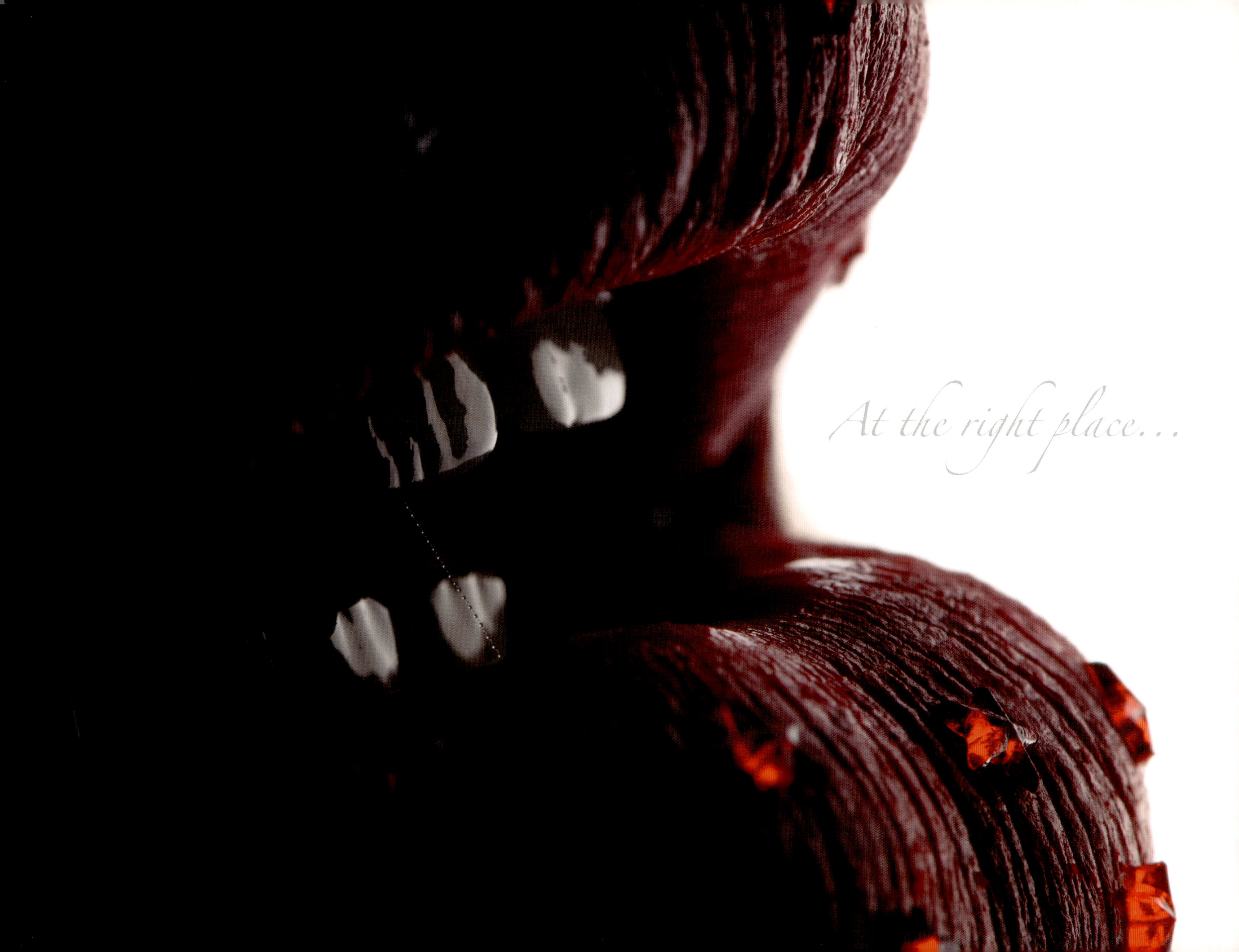
At the right place…

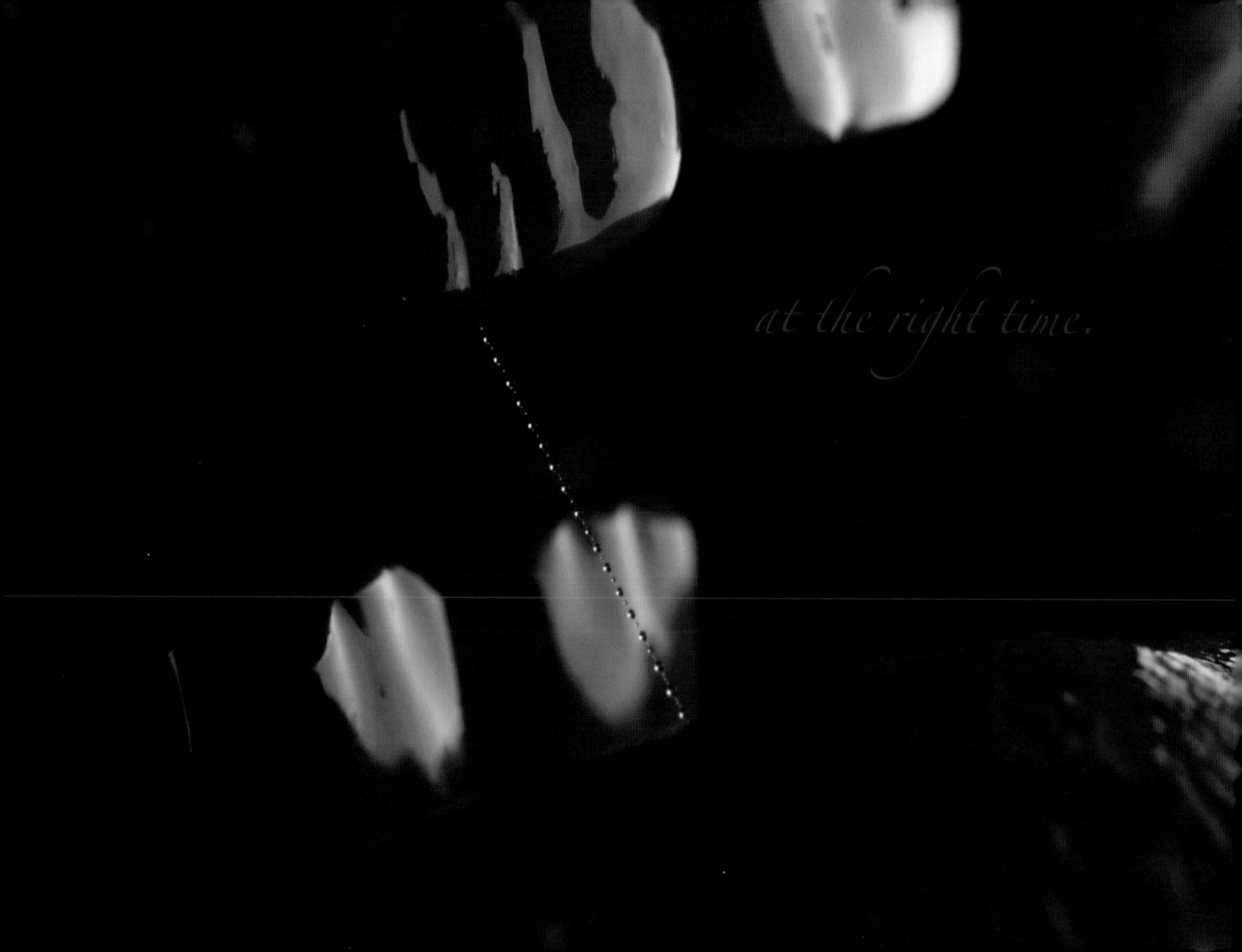

at the right time.

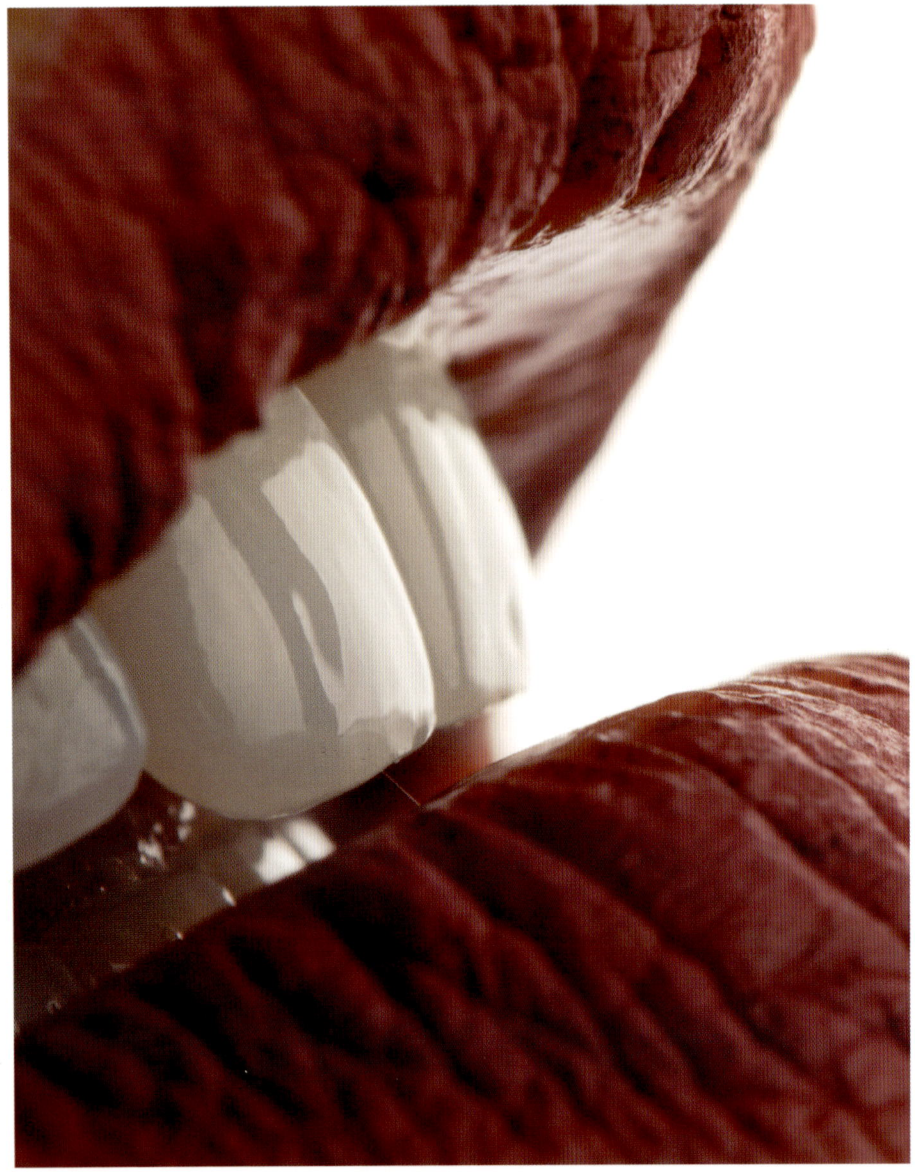

Dental Photography and Communication with the Dental Laboratory

I would like to talk with you about communication with the dental laboratory.

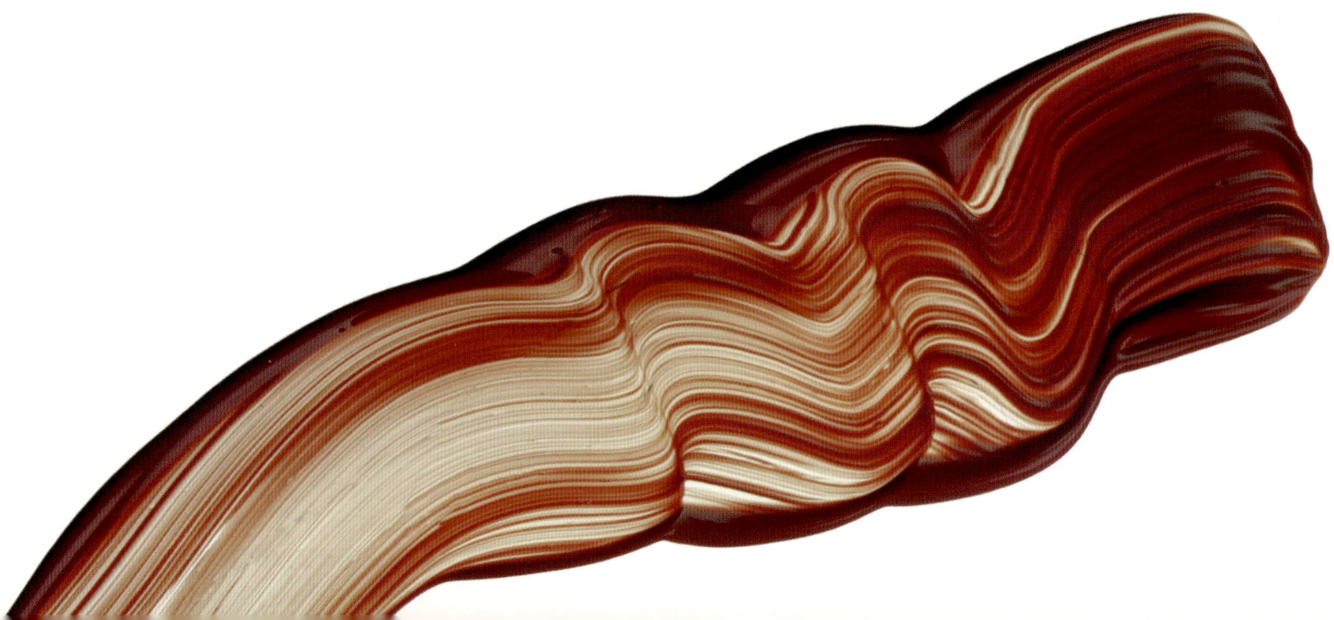

From the Office to the Lab...and Back

How many times have you heard people in our profession say things like, "Communication is the key factor in the relationship with your dental laboratory and it is essential for success"? I hear it all the time. The interesting detail that inevitably arises is that most, if not all, dentists express that they have great communication with their laboratories. However, if you ask most dental laboratories, the answer is unanimous: Communication with the dentist is almost nonexistent. How could this be? Why is there such a disconnect?

I believed that in order to bridge that gap we needed to ask questions, so I did. I started calling friends, dentists, and technicians. I asked them how the communication was with the other party. I did not stop there. I asked the dentists who said their communication was great to describe that communication to me. Then I asked the laboratory technicians who expressed concern about their communication with the dentists to explain to me how they would want that communication to change or improve. Most of the answers were similar in nature.

Dentists described how they always fill the prescription in detail and how if they have a complex case they call the laboratory and explain what they want or expect on that case. However, when asked, dentists reported that most of the problems they have with laboratories are restorations not fitting properly, shade matching issues, and case turnaround time that does not satisfy them. It is here that I realized that the disconnect is clear. None of the major problems a dentist has with a dental laboratory can be solved in a prescription paper or a phone call. But if communication really is key and writing and talking cannot fix it, how can we solve this problem? Well, let us see what the dental technicians had to say.

In most cases, laboratory technicians agreed that the problem arises not from being unable to talk or reach the dentist to discuss a case but with the quality of the work that they receive. In relation to poor restoration fit, they argue that most impressions they receive from their dentists are not up to standard, leading to poorly fitting restorations.

I had the pleasure of being a dental technician for almost a decade before becoming a prosthodontist. I hear you fellow technicians, I really do. I used to spend hours trying to decipher some impressions where the margins were nowhere to be seen. My fellow dentists might think that this is something that dental technicians face once in a while, but that would be wrong. What if I tell you that more than half of all impressions sent to laboratories in the USA are faulty? Yes, more than half. If you do not believe me, look at the literature.

The quality of fixed prosthodontic impressions*

In 2017, Rau et al* analyzed 1,157 impressions that reached a series of dental laboratories. Three prosthodontists independently evaluated each impression for critical errors. They found that 86% of impressions had at least one detectable error:

- 55% were critical errors to the finish line
- 49.09% had tissue over the finish line
- 25.63% presented with lack of unprepared stops in dual-arch impressions
- 25.06% presented with pressure of the tray on the soft tissue
- 24.38% had voids at the finish line

At this point, I want us to ask ourselves two very important questions: How do we expect our restorations to fit properly if half of all impressions sent to the laboratory are not up to standard? And how does this relate to having proper communication between the dental office and the laboratory? The first question is rhetorical in nature, but the second question goes to the heart of the matter. Laboratory technicians across the world will agree that they do not think they can call a doctor and tell them that the impressions they are receiving are faulty. Laboratories are afraid of losing the business.

Dental technicians also expressed that on occasions when they have called a dental office to indicate that a new impression is needed, they are met with anger, frustration, and denial. Often it has led to the dental office refusing to take a new impression. This is what lack of communication between a dental office and a laboratory looks like. This is exactly why there is a disconnect. The laboratory does not have the power or opportunity to express their opinions or suggest better approaches. Because dentists have the power in this scenario, improvement to communication comes by dentists allowing the dental technicians to judge, comment, and make suggestions on every aspect of the work they receive. Dentists should periodically ask their laboratories if there is something that they are doing that is leading to a lower quality of work being put out by the laboratory. Change will come when we dentists ask for and accept feedback. Then we must act on that feedback appropriately. And yes, it will mean that we might have to change how we do things in the office. If you are serious about good communication, accept it.

But how does research on bad impressions relate to dental photography? Read on.

*Rau CT, Olafsson VG, Delgado AJ, Ritter AV, Donovan TE. The quality of fixed prosthodontic impressions: An assessment of crown and bridge impressions received at commercial laboratories. J Am Dent Assoc 2017;148:654–660.

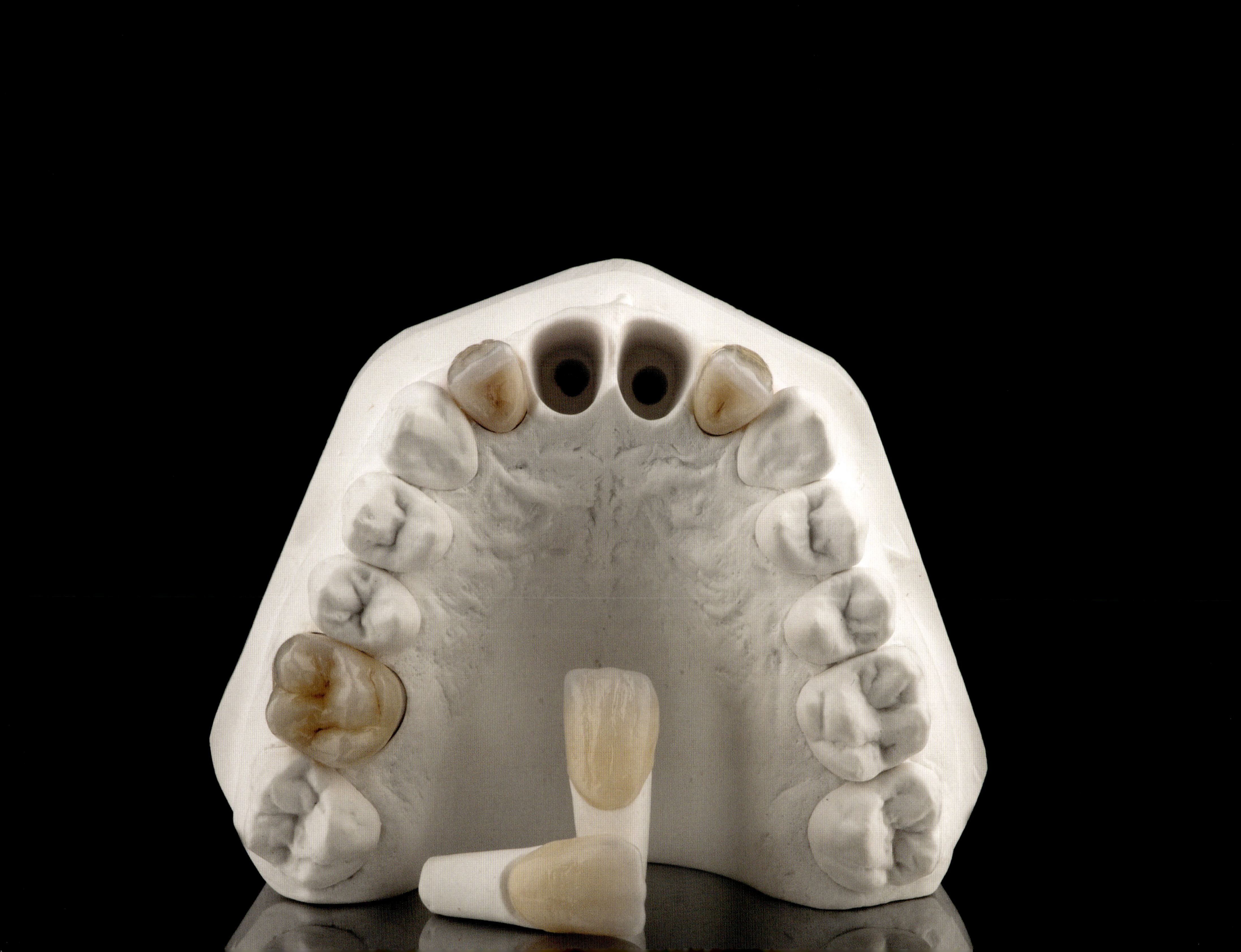

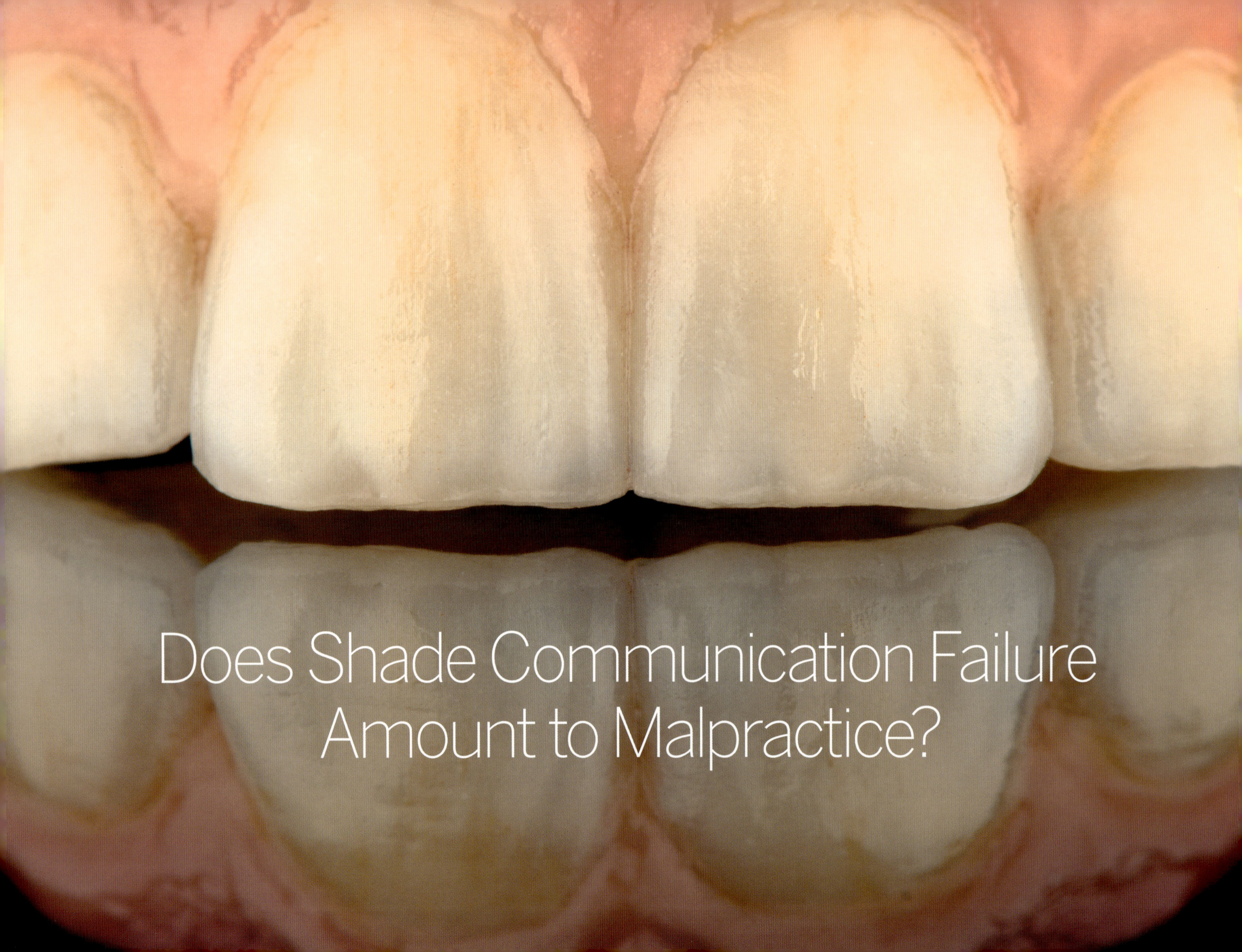
Does Shade Communication Failure
Amount to Malpractice?

Shade mismatch is the second big area of discontent among dentists and laboratories. Shade selection is undoubtedly a difficult science. However, shade selection and laboratory communication are almost the same thing. There is no way to escape this reality. The dental office must provide the laboratory with every tool necessary to succeed. The laboratory, on the other hand, must ensure that they have been properly and extensively trained to transform the information that arrives from the dental office into a piece of art.

Gone are the days where a dentist can write "Shade A2" on a prescription and expect a properly matched restoration in return. With the advent of affordable, high-quality dental photography equipment and many dental photography courses in existence, there is no reason for a dental office not to be trained on proper photographic protocols for shade communication. As I travel the world with my own dental photography course, I hear the same complaint from dentists over and over: "But Miguel, I do not have time to take photos." Or "My assistants do not know how to use a DSLR camera, so we have a point-and-shoot camera." Or even worse, "I use my phone to take shade photos."

All these excuses (yes I said it—excuses) could be considered, in my humble opinion, malpractice. Did I go too far? Well let me explain. I believe that as providers we are bound to treat every patient with respect. Part of that respect is to deliver the best service that is available for that patient. Some call it the standard of care. It is my belief that we must do everything in our power to have a restoration that has proper tooth preparation when it comes to retention form, proper reduction for the appropriate material of choice, adequate marginal seal, and yes, adequate color matching. It is our responsibility to match the shade as best as possible. Just as having the right tool to prepare the tooth is important and necessary, having the right equipment and training for shade taking and communication with the laboratory is part of the standard of care. If we decide not to invest in training and equipment for such a purpose, we might be engaging in malpractice by delivering treatment that is below the standard of care. No more excuses. Your patients deserve better.

In the next section, I share how I take shade measurements and how I use photography to communicate with my laboratory. Let me share with you a few tricks that I use.

Shade Evaluation and Photographic Acquisition

Shade evaluation is a science, but most of us in dentistry have not fully mastered all aspects of it yet: value, hue, chroma, translucency, opalescence, internal staining, texture, shape, size, etc. All of it contributes to shade evaluation and subsequent matching. That is not all. That is just the tooth itself. Then the environment comes into play: light conditions, color temperature, surrounding structures, colors, clothing, makeup, skin tone, etc. It never ends. As if that is not enough, we then need to capture all that information, possibly in a photographic manner, and transfer it to the laboratory. If we are successful at doing all that, the laboratory then has the job to create a restoration that matches the desired features. It is indeed a daunting task.

Undoubtedly, shade matching in the esthetic zone is one of the hottest topics when it comes to laboratory communication. First, if you are sending esthetic cases to your laboratory and you are never happy with the results, you must ask yourself a few questions: Is your laboratory capable of performing the kind of restorations that you are requesting? Does your laboratory have the talent to create such restorations? How much are you willing to spend to have a restoration that matches your expectations?

Most of us know the answer to these questions. If you are the kind of person that prefers to keep money in your pocket rather than put quality in your patient's mouth, then I do not have much to say to you. A very select group of ceramists can achieve top-notch restorations. These professionals have spent a lifetime of training to be able to perform at a high level, and you should expect their work to be properly compensated. Let us now continue on to communication with a talented team of technicians.

It is time to dive into how to use photography to transfer color information to the laboratory. Although this book is not intended to cover all aspects of color science, I will show you some techniques that might come in handy. The intent of this chapter is to examine the photographic considerations that are needed when capturing and transferring the information to the dental laboratory.

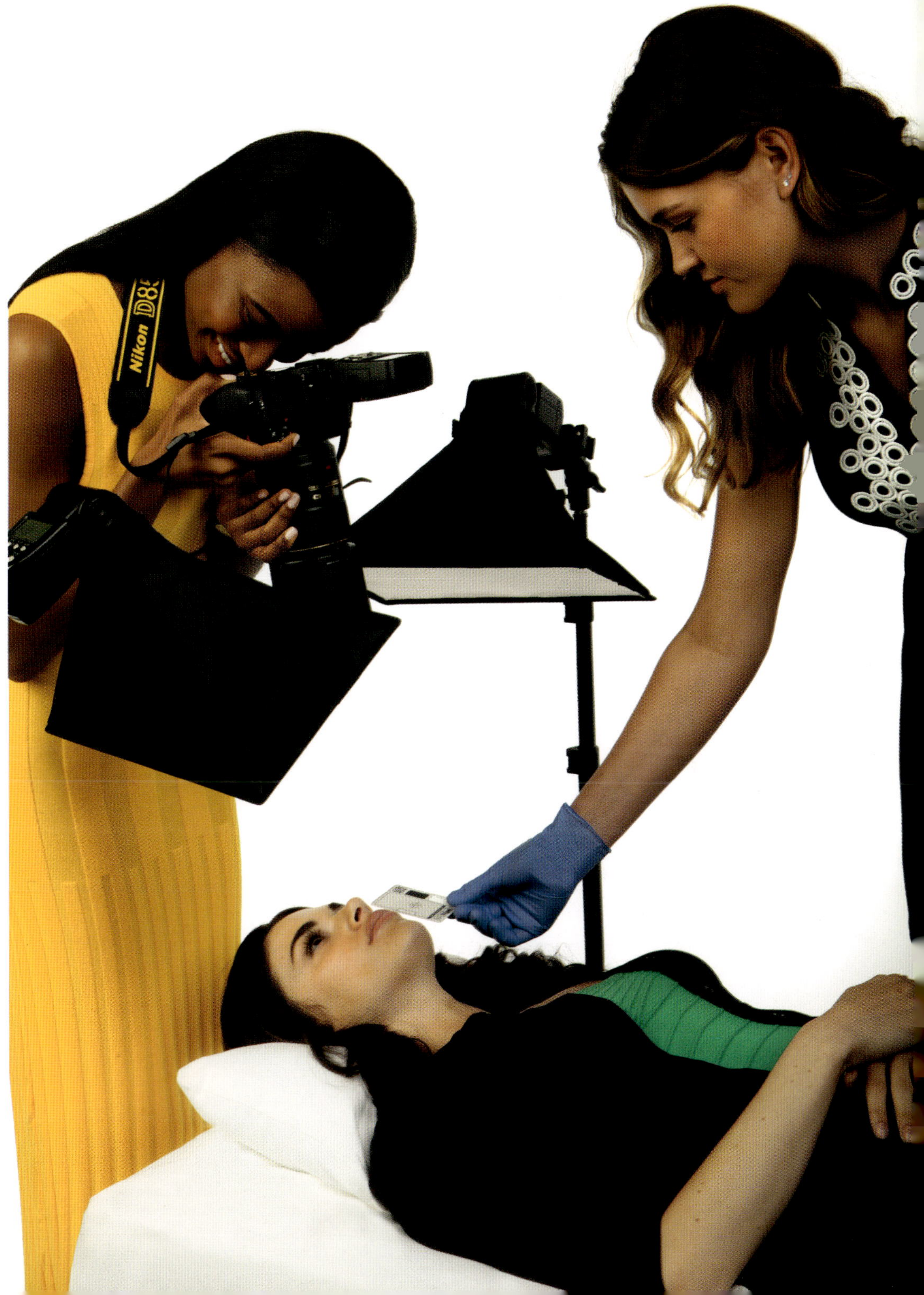

Gray card shot for white balance color correction.

Considerations when evaluating tooth shade

Lighting and white balance

The nature and color temperature of your light source is important. As discussed in one of my previous tips, knowing the color temperature of your flash units is not only important but necessary. One way to determine that is to take a series of photos of a gray card while changing the custom white balance. For example, you take the photo with a custom white balance of 4,000K, then 5,000K, then 6,000K, etc. Then in Photoshop, you can measure the red, green, and blue (RGB) values of the pixels on the gray card. The values should in theory be all the same. Choose the K value in which the RGB values are closer to each other. If that is, for example, the photo taken at 6,000K, then go back and take another set of photos, this time under values of 5,800K, 5,900K, 6,000K, 6,100K, etc. Go back to Photoshop and look at the RGB values once again. Doing this will allow you to narrow down to the real color temperature of your light source. My speedlights with the diffusers on have a temperature of 6,950K. Without the diffusers on, the value drops to 6,500K. The manual said the flashes were calibrated to 5,500K. I do not trust the manuals any longer. Ever since I calibrated my white balance this way, my post-processing color-correction calibration is almost nonexistent.

The process just described does not replace the use of a gray card, even after you have set your white balance. Finding the true color temperature of your flashes is something that you do once and then you have it, until you change your gear. I still use a gray card at every session in order to fine-tune the color correction prior to sending the photos to the laboratory.

Ideally you want to have color-calibrated lights in your operatories as well. These are referred to as *daylight color temperature lights*. They often come in 5,000K or 6,500K. The cost is similar to regular lights of different color temperatures. Having the lights calibrated will help you immensely when selecting the right matching shade tab and also by not mixing different color lights in your photos.

Diffusers will alter the color temperature when compared to direct light. However, diffusion is an asset when used accordingly, because it will reduce glare. Glare can cause areas of the tooth surface to depict no color at all.

Lastly, the color of surrounding walls, furniture, and patient clothing is important. Light from the room and the flash will bounce on the furniture, walls, and clothing and come back to your subject with a different color temperature. For example, green walls, brown furniture, and red lipstick will all taint your light and result in a photo that does not depict the intrinsic color characteristics of the teeth.

Shade selection

We are all used to taking shades using shade tabs. However, most of us do it wrong. I have spent years trying to get better at it, taking into account every variable that I could control. However, every time that I believe I have got it down to a science and I am finally doing it right, I realize that there was one more thing I was unaware of. Then I improve my protocol. In essence, it means I am always evolving and learning, which is important in our daily practice. I will share with you several items that need to be considered when using tabs to take a shade measurement.

Limit the time you look at the shade tabs intraorally to less than 7 seconds—yes, just under 7 seconds. If you stare at them longer, your eyes adapt and shade differentiation becomes less accurate. Rest your eyes on a neutral surface, such as a gray card, and come back to refine your shade selection, eliminating each time those shades that are obviously not right.

Select value first, then narrow down the chroma. Using the VITA Linearguide 3-D Master will help you a long way with that. It is already designed for you to pick value first, then chroma. I use this system every day. I find it easy and reliable. I have gotten great results with it, and I do not see myself changing anytime soon.

I complement the shade measurement protocol with the VITA Easyshade system. Gone are the days in which I start with the whole gamut of shade tabs and then, step by step, narrow it down to a couple tabs. Nowadays, I will start the process with the VITA Easyshade system. I use the shade measurement that it gives, and then I pick up that tab to reconfirm intraorally. It is consistently within one shade value, if not right on. It saves me time and, most importantly, it allows my eyes to be rested when it comes to looking at the last two to three tabs. I recommend you look into it. It is worth every penny.

Note that you should not use a black constraster while taking shades. Let the natural background in the mouth be present in its natural form. A black contraster lowers the value of the teeth and the shade tab. The shade tab itself has a metal backing, and some dentists recommend picking one shade value higher to compensate for that. I do not do it, but I do not have an argument against it either.

Lastly, use the same tabs as the laboratory's porcelain system. Ask your laboratory what kind of porcelain they are using, then make sure your tabs are from the same manufacturer. If you are using the Noritake shade tabs and your laboratory uses VITA porcelain, you will not get the same result.

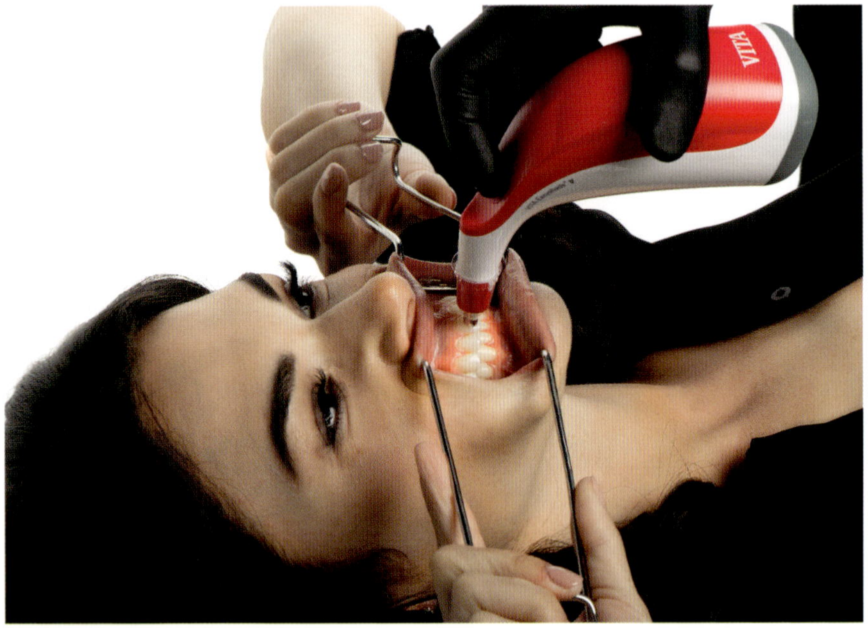

VITA Easyshade V

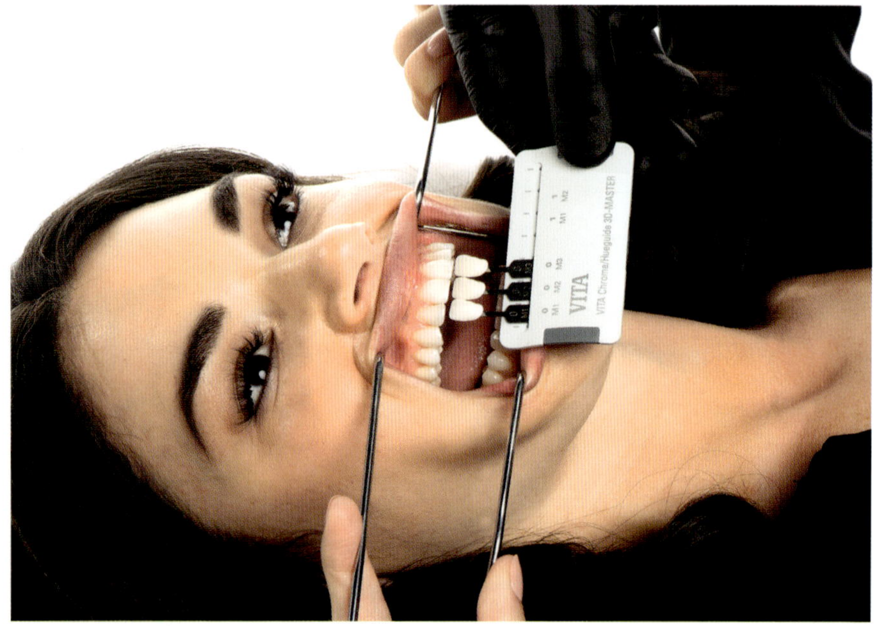

VITA Linearguide 3-D Master

Polarization

A polarization system as part of your armamentarium is a must, in my opinion. I started using them several years ago, and the results were evident. It all comes back to the same basic principle. If you are working with skilled ceramists with proper training, the more information you get to them, the better your results will be.

Polarization is all about that—information. It allows for the removal of all glare from your image. Without glare, chroma comes to life like you have never seen it before. A well-balanced and exposed photo will give you proper value measurements. A properly polarized photo will give you helpful chroma information.

It is not only chroma that you obtain from a polarized photo. The second set of data that you will obtain is that of characterization. Minor craze lines, white stains, decalcifications, translucency, and opalescence will all show up better once the glare is removed. When matching anterior teeth, polarized photos should always be included.

There are several systems in the market. I use the Polar Eyes cross polarization filter from PhotoMed. It is specifically designed to fit onto my ring flash. The picture quality is fantastic.

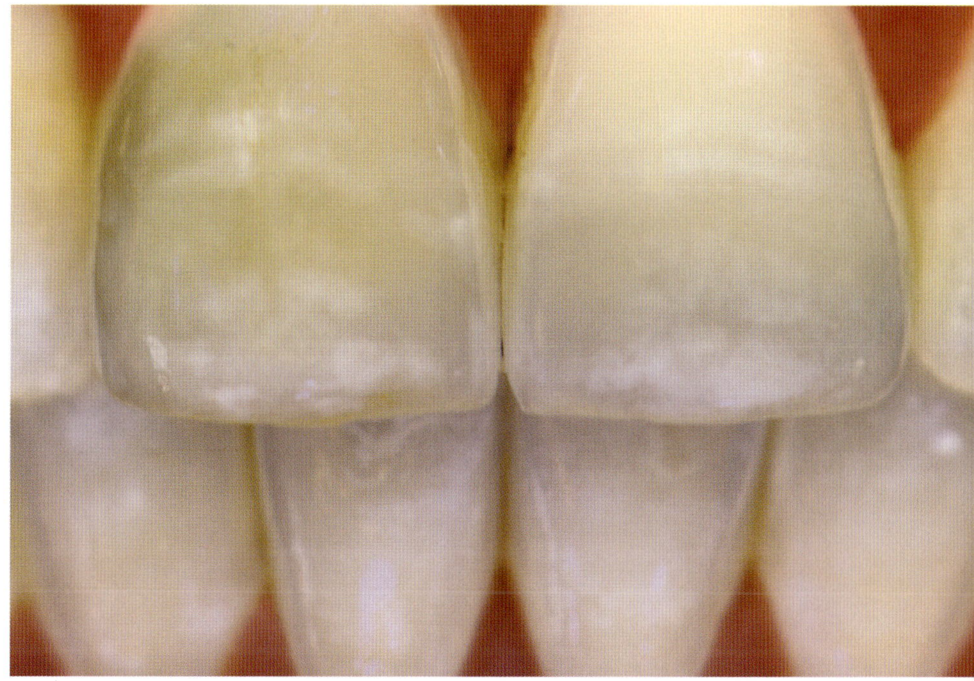

Polarized image taken using Smile Lite polarization filter (Smile Line). Notice the presence of high chroma regions, calcification, translucency, and opacity.

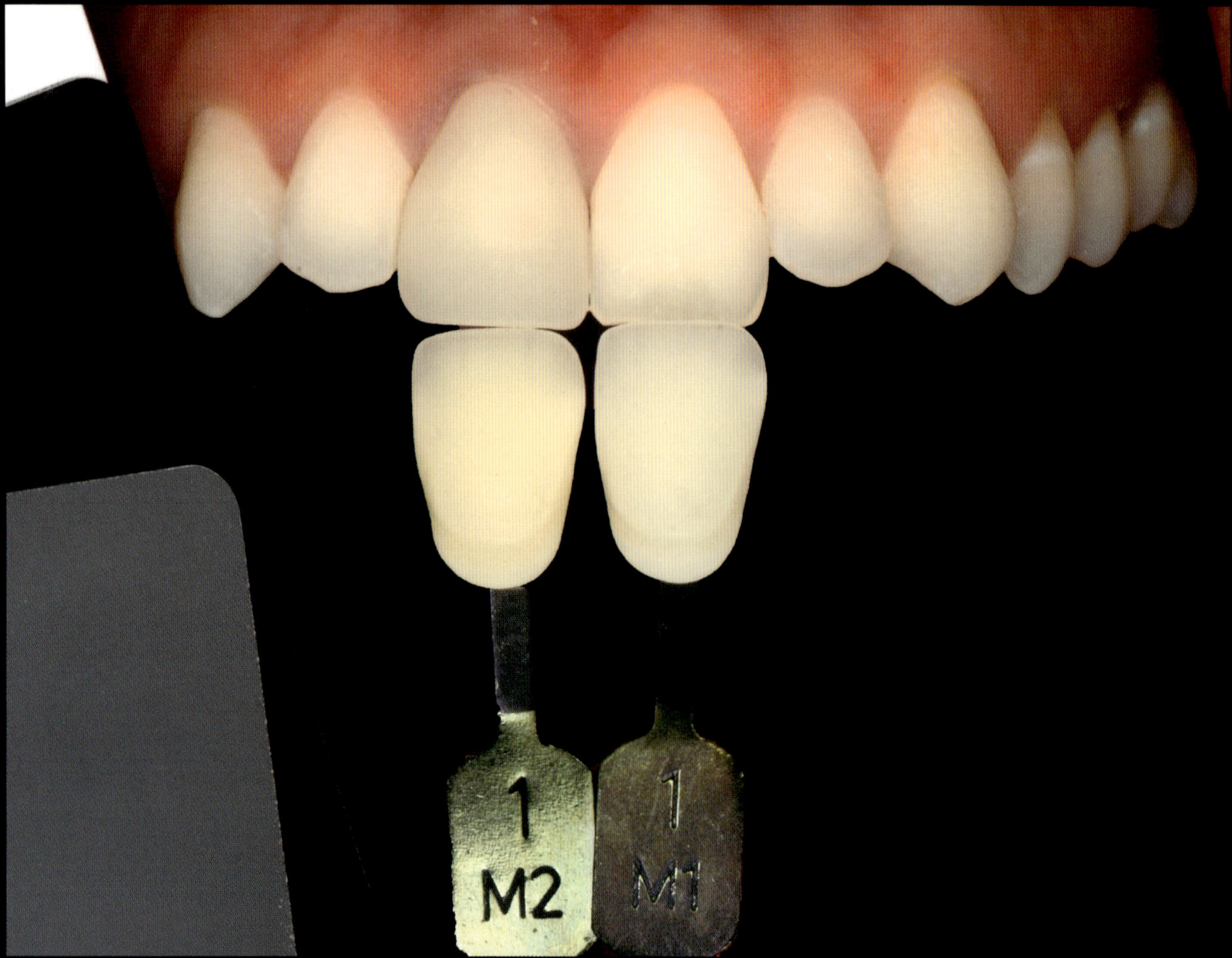

Polarized image with white balance cards for color correction

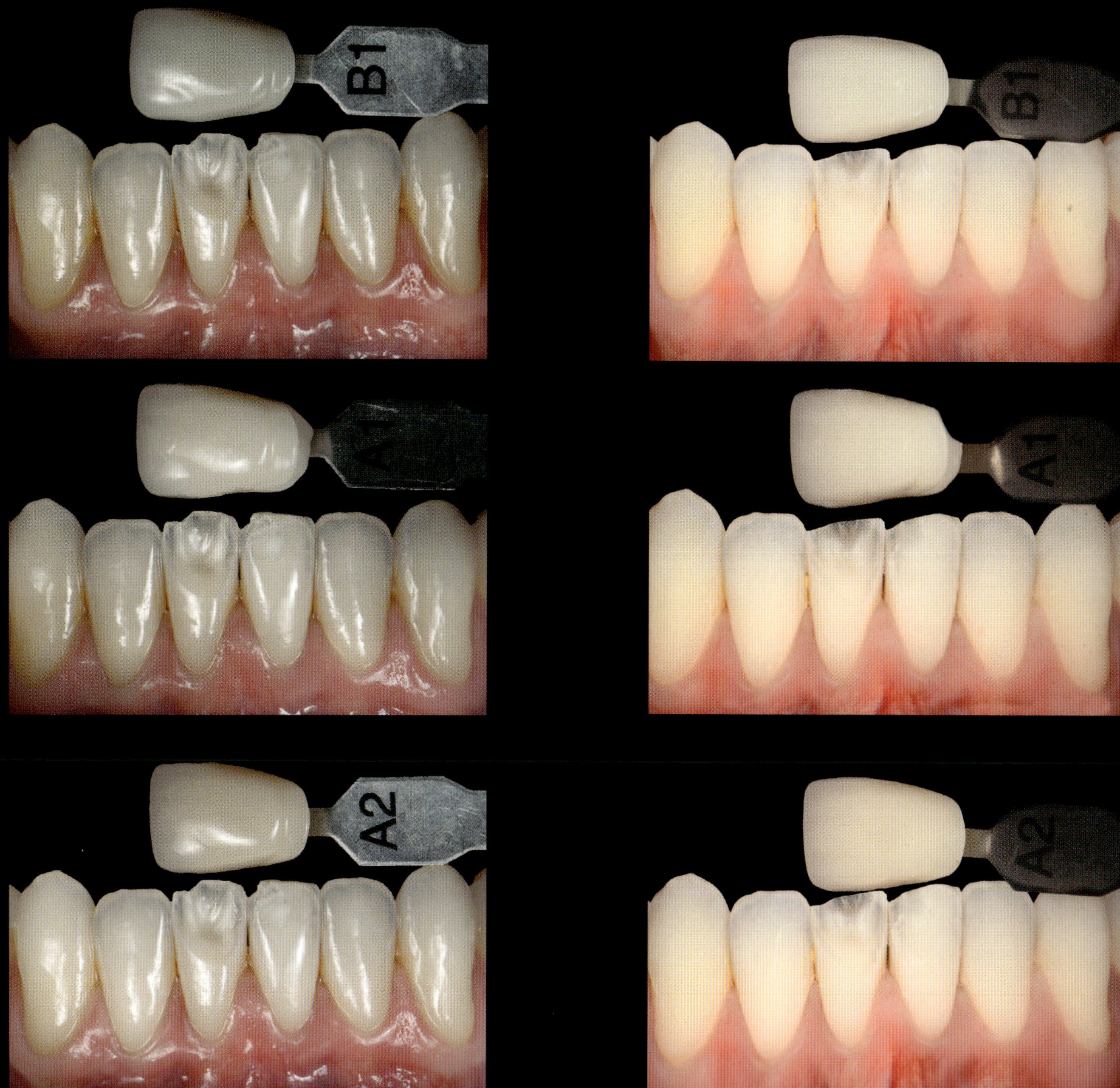

Nonpolarized

Polarized

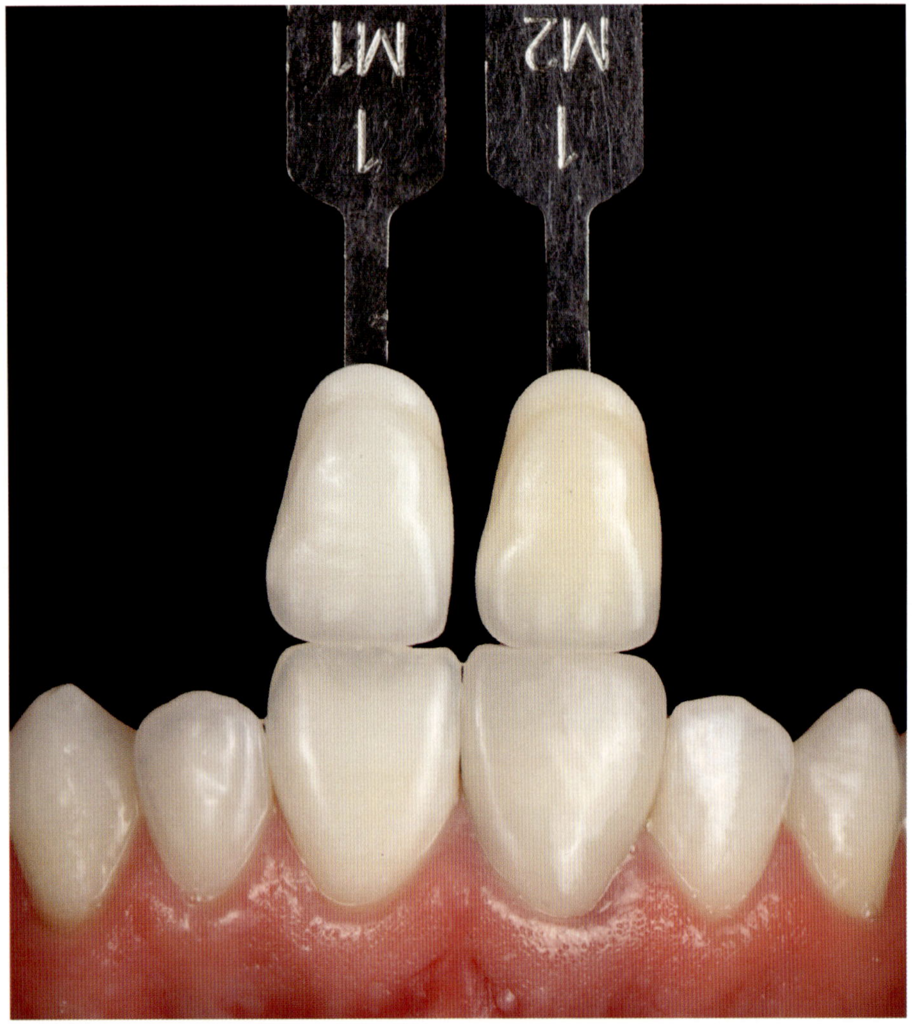

Placing a higher chroma tab next to the chosen tab will help your ceramist evaluate chromatic regions better.

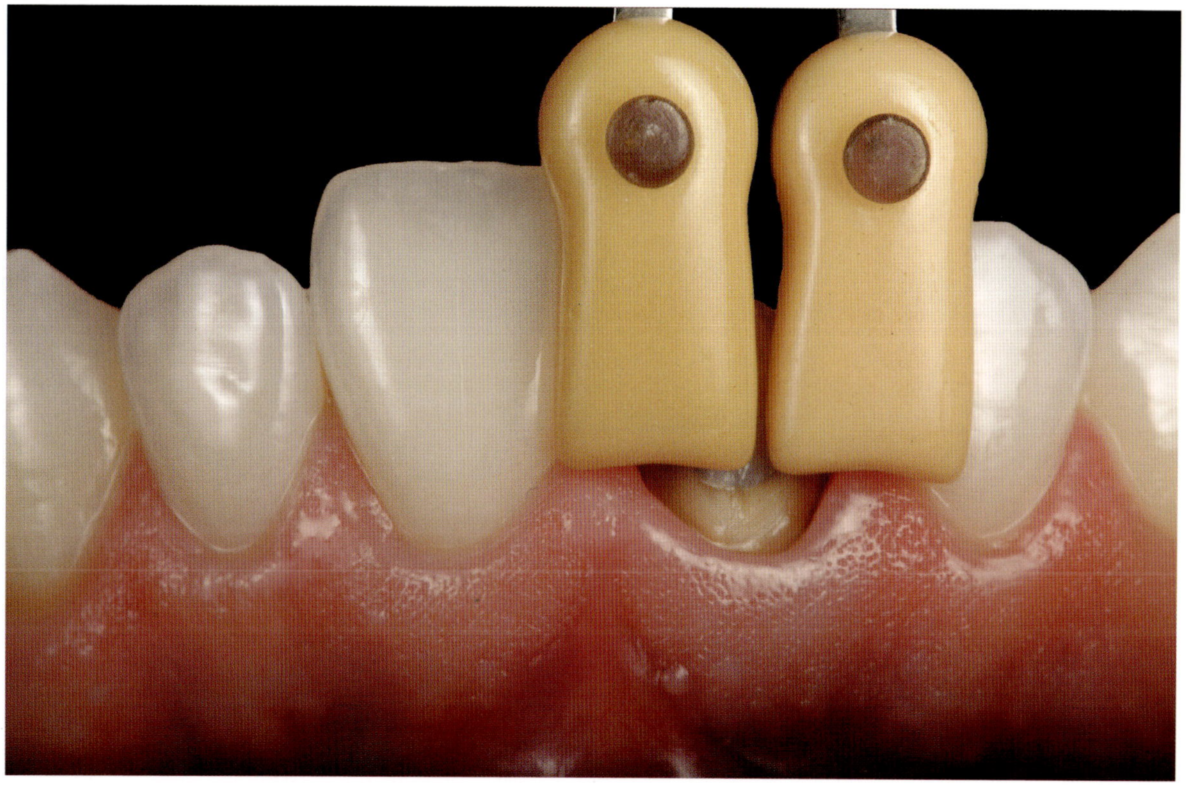

Stump shade measurements are indispensable in the era of all-ceramic restorations.

Dental Laboratory Photography

Simple and Inexpensive Setup for Dental Laboratories

- A portable photo studio box
- 3 speedlights
- 1 commander
- 3 tripods with flash brackets
- 2 softboxes or umbrellas
- A medium/large front-surface mirror
- A set of 16 to 24 rechargeable batteries with a large charger

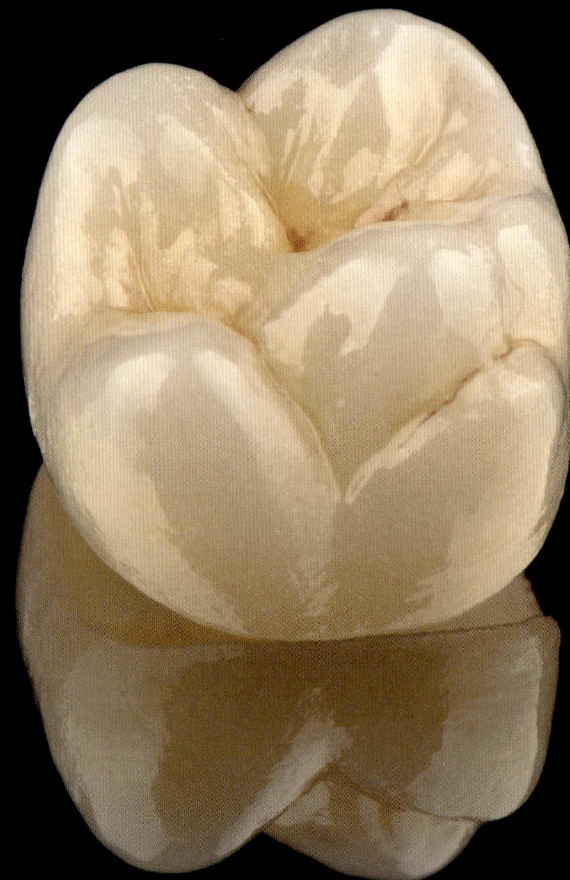

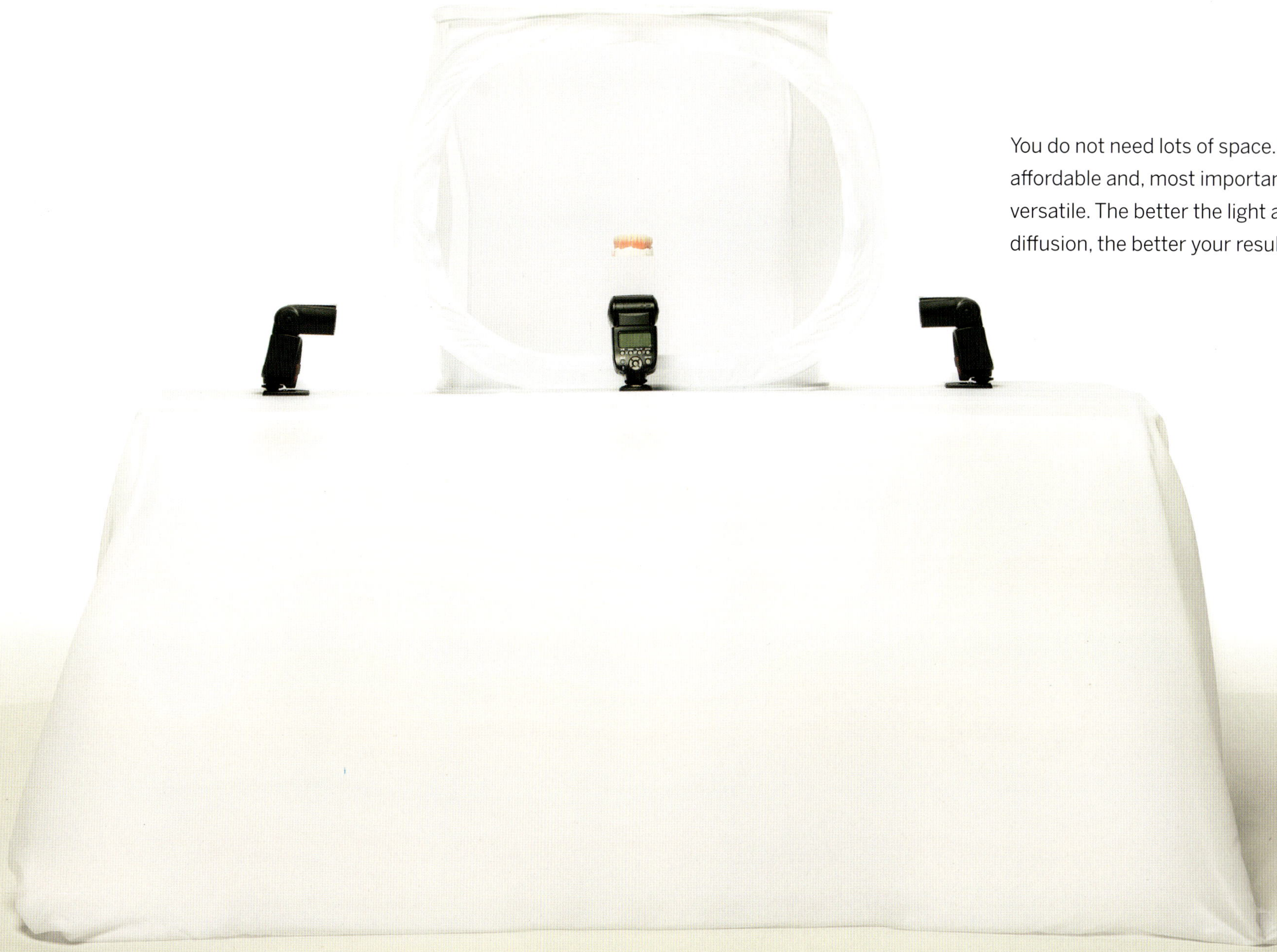

You do not need lots of space. It is affordable and, most importantly, versatile. The better the light and the diffusion, the better your results.

Using speedlights will give good battery life and flexibility of movement. The light box could be used as a diffuser, but it might not be enough to achieve all the desired effects.

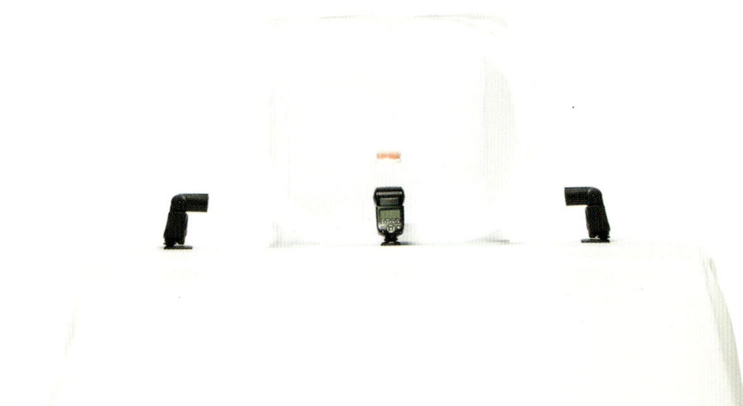

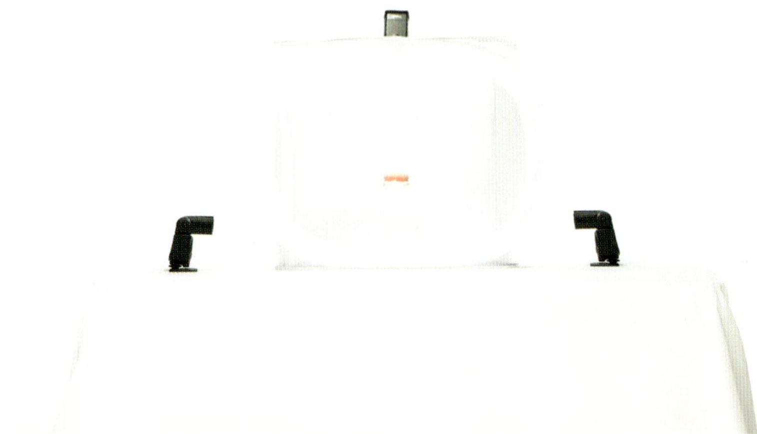

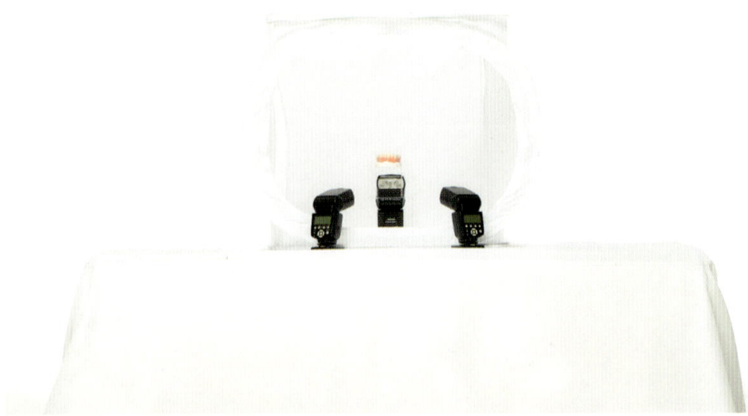

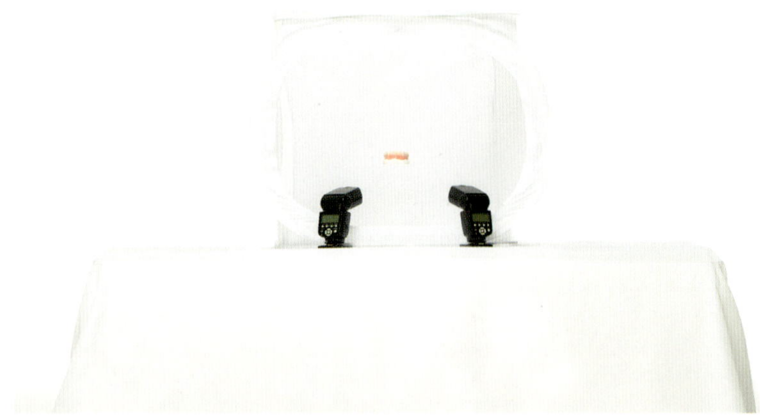

SEVEN

Speedlights with no diffusion

Front

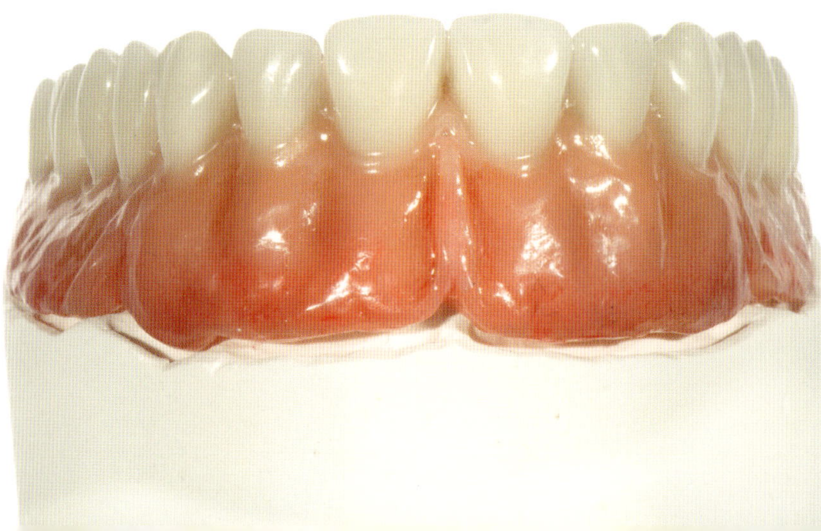

Side

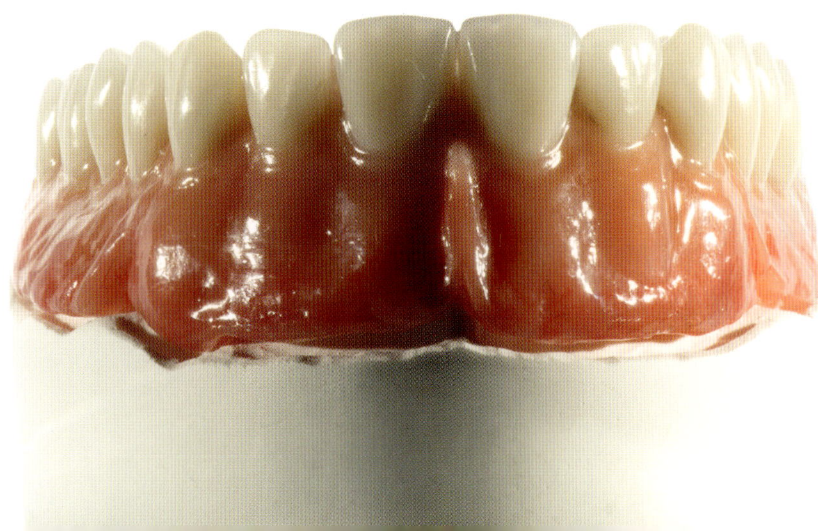

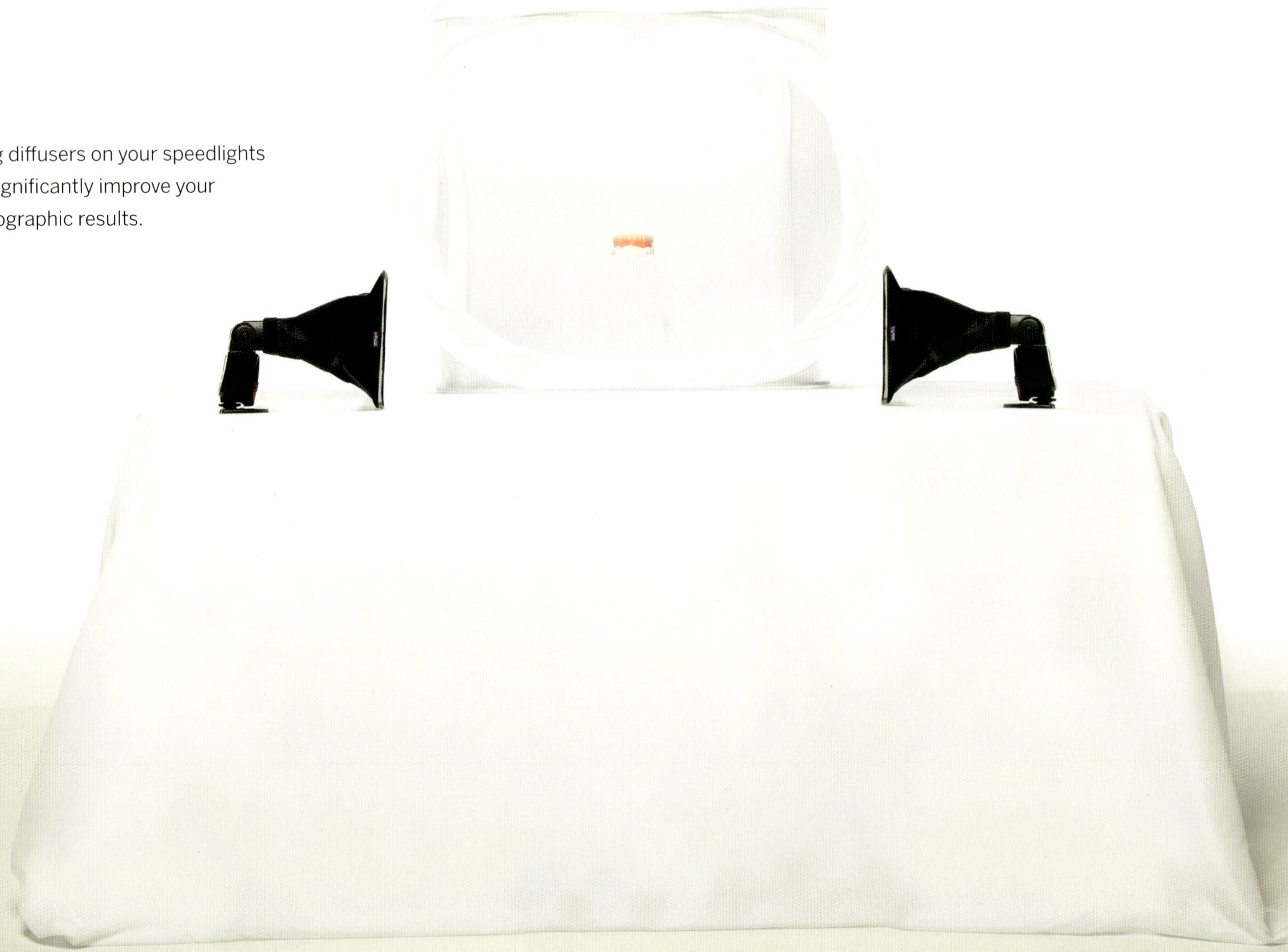

Using diffusers on your speedlights will significantly improve your photographic results.

Speedlights with diffusion

Front

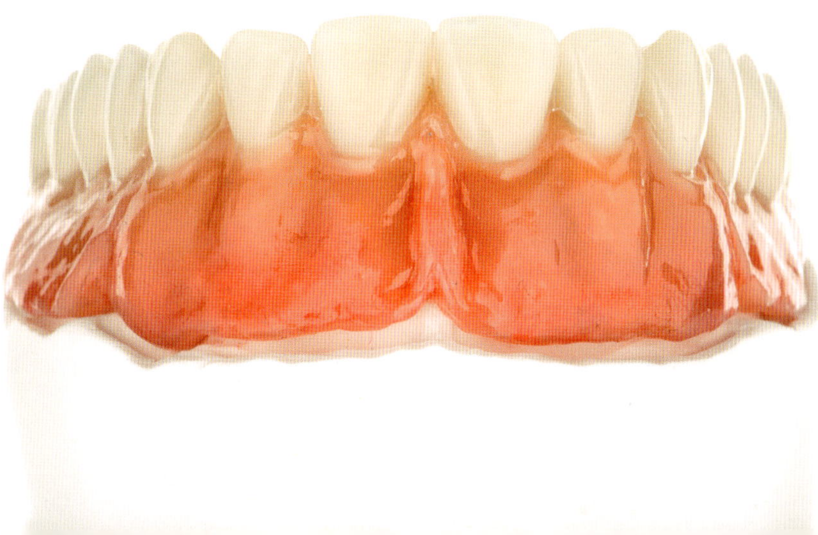

Side

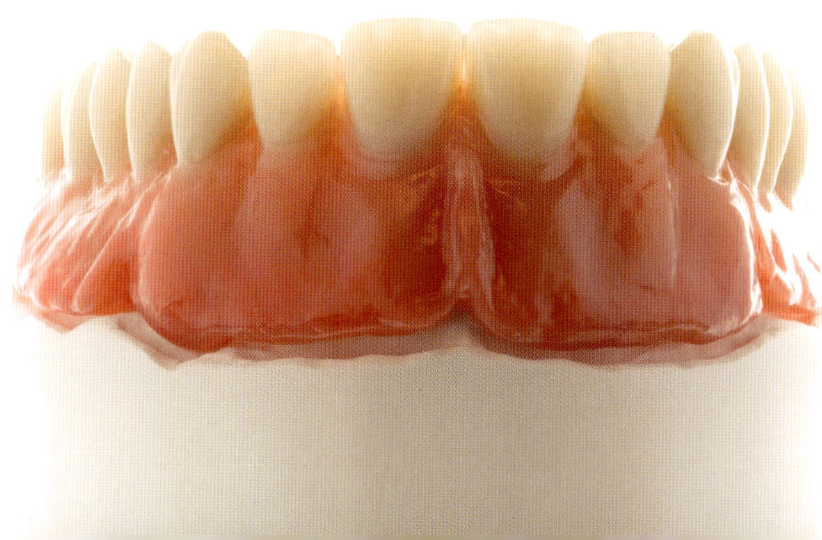

The Nikon SB-R200 dual flashes can be used as well. However, battery life is not ideal and recycle time can be frustrating.

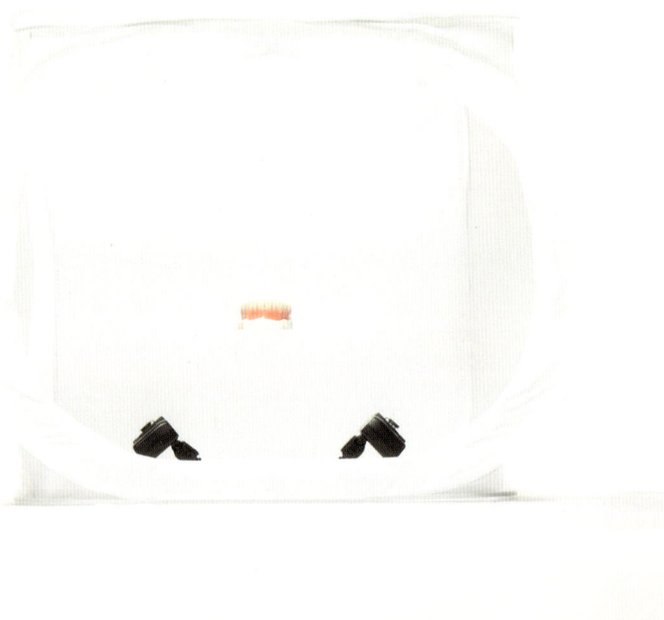

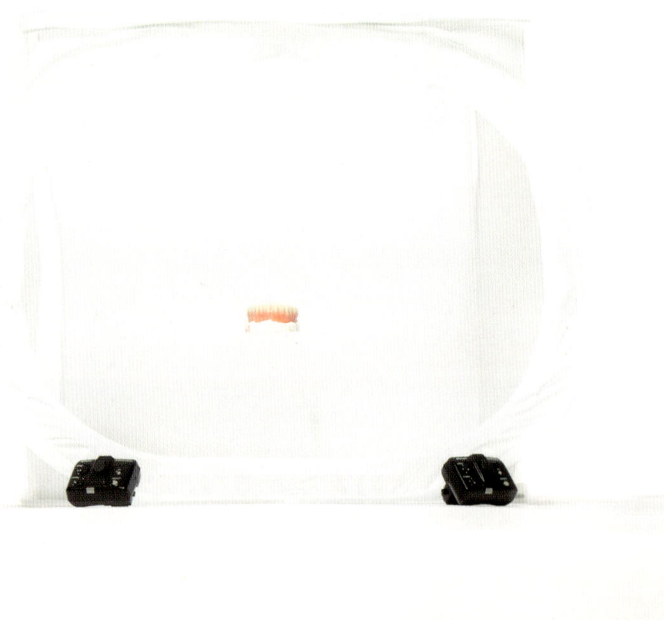

Adding the bouncer/diffuser to the Nikon SB-R200 dual flashes will give you better results at a very low cost.

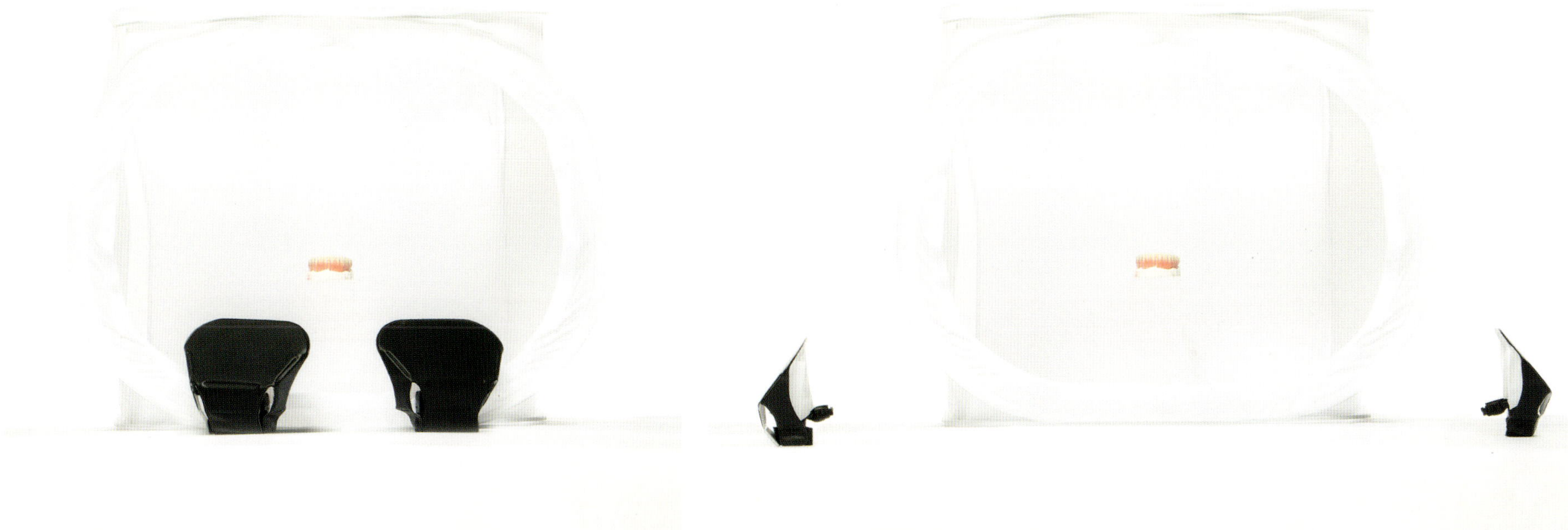

Dual flashes with no diffusion

Front

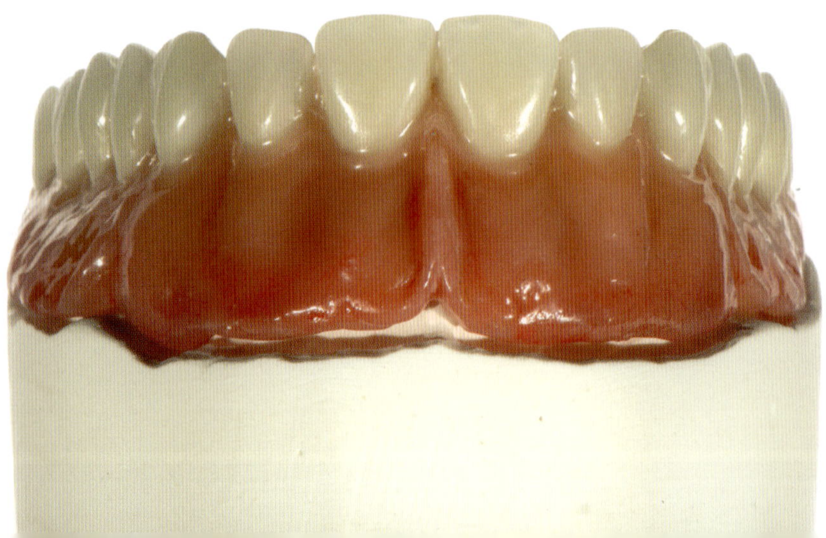

As always, if you have the means and the space, strobes will give you the best results. A light box might not even be needed.

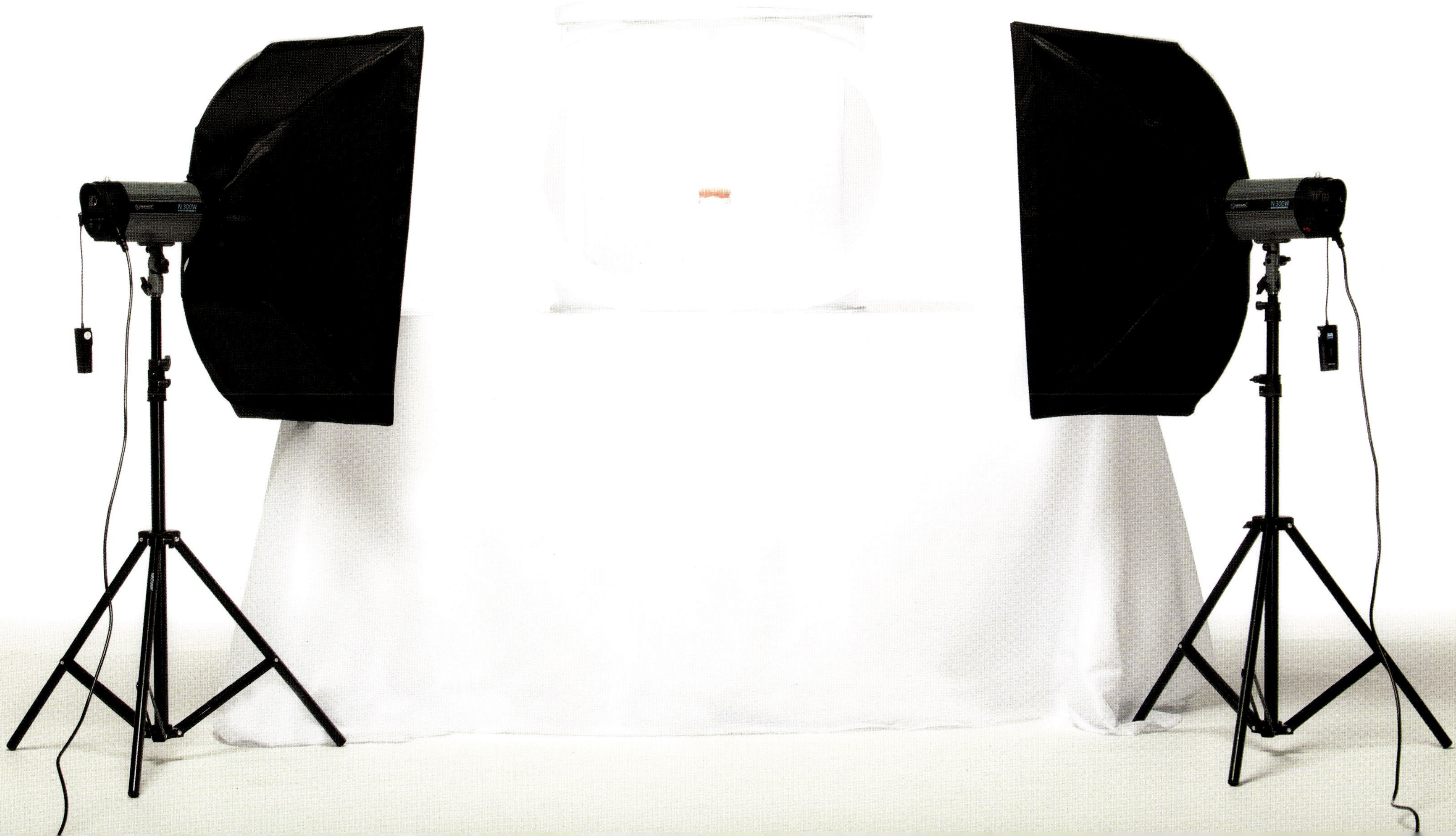

Strobes with softboxes

Front

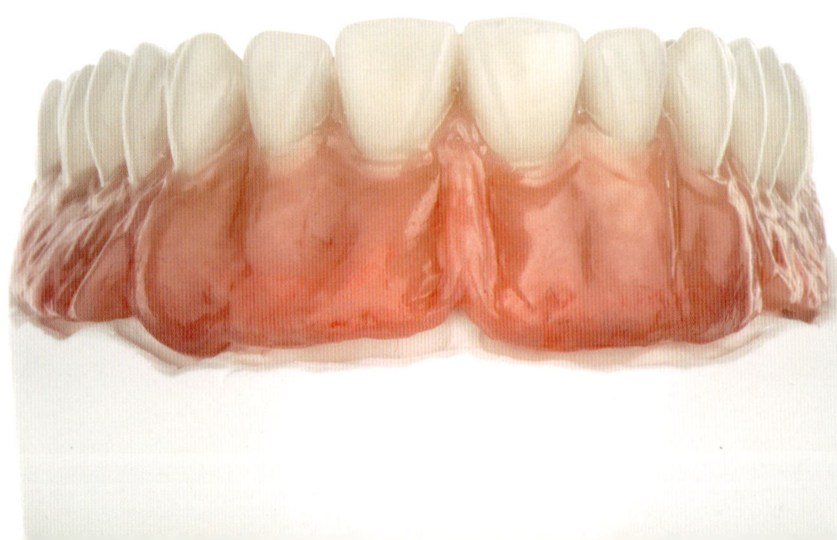

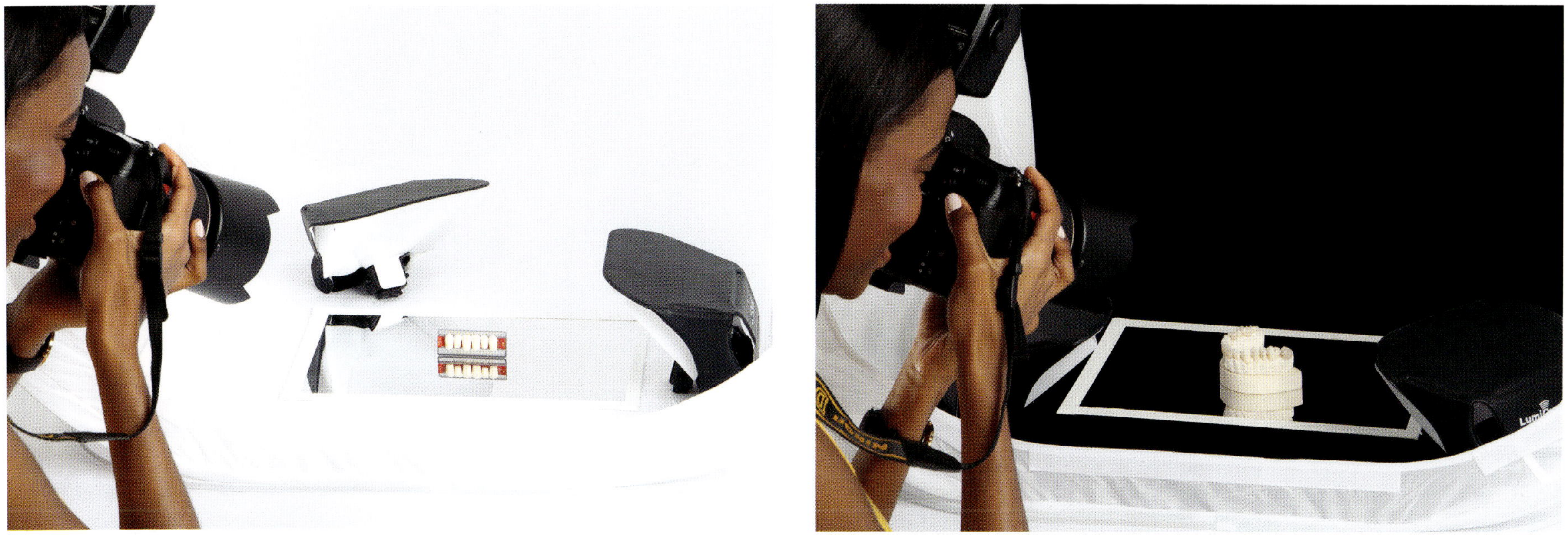

Front-surface mirrors, backgrounds, and light modification

Photographing Small Elements

Photographing small elements has its tricks. I learn new ones every day. My intent is to save you some of the trial-and-error time so that you can get right to the shots you always dreamed of taking.

Get a macro lens.

As discussed earlier, a macro lens will allow for reproduction ratios of 1:1, which is extremely important when photographing small elements.

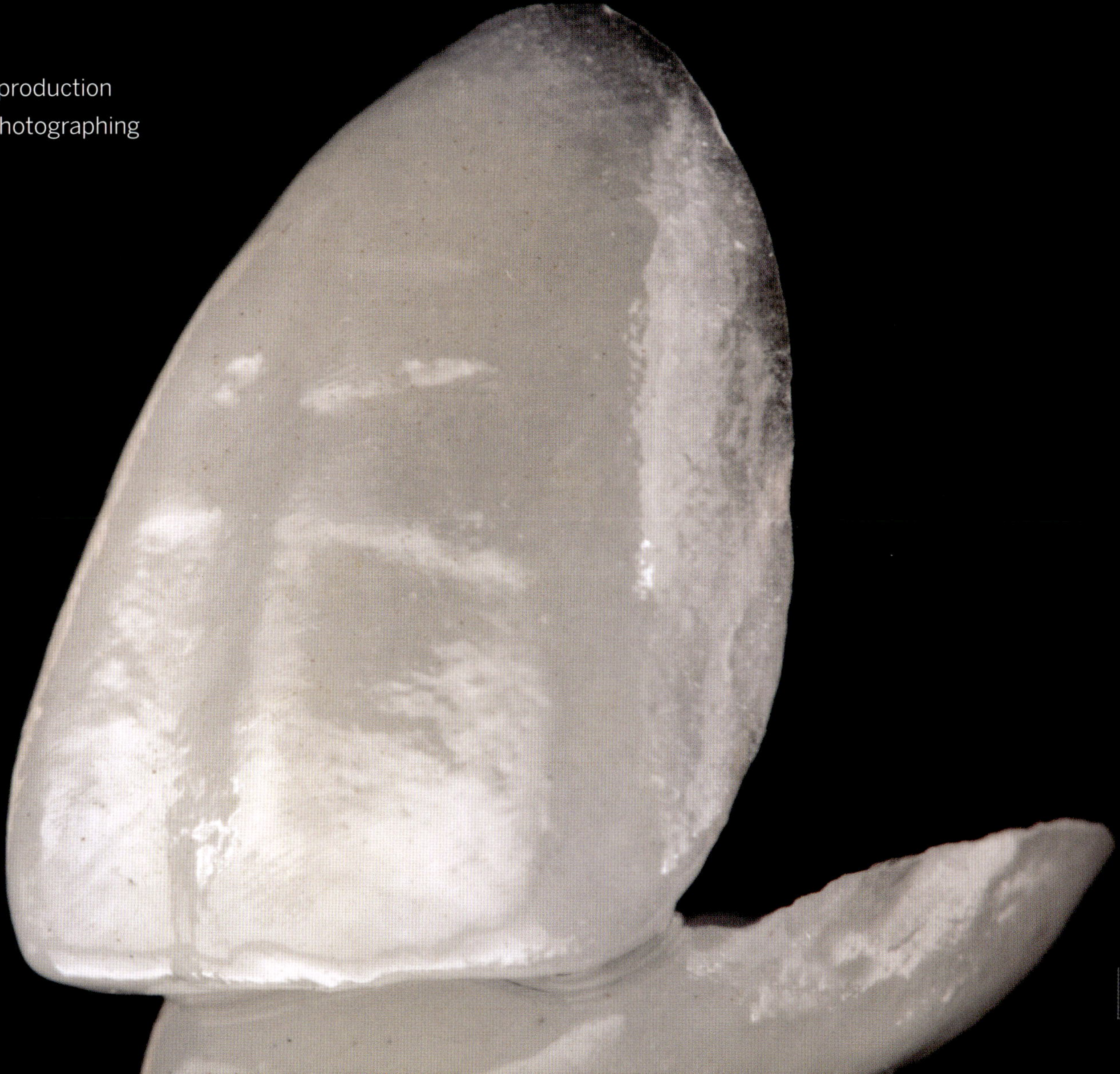

The use of plain backgrounds, such as black or white (colors are an option as well) will give you a clean look.

Remove distractions from your composition.

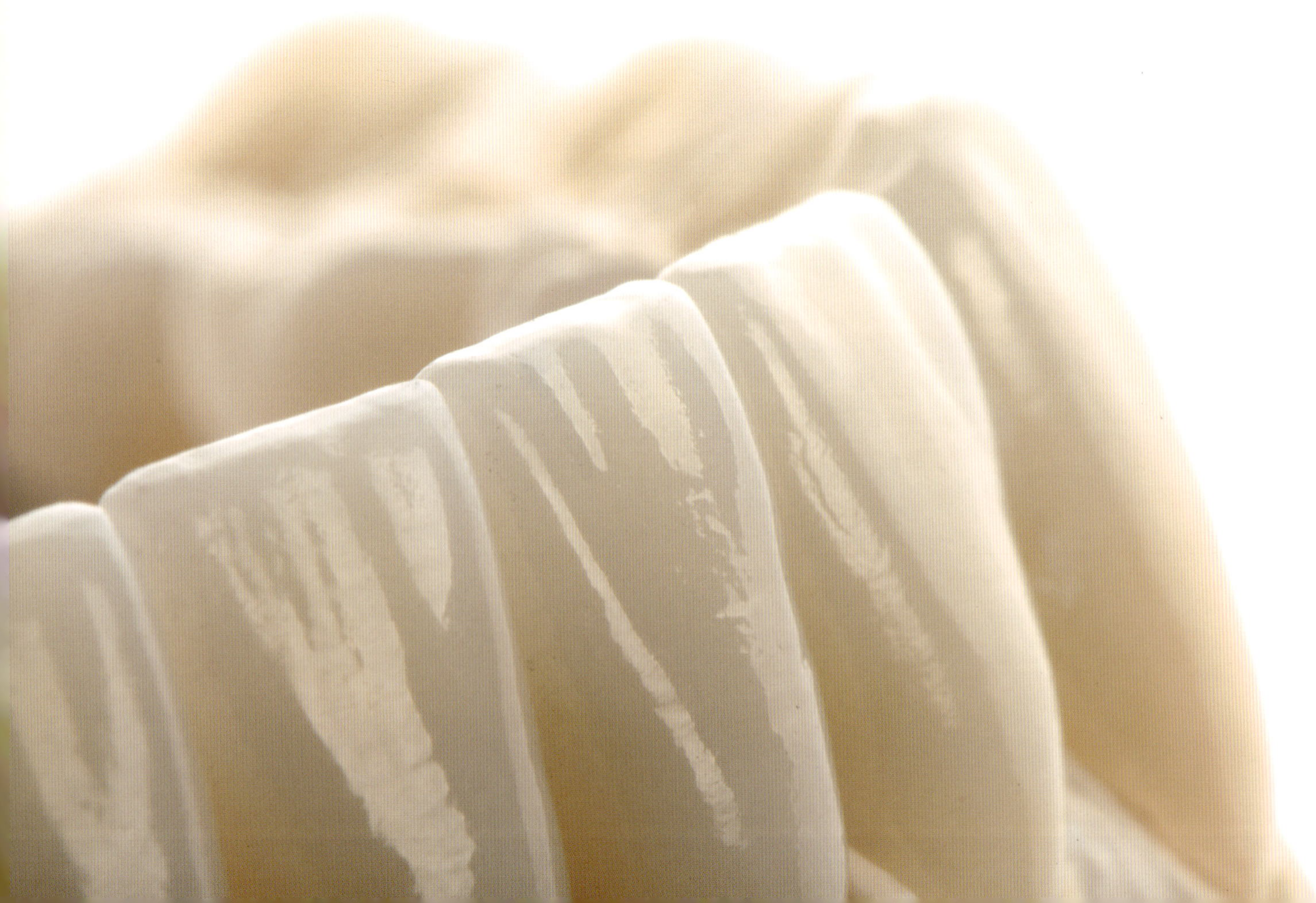

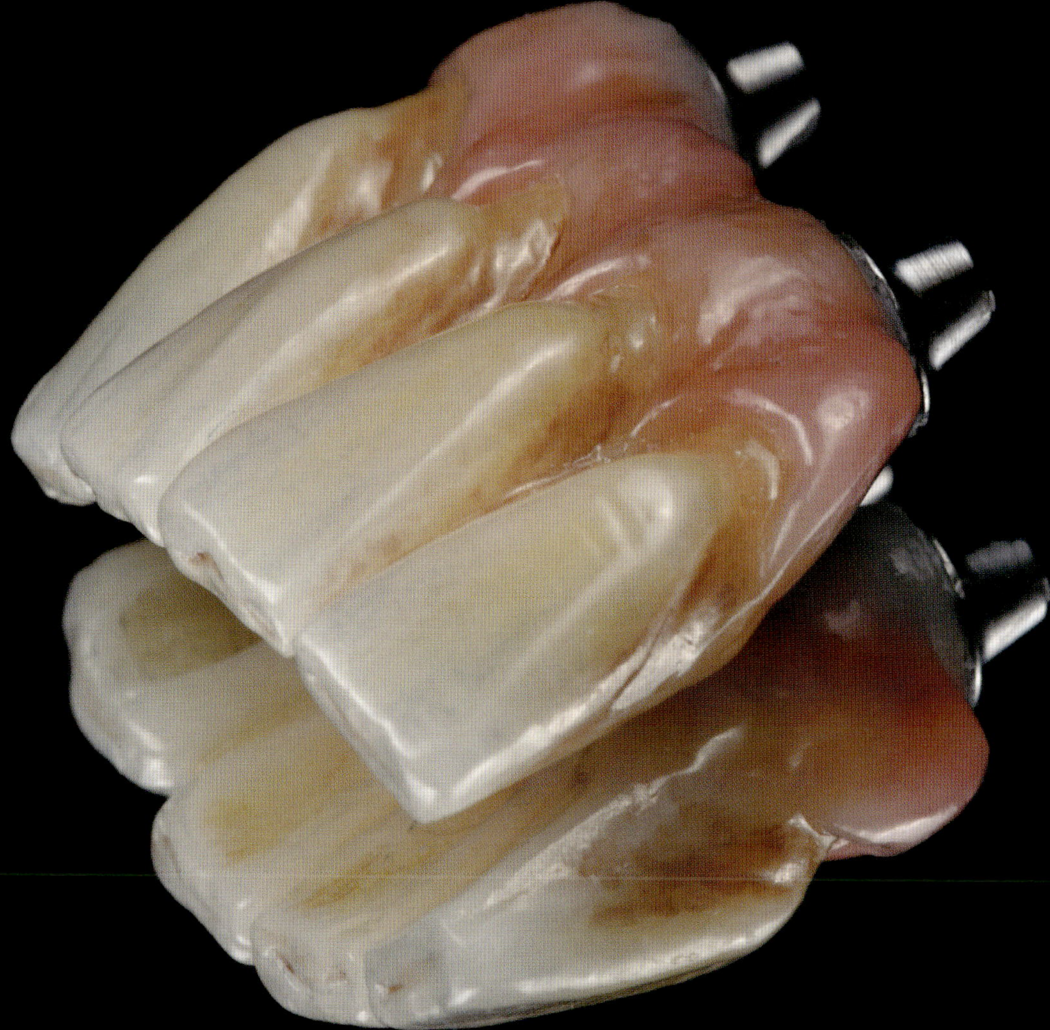

Use the histogram to evaluate exposure.

The screen on your camera tends to show an image that looks more exposed than what it will appear in the computer later on. Use the histogram to corroborate, in an objective manner, if you have the exposure levels that you intended.

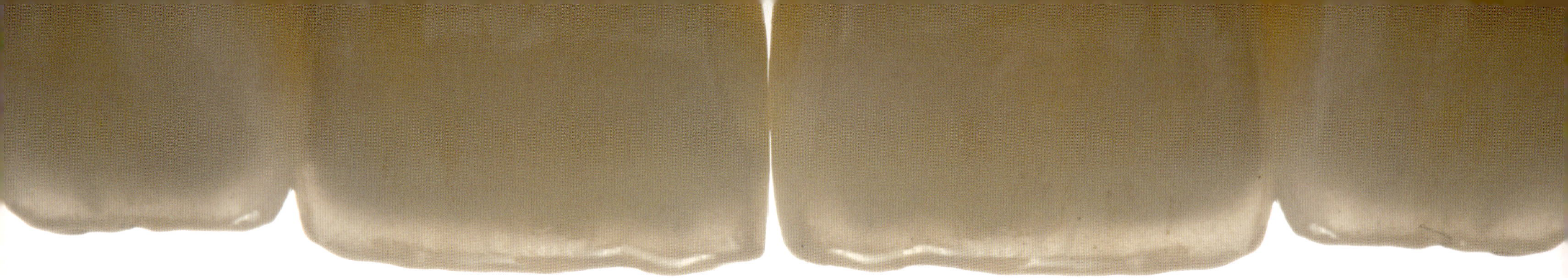

Be aware of your aperture settings.

In the laboratory, we tend to get pretty close to the subject. It is important to remember that the closer you get to the subject (everything else unchanged), the narrower your DOF. Things will quickly get blurry. If this is the effect you want, then it is okay. But if you took a picture from 20 inches away and it looked just as you wanted, getting closer on the next shot might get you in trouble. Your DOF will be reduced dramatically.

Pay attention to your focus point.

This is the same reasoning as with aperture and DOF. In macro photography, we position ourselves so close to the subject that our DOF is narrow. Thus, the focal point has to be carefully chosen. A small discrepancy can result in your shot being completely out of focus from what you intended.

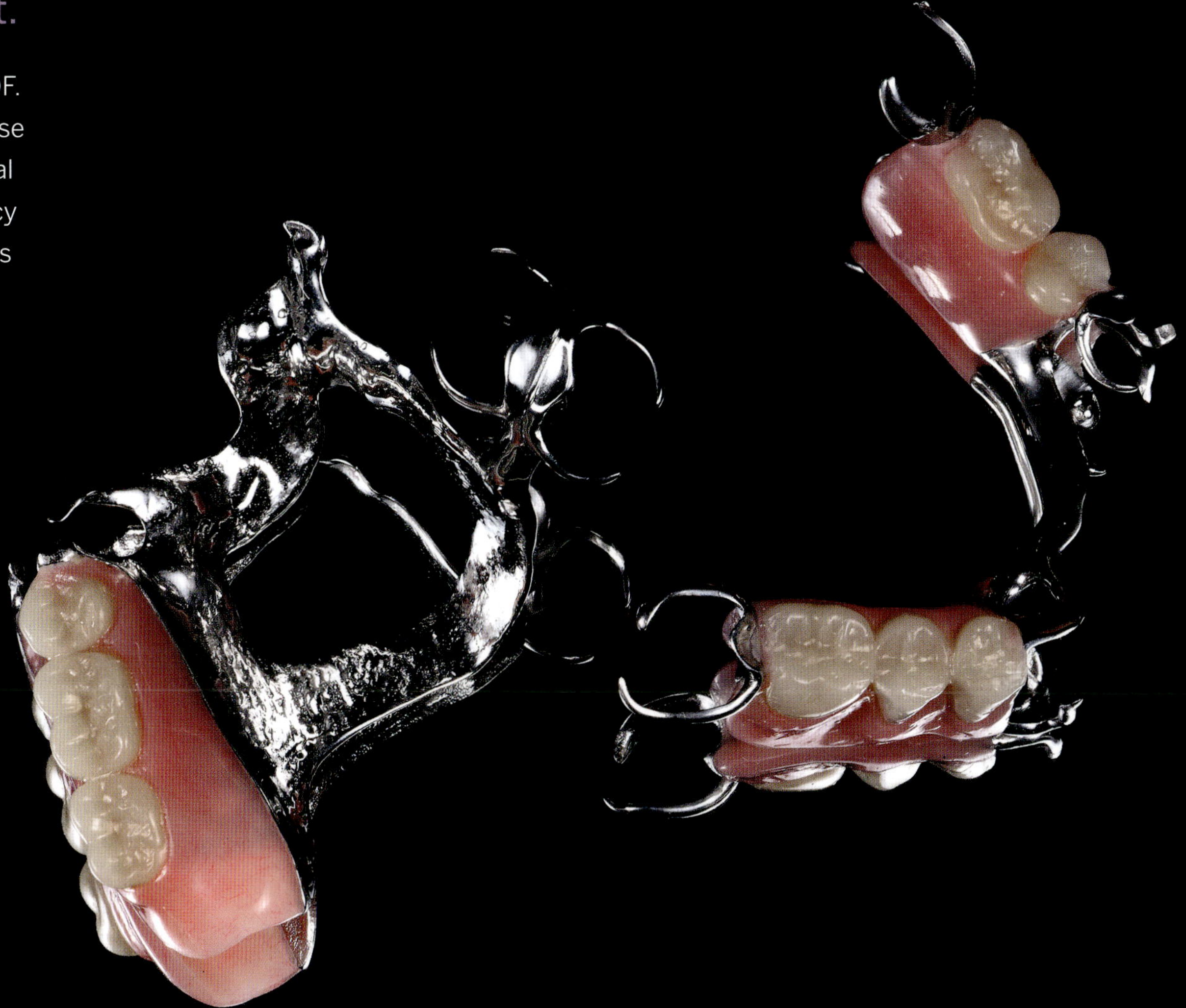

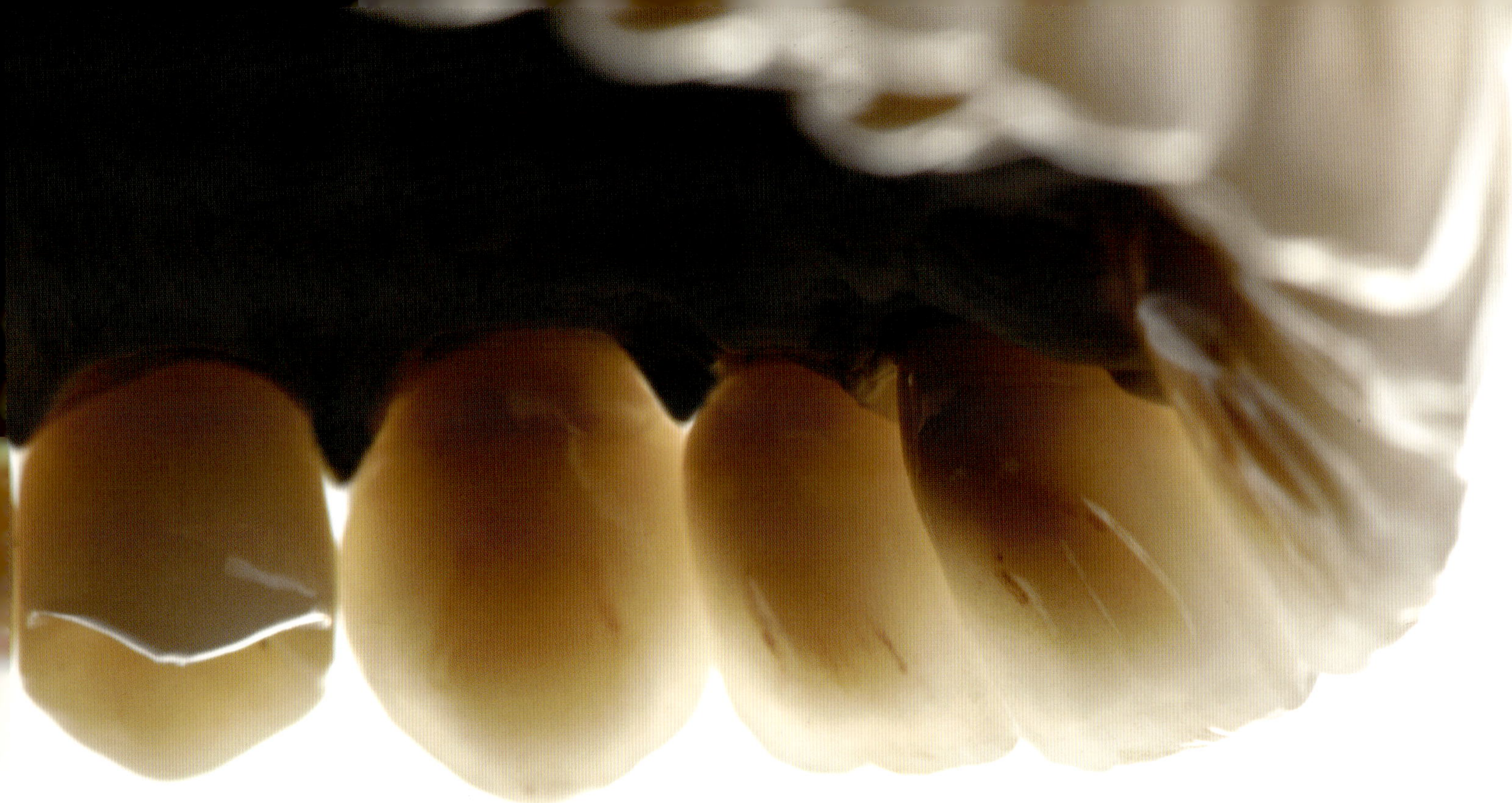

Consider single point and continuous autofocus camera features.

As our DOF becomes narrower, getting the right focus point becomes hard. Tiny camera movements will put the subject out of focus. Continuous autofocus continues to adjust the focus, so those tiny camera movements will be accounted for.

You can also try single point autofocus for macro photography. Single point allows you to choose exactly the place you want to focus, allowing your composition to be sharp exactly where you want it.

If you prefer manual focus, there is something for you too.

Manual focus is often best when shooting subjects that are 1:1 or even closer. Instead of continuing to adjust the focus ring, move yourself and the camera back and forth slowly until the subject is in focus. You can go farther by setting your desired reproduction ratio on your lens manually, then moving back and forth until the subject is in focus. This creates a pseudoreproducible scenario in which, if everything else remains the same, you are always at the same distance from your subject in consecutive shots.

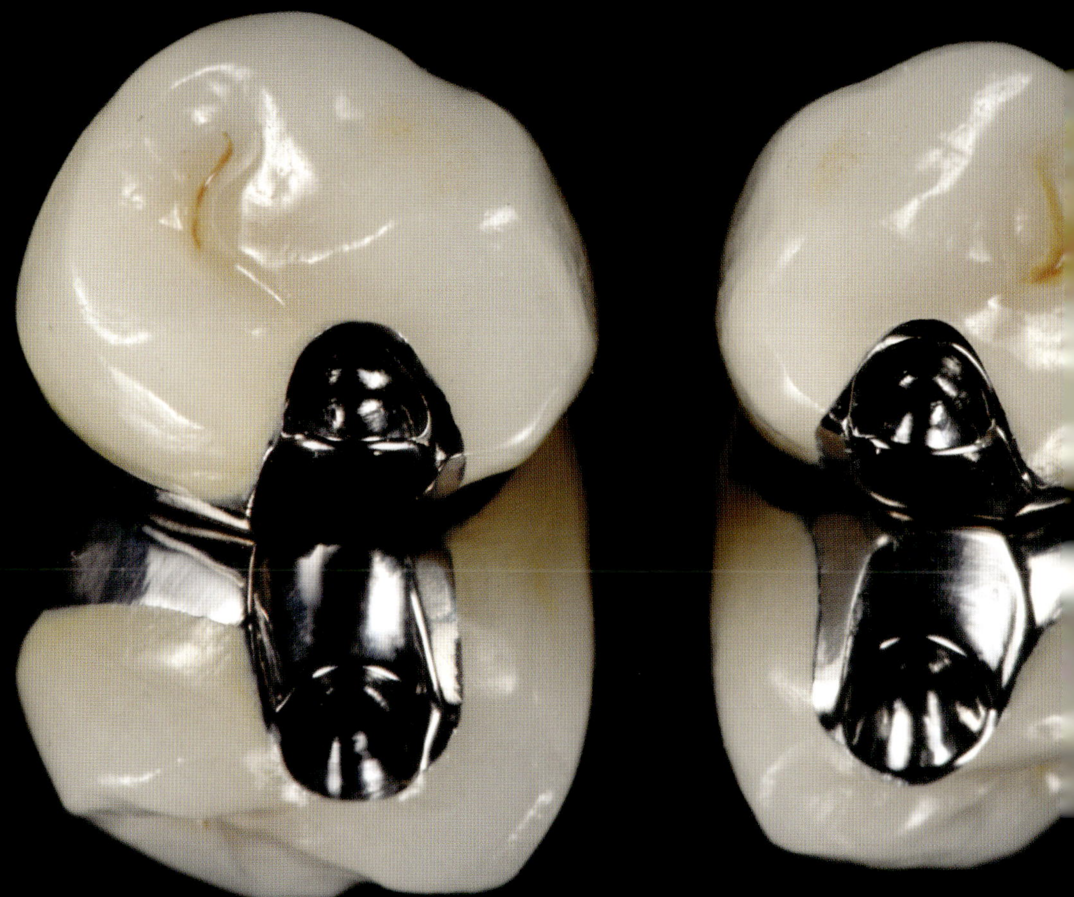

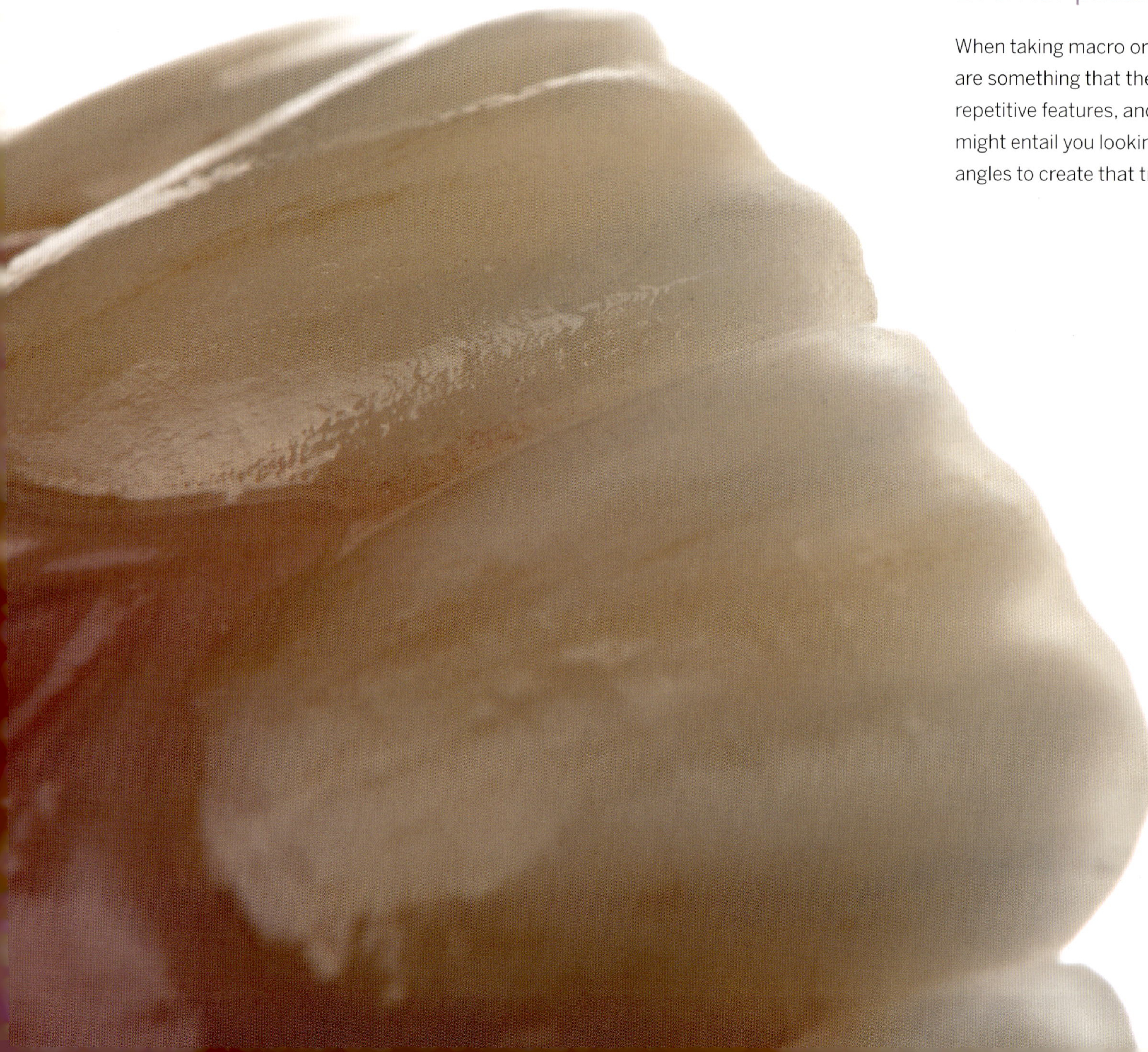

Look for patterns in your composition.

When taking macro or any other photography, patterns are something that the brain enjoys. Look for parallel lines, repetitive features, and congruencies in your subjects. This might entail you looking at your subject from many different angles to create that truly marvelous shot.

Front-surface mirrors are a must.

Front-surface mirrors are the best friend of the laboratory technician when it comes to taking photos of your work. It is not the only way to photograph your work, but it certainly is one that is pleasing to the eyes. You must be very careful. Most things that we place on that mirror will scratch it. Front-surface mirrors are expensive, so care for them accordingly.

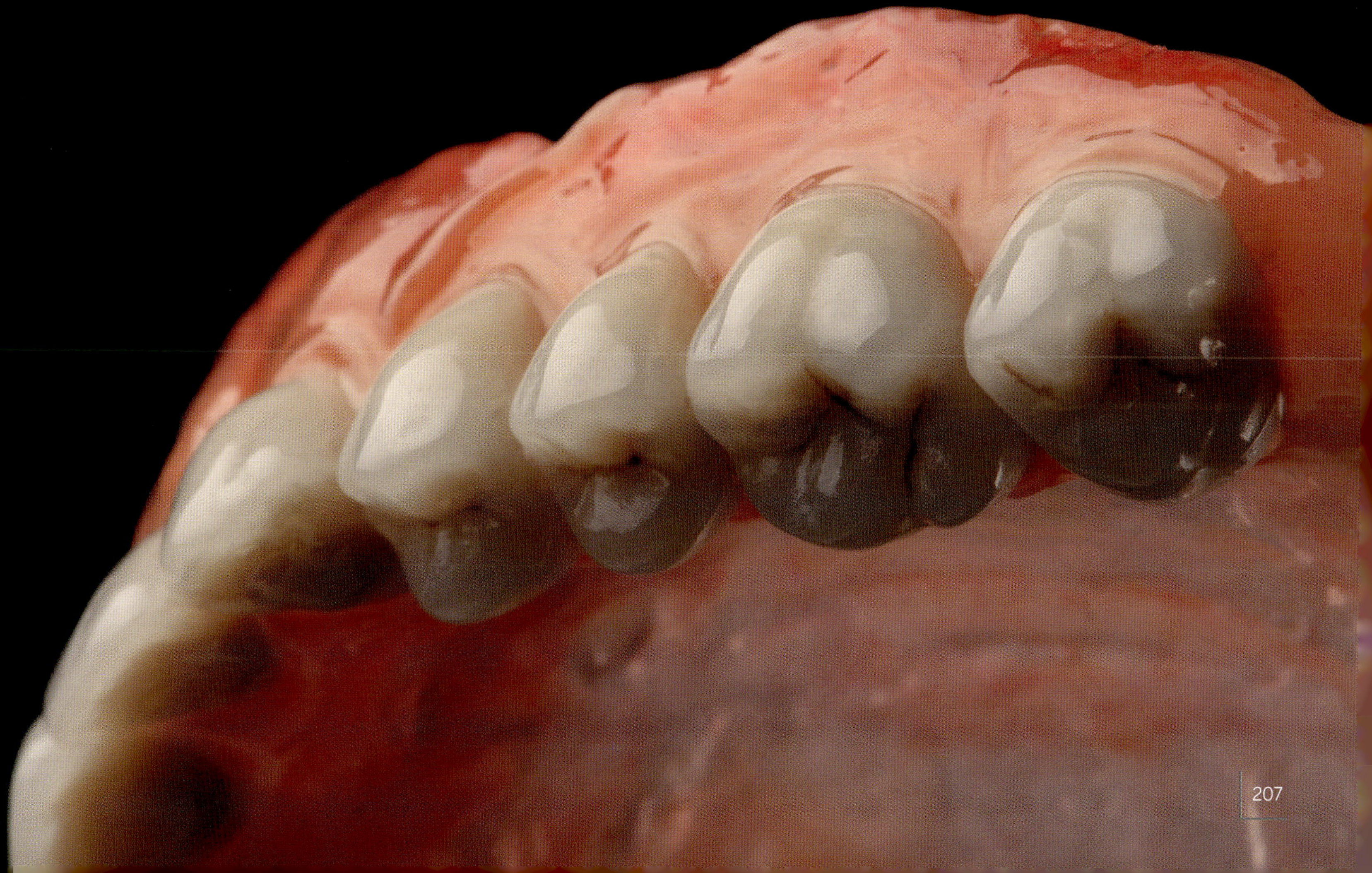

Backgrounds are also part of the composition.

The classic black background is a must have. Separating the object from the background as much as possible will lead to "truer blacks." (I just made up that term, I think.) Pure white or variations of white backgrounds allow you to have more control over your composition. With white backgrounds, you can play with the light source in a way that is not possible with black backgrounds. You can use the white background to reflect light back at your subject. This will soften and disperse the light for a less harsh effect. You can also use the white light source, such as a softbox or a piece of paper in front of your speedlights, as the background. Once you discover the power of diffused light coming right at you, it will blow your mind. It takes time and imagination. It takes modifying the position and power of your light source several times, but the results are going to be worth the time.

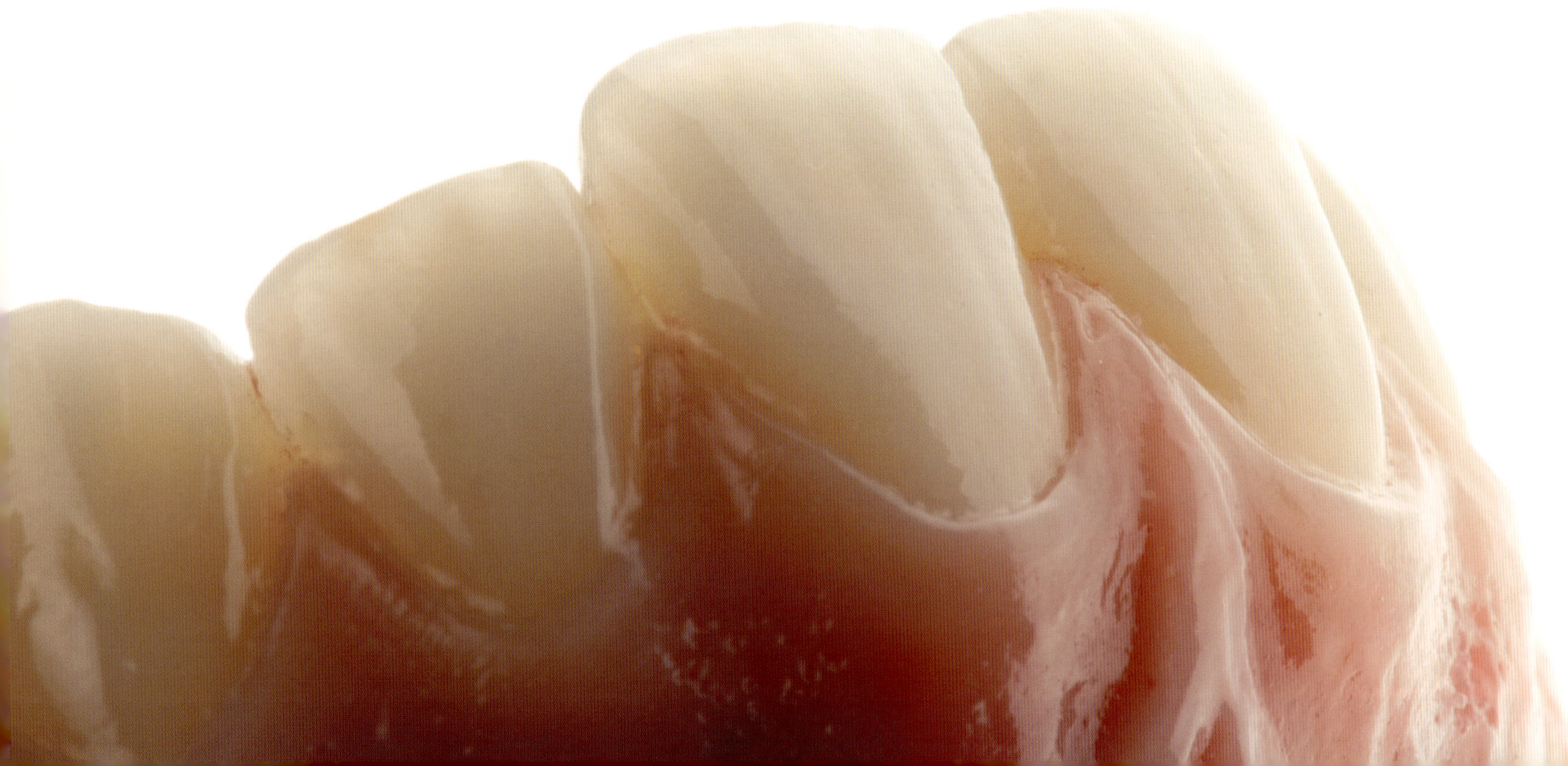

Capturing surface textures is a powerful tool to communicate emotion and creativity.

The number one mistake I see when people are trying to capture surface texture is the belief that getting closer and closer to the subject will allow you to capture more texture and detail. In a way it is true, but it is a very limited approach to obtain your goal. Texture can be captured and controlled best by modifying the position, nature, and power of the light source. Light source is the key element in photography, and once again it is the key element to capturing surface texture.

Make sure to consider the angulation of your light source with respect to your shooting position. If your light source is parallel and next to the axis of your lens (such as in a ring flash), it will be almost impossible to capture texture. However, if you increase the angulation of your light source with respect to your shooting position, you will be able to capture texture properly.

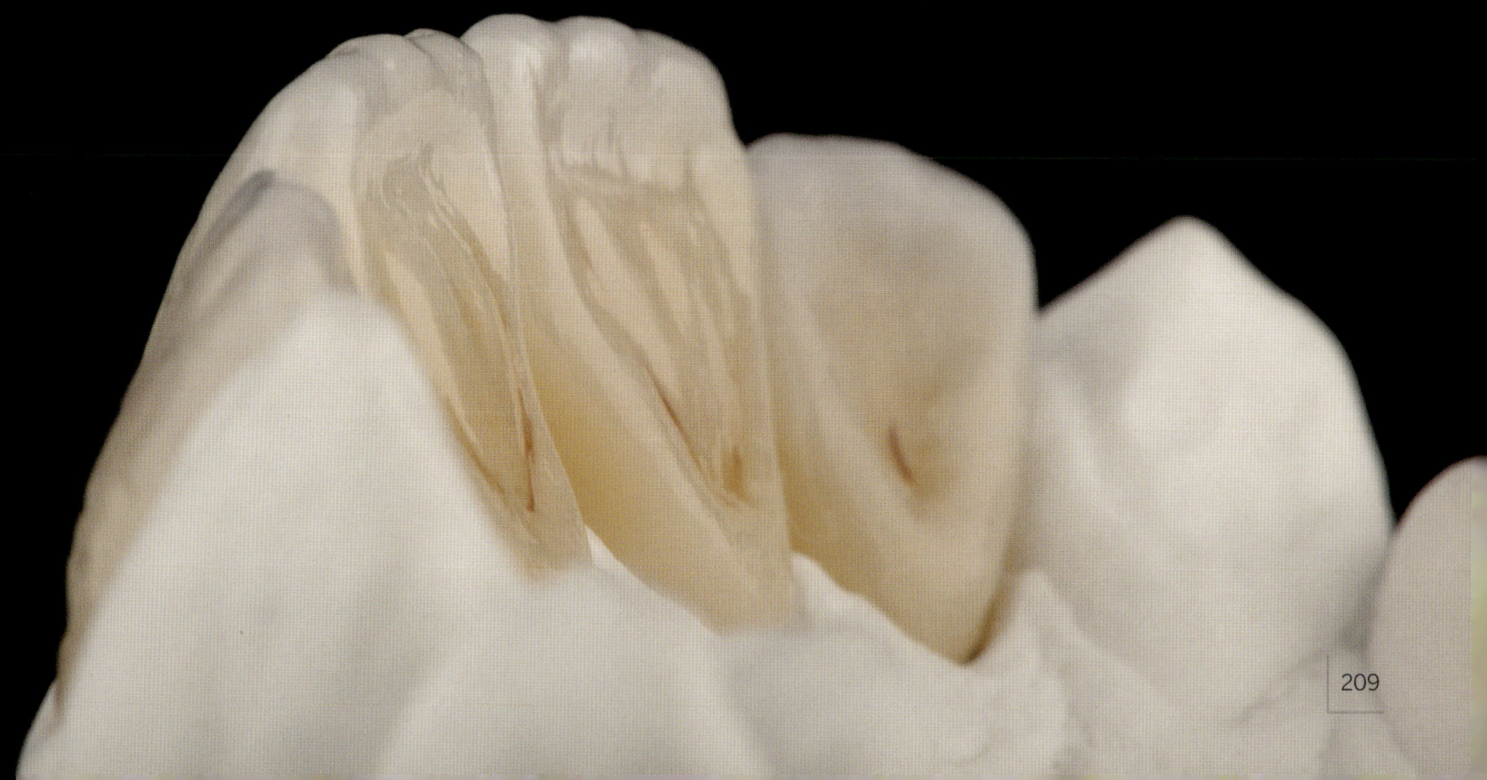

Embrace color.

Color is one of those things that captures our imagination. Color, if captured right, can take your composition to the next level. The same can be said about lack of color, but in my opinion, we are still talking about color even when it is lacking. More color does not mean a better composition. There are no hard rules about what to do with color and what not to do with it. If you look in social media, it is very clear that different cultures will have a different sense of what is a "beautiful" composition. Different tastes in composition does not mean that one is right and the other is wrong. It just illustrates that there is no right or wrong way of framing your shot. But you might want to think of your audience when creating it, if the audience is of importance to you.

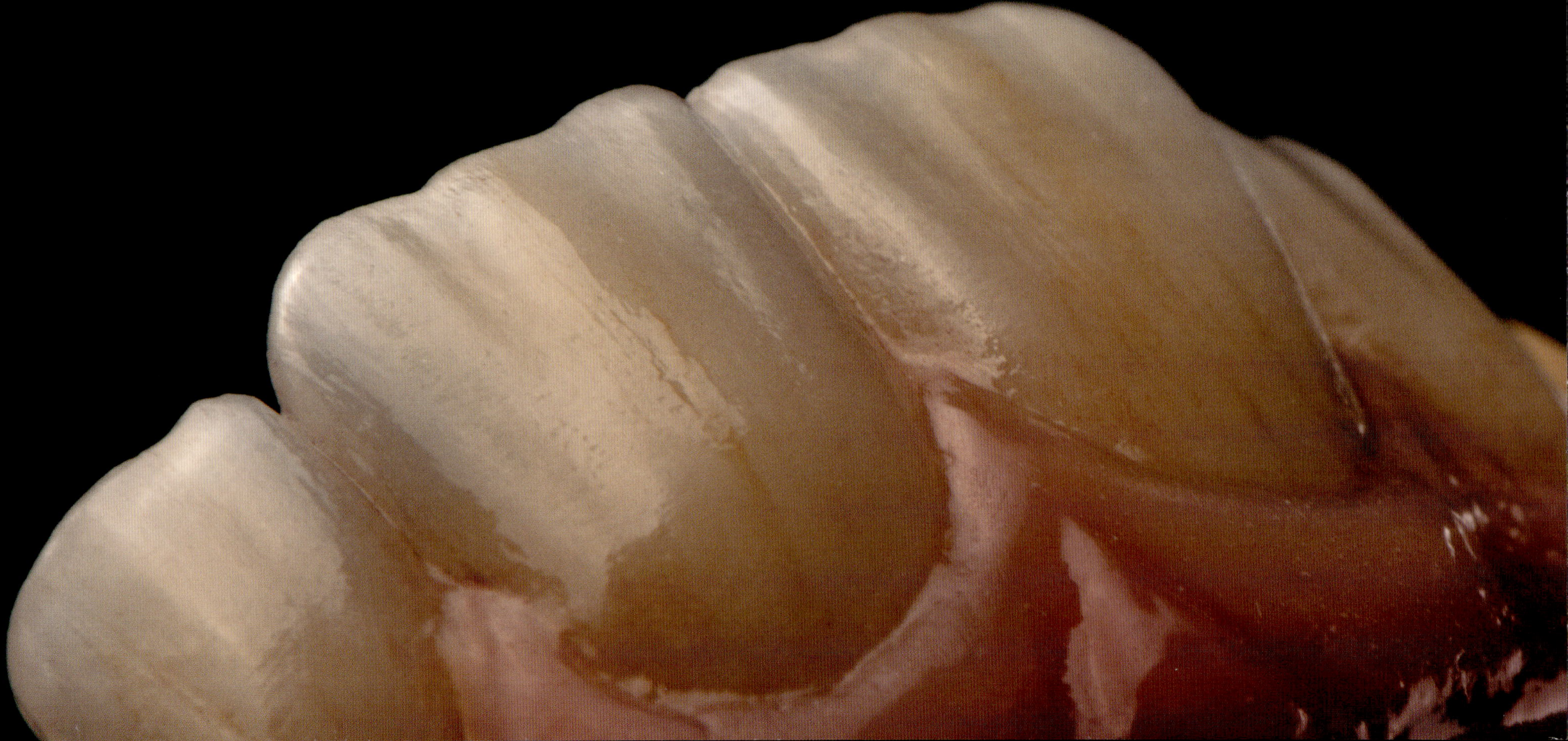

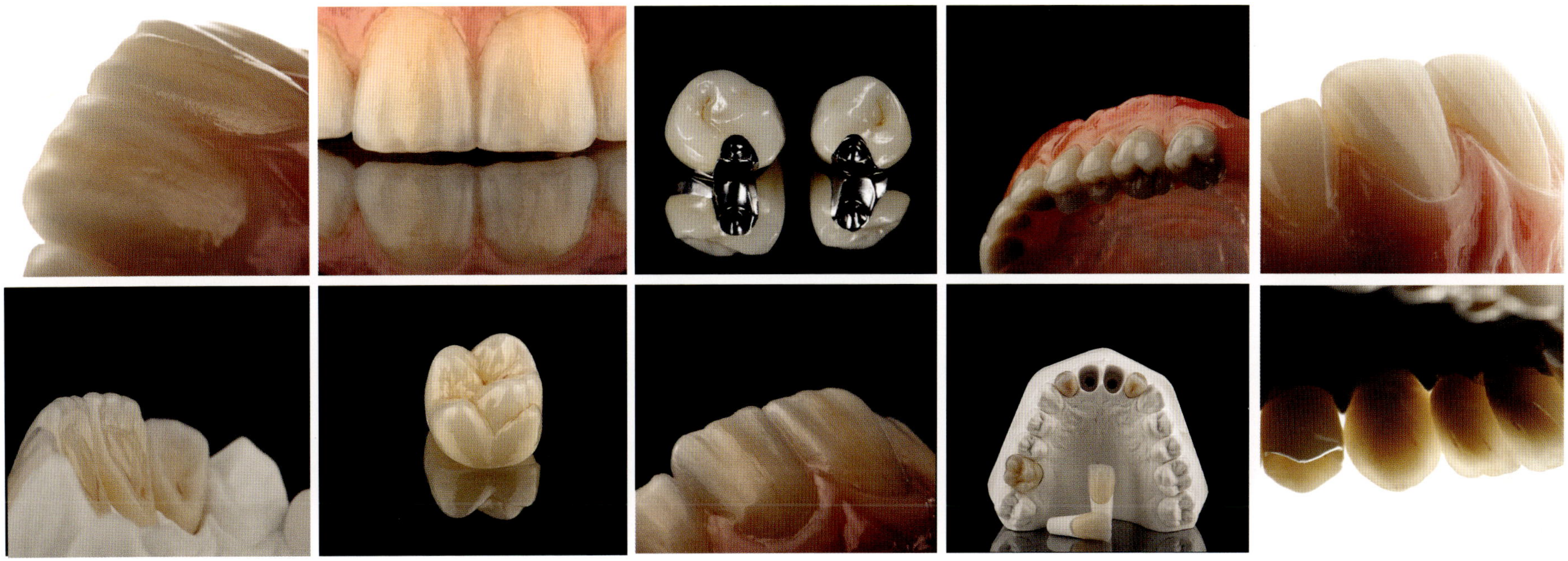

I would like to thank TPD Carlos A. Ortiz and the entire team at Ibiza Dental Lab. Without such a talented group of technicians, my patients would not have the quality of work they deserve.

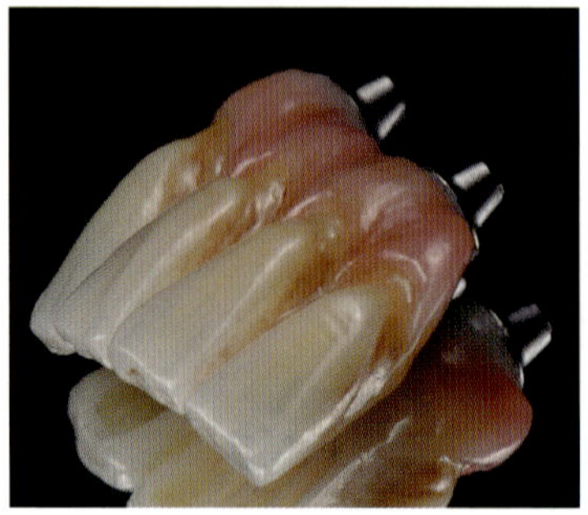

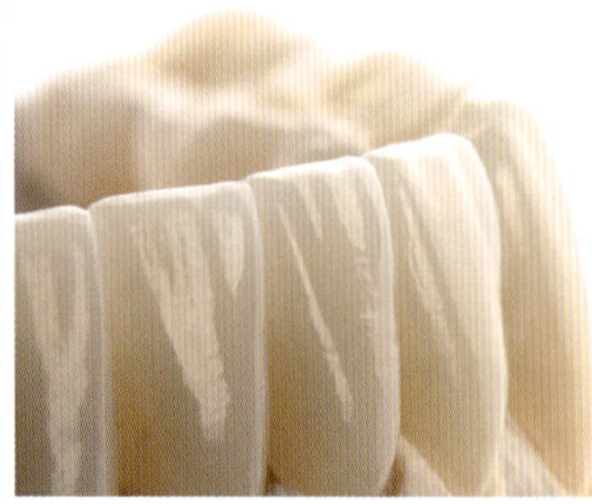

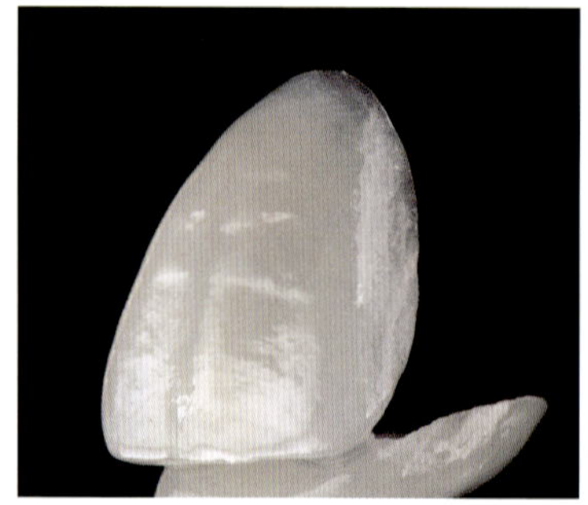

I would also like to thank Justin McElroy and the entire team at Midwest Dental Arts for their commitment to excellence.

8 Marketing and Social Media

Powered by Webistry

Dental Marketing Strategies and Social Media

After completing 8 to 14 years of schooling to become a dental professional, there is something that we can all agree on: Business and marketing strategies are nonexistent in every dental curriculum. It is an astonishing fact, considering that we are, as dentists, running a business.

For this last chapter of the book, I have partnered with WEBISTRY, a boutique agency that specializes in digital advertising and conversion rate optimization in the health sector. Together, we want to give you a glimpse into the ever-changing world of digital marketing in the dental profession.

Unfortunately, the fast-changing nature of advertising and social media creates an almost impossible area of discussion in textbooks such as this one. By the time this book is written, published, and released, the information might not be up-to-date or relevant any longer. This is a risk I am willing to take in order to bring you some insight in the subject.

Understanding SEO

Search engine optimization (SEO) is a long-debated and often-misunderstood topic. Because of that, dishonest service providers will take advantage of their clients. It is important to define SEO in an easy-to-understand fashion. I want to arm you with the knowledge for proper decision-making.

Google: Organic vs paid

SEO is the collection of strategies you can adopt to help you rank higher in Google's organic rankings, for specific terms. One common mistake is to confuse SEO strategies with paid strategies, such as Google Ads, which is an ads platform that allows you to rank high in Google's search engine results page on a pay-per-click basis (you pay only when a user clicks on your ad).

**Important Disclaimer: SEO strategies have evolved greatly in the last few years, let alone the past few months. What used to work at one time can now significantly harm your business. We recommend you exercise caution when dealing with an SEO provider.*

Pros and cons of SEO

SEO is important and should not be neglected. It is a long-term strategy that will allow your business to be found with a wide variety of search terms, both low intent (eg, "what are the benefits of implants") and high intent (eg, "best implant specialist in [city]"). When you rank high on Google, this basically means that Google deems you worthy of being in a search result for a specific topic. This means you have the potential of showing up on both Google Search and Google Maps. As Google makes technologic advances in voice through Google Home, this also means that Google may deem you worthy of showing up in a voice search. This is why SEO should not be ignored as a long-term strategy.

It is equally important to understand the limitations of SEO. For instance, did you know that Google Analytics will hide a large majority of the source of your traffic? In other words, you cannot see what keywords led to a majority of your site's traffic. Consequently, how can you know what in your strategy is working, and what is not? Furthermore, how can you scale that? How can you determine which keywords led to form submissions? You get the idea....

The Do's and the Absolute Do Not's of SEO

We mentioned that certain old SEO tactics used to work and now they do not. In fact, some of them may actually harm you. Let's go through the do's and do not's.

Back-linking

This is the practice of creating links on other websites that would direct the user to your website. Google used to treat this as a measure of your authority online. If lots and lots of other sites mention you, then you must be a trusted business, right? Not anymore. The strength is no longer in the numbers (or volume) but in the quality. Think of this as your typical high school, with the "cool" kids and the "not-so-cool" kids talking to each other about who's the most popular kid in town. Who has more say? Now in the real world, that's not such a good thing. However, in Google's world, it is a necessary measure. Imagine all the illegitimate and undeserving businesses creating a ton of fake websites mentioning their real website. Now imagine others paying third-party sites that bring absolutely no value to the web, just to have their names listed on their sites. Do you want to live in a world where any dentist can show up first with tactics such as these? Of course not.

So how does it actually work? Google now looks at the quality of the back-link. They will analyze and ask questions like:

- Who is mentioning you?
- Are they popular or trustworthy?
- Are their websites frequented by many?
- Do people visit their site more than once and keep coming back for more?

Does this remind you a little bit of traditional public relations (PR) work? That's exactly what it is. This is why we like to say that back-linking has now actually been replaced by digital PR.

GET TRUSTWORTHY SOURCES TO TALK ABOUT YOU, AND GOOGLE WILL REWARD YOU. IT'S THAT SIMPLE.

On-page keyword optimization

This is the practice of repeating a desired keyword as much as possible on your site so that Google rewards you for it in the results page. You need to be careful for this one. You absolutely should have a single page for every service you offer. On that page, for instance the implants page, you should make sure to mention the word *implants* in your titles, subtitles, and body paragraphs. There are easy-to-use tools that can help guide you in this process, such as Yoast SEO.

Just be careful. The free-for-all keyword-jamming days are over (at least we hope so, for you). Google now optimizes for user experience and relevance more than they do for keywords. Google also has a deep understanding of what makes sense and what does not. If they feel like your hyper-jammed keyword has been used in an attempt to cheat the system, they will demote you. This means Google wants to make sure that once a user lands on your site, they are actually finding what they want. How can they do that? It's simple really. Is your website mobile friendly? Do people come back to your site after their first visit? What's your bounce rate like? For how long does a user stay on your site? The list goes on and on.

Reviews

You know what those are, but did you know that Google cared about them? Remember, Google is trying to determine who deserves to be found and who does not. If your competitor has a 4.5 average on Google Reviews with 126 reviews, and you have a 2.4 average, who do you think Google will choose? To increase your odds, try to get as many reviews as you can on platforms such as Google, Yelp, and others.

While the practice of repeating a desired keyword as much as possible on your site is no longer effective for Google to rank you higher, reviews are increasingly important.

Google Ads

How does Google Ads charge you?

Many get confused about how Google's mechanisms work. For instance, you do not pay Google to show up as the first result on the first page, at least not directly. In reality, you only pay when someone clicks on your ad.

Google Ads will determine the cost of this click based on an auction-style bidding. If you are willing to pay even a cent less than your competitor, your rank on the results page will be lower.

Many factors determine the ideal cost-per-click. Here are some of them (keep in mind Google does not tell us everything and so we only have access to some of their decision-making variables):

- Search volume: How many people search for your keyword on average?
- Competition: How many competitors are bidding on that keyword AND how much are they willing to pay for that keyword?
- Quality score: This is a score that Google Ads attributes to your ads on a scale of 1 to 10; the lower the score, the more you will need to pay for your keyword.

What is a quality score?

A quality score combines a ton of factors. What we do know are the main three factors that matter most:

- Click-through rate (CTR) on your ads: For every 100 people who see your ad, how many of them end up clicking on it? The average CTR on Google is 2%. If you're getting a 5%, this will contribute to a Google quality score.
- Ad relevance: Is your ad relevant to your audience? Do they stop to read it? Do they click-through? Is it as specific as possible to the keyword that leads to it? If I search for "dentist for implants" and your ad copy reads "best dental clinic in NYC," chances are your ad relevance will suffer. Instead your ad should read "dentist for implants."
- Landing page relevance: Google goes as far as to make sure the page you send your traffic to is relevant to your ad. If you send people who searched "dentist for implants" to your home page, your score will suffer. Furthermore, if your site is slow to load or not mobile friendly, your score will also suffer.

Keywords research

When I started working with Webistry, I realized that while I might know a lot about dentistry, I have no idea about marketing. It is a good thing that they know dentists have a type A personality, and they took the time to guide me away from rookie mistakes.

You will possibly be tempted (just as I was) to use your own instincts when deciding what keywords to use in Google Ads. Don't. Always start with keyword research. Why? Research will allow you to find opportunities you may not have considered. Most importantly, good keyword research will enable you to make decisions based on data. When conducting thorough keyword research, you can find hundreds of keywords for every service you offer. For every keyword, you will get data such as search volume, competition, potential clicks, average cost-per-click, average CTR, and much more. The same exact keyword can have completely different data in any two markets, which makes this exercise essential. Google has a free tool you can use for this called Google Keyword Planner.

Campaign structure

Campaign structure is the most important "best practice" that is often overlooked, even by so-called experts. When building a campaign on Google Ads, it is not enough to simply put in your keywords, write up an ad, and click "GO." Google Ads has three layers of hierarchy for your campaigns, and they go as follows:

1. Campaign
2. Ad group
3. Keyword

Most people create one campaign, then an ad group for every service or concept they want to advertise for, and within that ad group add a ton of keywords. This is not a good campaign structure.

SKAG: Good campaigns vs bad campaigns

The correct way of going about your campaign build is by using a structure called *single keyword ad groups* (SKAG). In this structure, you create a campaign for every service you offer. On the ad group level, every keyword gets its own dedicated ad group. In other words, you would create as many ad groups as the amount of keywords you have.

On the keyword level, you would include three "match types" for your keyword. Match types are ways of telling Google how specific you want to be with your keyword. There are three main match types:

1. Exact match: You want to appear for the exact words you chose.
2. Phrase match: You want to be found for slight variations of that word (eg, you bid for "best implant dentist" but are found for "best implant dentist in Boston").
3. Broad match: You want to be found for larger variations of that word (eg, you bid for "best implant dentist" but are found for "best implant specialist").

Example of a bad campaign structure:

Campaign > Cosmetic dentistry

Ad Group > Implants

Keyword > Best implant dentist
> Dental implant clinic Boston
> Dental clinic for implants

Example of a good campaign structure:

Campaign > Implants

Ad Group > Best implant dentist

Keyword > Exact match best implant dentist
> Phrase match best implant dentist
> Broad match best implant dentist

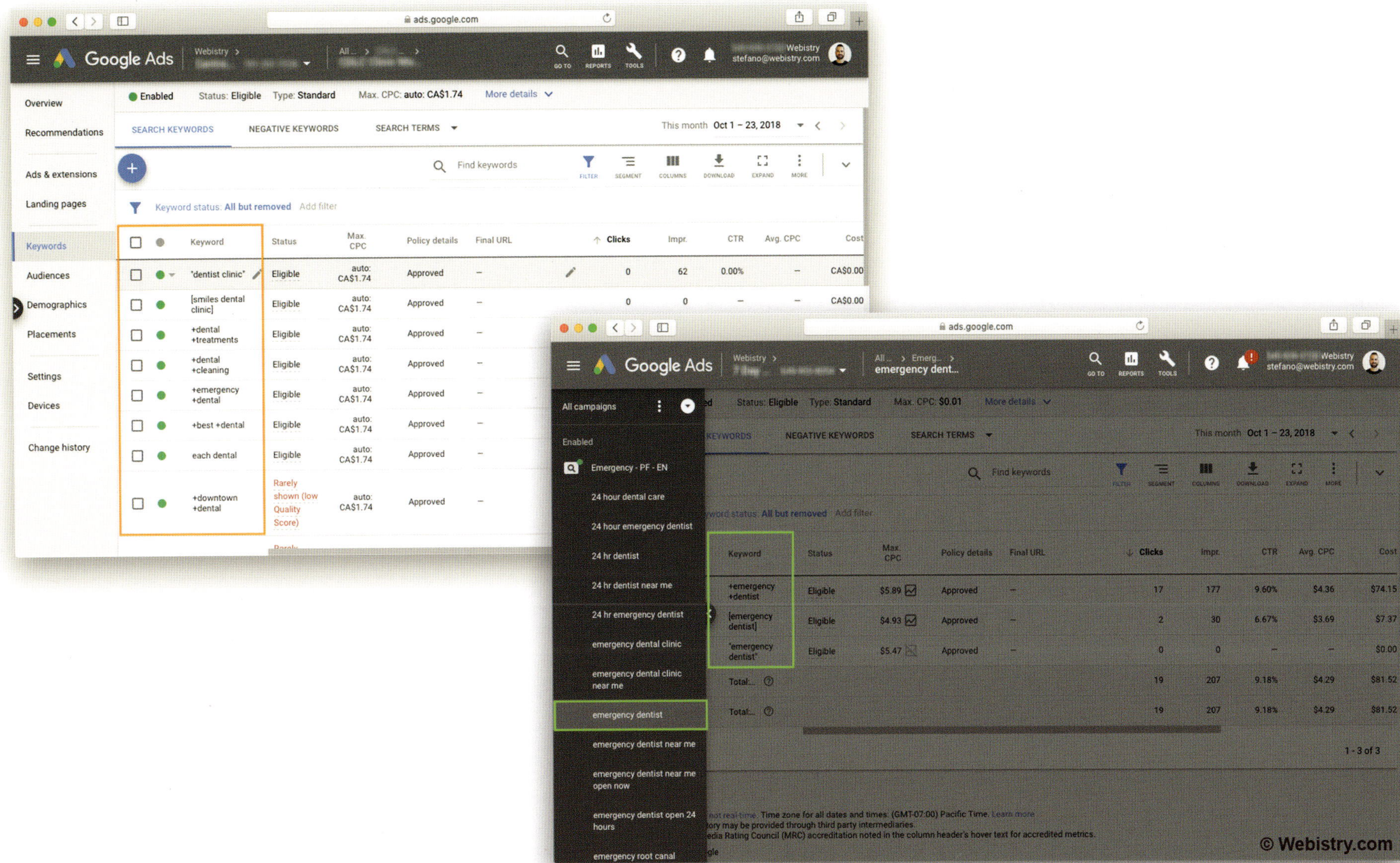
ads.google.com
Google Ads
Enabled
Status: Eligible
Type: Standard
Max. CPC: auto: CA$1.74
More details
Overview
Recommendations
Ads & extensions
Landing pages
Keywords
Audiences
Demographics
Placements
Settings
Devices
Change history
SEARCH KEYWORDS
NEGATIVE KEYWORDS
SEARCH TERMS
This month Oct 1 – 23, 2018
Find keywords
Keyword status: All but removed
Add filter
Keyword
Status
Max. CPC
Policy details
Final URL
Clicks
Impr.
CTR
Avg. CPC
Cost
"dentist clinic"
[smiles dental clinic]
+dental +treatments
+dental +cleaning
+emergency +dental
+best +dental
each dental
+downtown +dental
Rarely shown (low Quality Score)
Approved
All campaigns
Enabled
Emergency - PF - EN
24 hour dental care
24 hour emergency dentist
24 hr dentist
24 hr dentist near me
24 hr emergency dentist
emergency dental clinic
emergency dental clinic near me
emergency dentist
emergency dentist near me
emergency dentist near me open now
emergency dentist open 24 hours
emergency root canal
emergency dent...
Max. CPC: $0.01
+emergency +dentist
[emergency dentist]
"emergency dentist"
Total
1 - 3 of 3
© Webistry.com

Benefits of using SKAG

There are very logical reasons for using SKAG, and the benefits include quality score, tracking, and building strategy.

Quality score
By using SKAG, you are able to match your ad copy dynamically to every single keyword. In this instance, your Headline 1 copy, the first line of text, will match word for word the keyword that is searched before your ad is seen. Like we saw earlier, matching ad copy to keyword will increase your quality score. That happens mainly due to your ad relevance score but is also due to a consequent increase in CTR.

Tracking
Using SKAG also enables you to track on a more granular level. You will be able to know what every match type, every keyword, and every ad group was able to generate for you, including leads.

Bidding strategy
Thanks to better tracking, you will be able to better optimize your bidding strategy, or your cost-per-click. For instance, you should be willing to pay more for an exact match keyword, given that you know for sure that this is the highest-quality search for which you can appear. On the other hand, your bid should be the lowest for a broad match keyword, because this type of keyword can result in wide variations of itself.

Bottom line
There are so many reasons to be using SKAG, but the most important one is also the simplest one: Google wants you to. Using SKAG almost always leads to an increase in quality scores, lower cost-per-clicks, and overall better results!

Ad copy

Google Ads gives you other opportunities to write compelling copy. What is so alarming about this step is the number of businesses that forget most of these (or simply do not know about them)! The more copy you include in your ad, the more real estate or space you take up on the results page. There is absolutely no reason you should not be utilizing all of these.

Ad copy opportunities include:

- H1 (headline 1): 30 characters allowed
- H2 (headline 2): 30 characters allowed
- H3 (headline 3): 30 characters allowed
- Description 1: 2 lines of text below the H3, 90 characters allowed
- Description 2: 90 characters allowed
- Ad extensions: A set of predetermined snippets of information, such as location extensions, callout extension, call extensions, sitelink extensions, structured snippet extensions, price extensions, and promotion extensions

Testing copy

Google highly recommends you test 3 different versions of your ads at all times. This allows you to find the winning ad copy, but most importantly, it will actually act in your favor with Google's algorithm.

Tracking Calls

Most of your new patient requests will come through telephone, not web forms. Whatever strategy you are investing in, tracking phone calls is the only way to measure the fruit of your efforts.

Attribution

It is important to specify what we mean by "tracking." Simply keeping track of how many phone calls come in is not enough. It is essential to know exactly where calls originated from. Was it from your implants campaign or your emergency campaign? Taking it a step further, not only do you want to know what campaign generated that call but also which ad group and which keywords. Tools such as Callrail even allow you to see this conversion data directly in your Adwords dashboard itself. This is probably the most important part of it all.

Think about it: If you cannot see which keywords led to your incoming calls, how can you truly optimize your ad spending? You want to allocate your budget to the best-performing keywords and spend as little as possible on the low performers. If you are not tracking and attributing your calls on the ad level, then you are simply optimizing for clicks, not calls.

Recording and lead scoring

Now that you are attributing your calls and measuring the success of your campaigns, you also want to measure the quality of these calls. Furthermore, you want to learn which calls converted into visits to the clinic. Recording your calls will help you do both. It will also enable you to optimize the way your front desk handles questions, objections, and sales. Certain tools can automate some of this process, by listening to specific words in the conversation and tagging the call. These tools can also automatically transcribe the conversation for you to review on the go. Notice that you are still attributing these calls to the right campaign on Adwords, allowing you to focus your efforts on what brings you the most patients versus the most clicks.

Tracking calls might be as important as any other aspect of your marketing strategy.

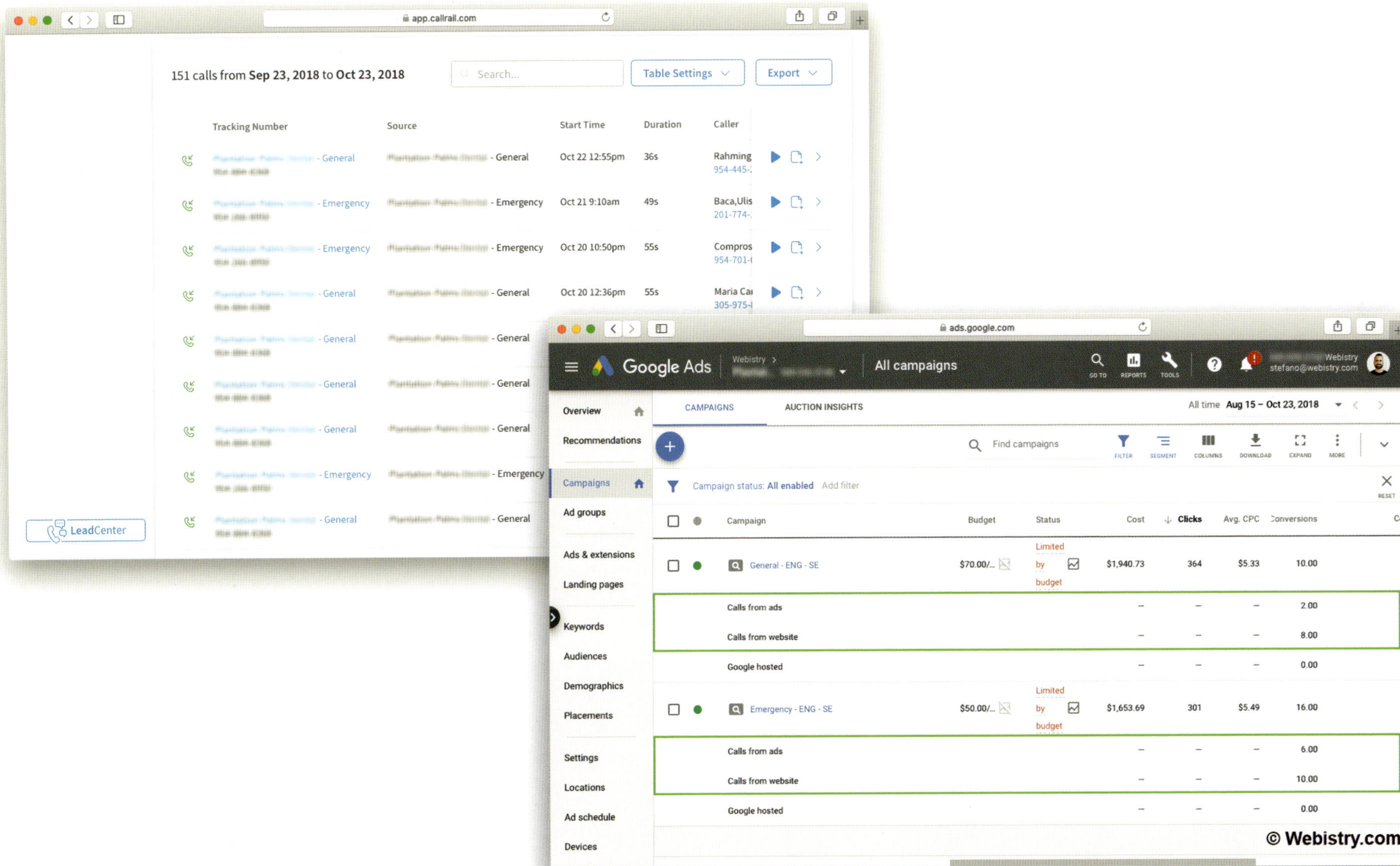
app.callrail.com
151 calls from Sep 23, 2018 to Oct 23, 2018
Search...
Table Settings
Export
Tracking Number
Source
Start Time
Duration
Caller
- General
- General
Oct 22 12:55pm
36s
Rahming
- Emergency
- Emergency
Oct 21 9:10am
49s
Baca,Ulis
- Emergency
- Emergency
Oct 20 10:50pm
55s
Compros
- General
- General
Oct 20 12:36pm
55s
LeadCenter
ads.google.com
Google Ads
Webistry
All campaigns
stefano@webistry.com
Overview
Recommendations
Campaigns
Ad groups
Ads & extensions
Landing pages
Keywords
Audiences
Demographics
Placements
Settings
Locations
Ad schedule
Devices
CAMPAIGNS
AUCTION INSIGHTS
All time Aug 15 – Oct 23, 2018
Find campaigns
Campaign status: All enabled Add filter
Campaign
Budget
Status
Cost
Clicks
Avg. CPC
Conversions
General - ENG - SE
$70.00/...
Limited by budget
$1,940.73
364
$5.33
10.00
Calls from ads
2.00
Calls from website
8.00
Google hosted
0.00
Emergency - ENG - SE
$50.00/...
Limited by budget
$1,653.69
301
$5.49
16.00
Calls from ads
6.00
Calls from website
10.00
Google hosted
0.00
© Webistry.com

Facebook and Instagram: Intent

You cannot ignore them when they own more than 50% of the market share. But they are not Google. There is one core difference between search and social, and it is called *intent*. You have to look at both channels as two completely different universes.

On search, most individuals are looking for something specific. When you pick the right keywords, you can even focus on getting traffic that is actually looking for your services and not just general information. You can say that traffic from search has a high level of intent. You know what they want, but you have no clue who they are.

On social on the other hand, you have no idea what the user wants. However, you know exactly who they are: their likes and dislikes, habits, age, gender, location, etc. Social is more about getting the click at a moment of curiosity, not intent. It is your job to turn this curiosity into intent and then into a measurable action.

When you understand these key differences, you can learn to better understand what service you should advertise on which channel. In Google you know what the person is looking for but not who they are. In social media you know a lot about them but not necessarily what they want.

Market share of social networking channels

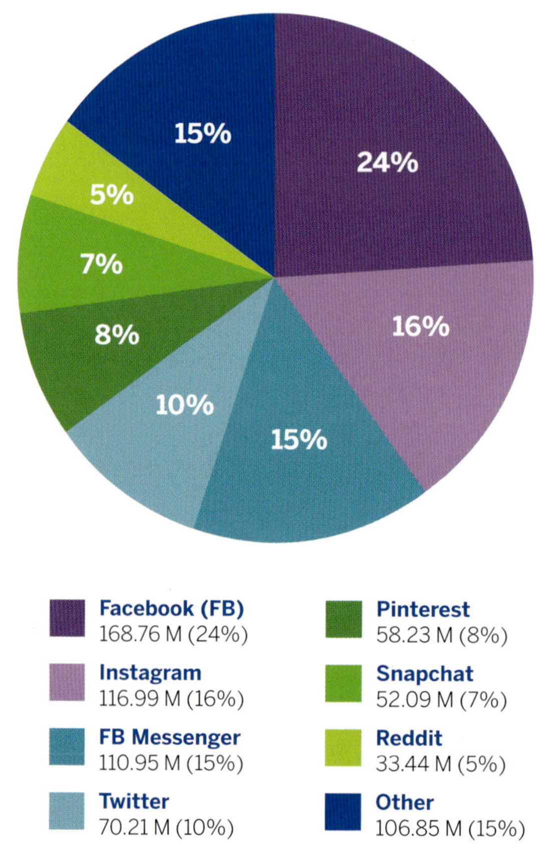

Facebook, services, and the Pixel

Now that we understand the main difference, it stands to reason that it would be hard to find the exact people on Facebook that happen to be looking for a root canal or implant treatment. However, with a bit of creativity you can get amazing results on social media.

First you need to ask yourself this question: What service is desired or needed by a big proportion of a specific demographic? For example, do engaged couples have a bigger assumed need for whitening or Invisalign, given that their wedding day is coming up? Are parents of children aged 17 to 25 more likely to be interested in wisdom teeth extractions? Our experience has taught us that a bit of creativity, mixed with some aggressive pricing, can yield some impressive results.

We have also learned that some services tend to do very well on Facebook or Instagram. These include, but are not limited to, Invisalign, tooth whitening, cleanings, and exams. If you are able to offer compelling pricing and great before-and-after shots, all while creating trust, these can be big winners.

Measuring your Facebook ads success is important. The Facebook Pixel can help you with that. The Pixel is a piece of code that you can simply copy and paste into your website. It will help you capture and measure a wide variety of actions that take place on your site, as well as the source of these actions. With the Pixel, you can tell which campaigns generated specific page views, form submissions, phone calls, and more. The Pixel also allows you to capture these users, so you can then create retargeting and lookalike audiences.

A *retargeting audience* allows you to target content (ads) to people who have already interacted with your business. For instance, you can retarget individuals who have been on your website three or more times. You can also control the frequency at which they see your ads, to avoid giving off the wrong impression.

A *lookalike audience* basically takes a basket of individuals, such as those who have been on your website, and utilizes Facebook's enormous database of users to find others that share the same traits. It is a powerful tool that allows you to expand your target audiences without necessarily knowing what similarities your ideal clients share.

Your Website and Landing Pages

A *landing page* is—drumroll—the page that a user lands on, but no that's not all! In theory, it is much more than just that. In the world of digital advertising, a "true" landing page is a standalone page, separate from your site, without any link-outs, that is entirely focused on selling one thing. Only a few actions can take place on a landing page: closing the window, making a call, or filling out the form. In essence, every campaign should always get its very own landing page. It is an environment that gives you full control on what a specific set of visitors see. It is your elevator pitch.

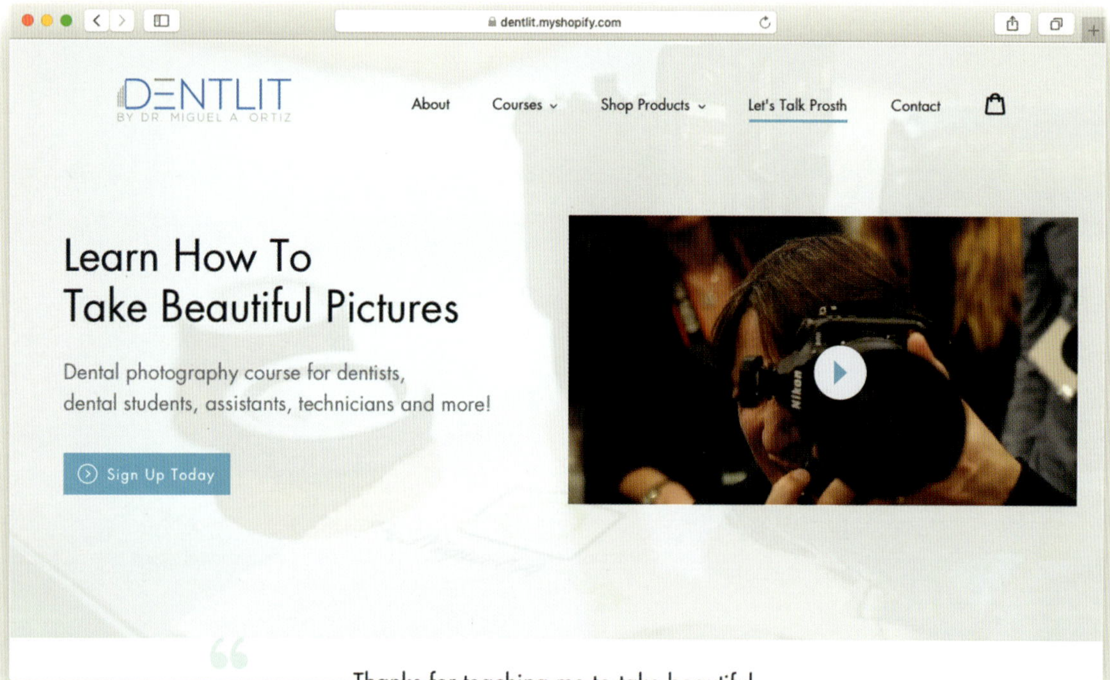

Landing pages have been proven to convert more traffic into conversions than your typical website home page or service page. The data is clear on that one. It is that simple. "How come?" you might ask. Well, we know a few things about average behavior on websites. For example, visitors tend to spend at most 20 seconds on any given website. In fact, you have about 5 seconds before a visitor decides if they will hang around or just close their window. Your typical website tries to increase the time spent on the site by offering up lots of information, educating the visitor, and providing them with tools.

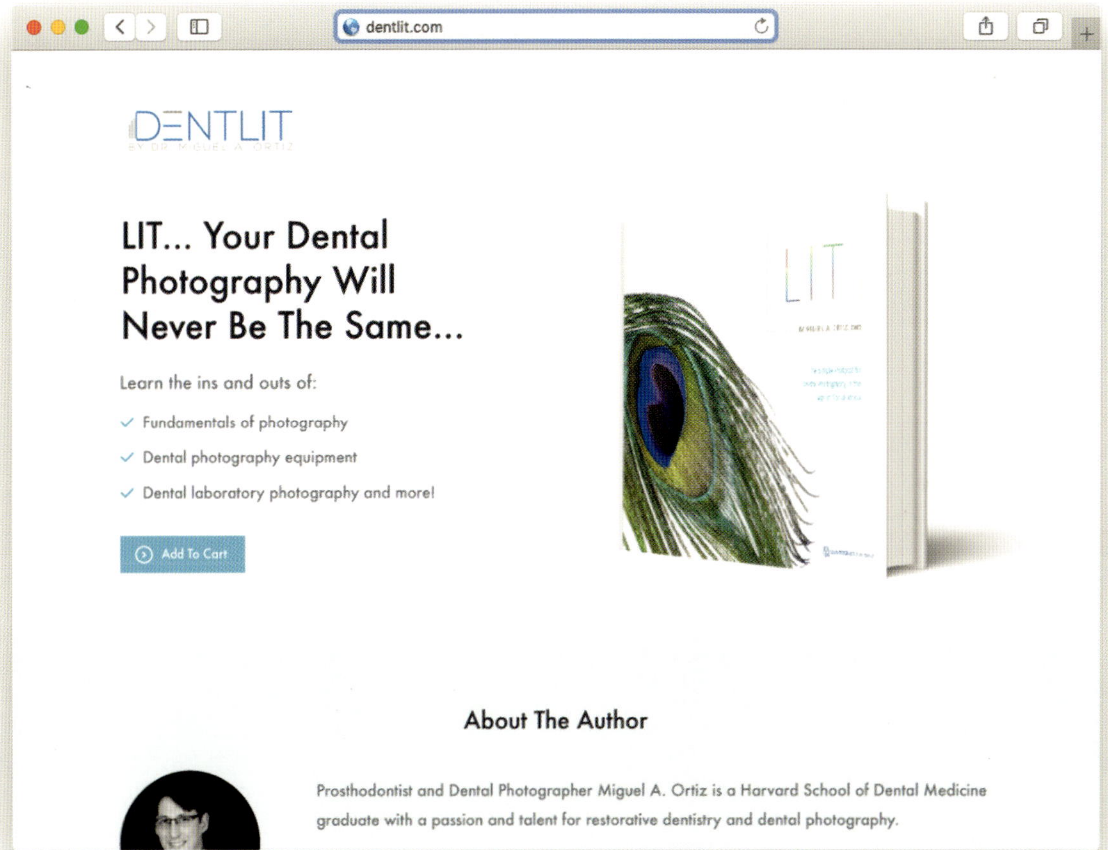

The importance of using landing pages

When you are paying for traffic, you know exactly what your visitor wants. Your goal should be to convince as quickly as possible, before you lose their attention. While working with Webistry, I learned about and experienced the importance of landing pages. The results were immediate and positive. A landing page is your opportunity to ask yourself, "If I were in front of this person, and I needed to convince them within 20 seconds that I am the right choice, what would I say?" Would you show them before-and-after photos? Would you talk about your accreditations? Would you showcase reviews you have gotten from other patients? Would you mention your flexible hours or years of experience?

A landing page is also an opportunity to provide a web experience that is both quick and concise. An Amazon study highlighted a 1% decrease in sales for every 0.1 second decrease in load times.*

*Kohavi R, Longbotham R. Online experiments: Lessons learned. Computer 2007;40(9):103–105.

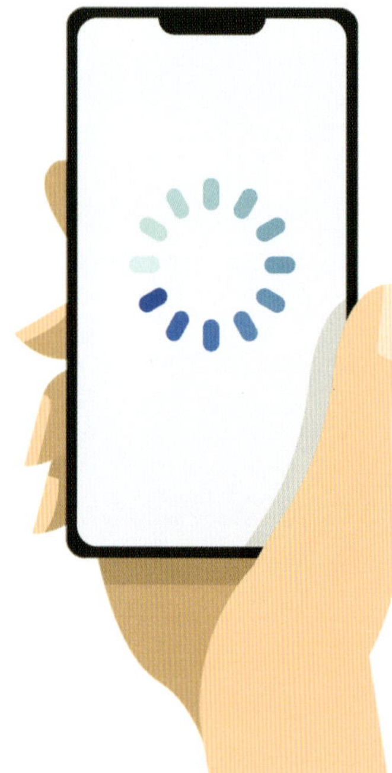

The probability of a mobile site visitor bouncing†

As page load time goes from...

1s to 3s
The probability of bounce **increases 32%**

1s to 5s
The probability of bounce **increases 90%**

1s to 6s
The probability of bounce **increases 106%**

1s to 10s
The probability of bounce **increases 123%**

†An D. Find out how you stack up to new industry benchmarks for mobile page speed. Think with Google. https://www.thinkwithgoogle.com/marketing-resources/data-measurement/mobile-page-speed-new-industry-benchmarks/. Updated February 2018. Accessed 18 March 2019.

AB testing

How can you optimize on-page experience? You have an idea of what it takes to optimize on the ad level, but did you know you can optimize at the landing page level too? The main way of doing so is through AB (or split) testing. This is the practice of splitting your traffic 50/50, simultaneously, and in a random fashion. Using this method, 50% of your traffic would be sent to version A of your page and the other 50% to version B. Both versions are almost identical, except for one key differentiator. This can be the photo you use in the header, the first line of copy, the position of the form, one element of design, and so much more. Because every campaign has its own landing page, and given that you are able to track both forms and phone calls for every campaign or landing page, you will be able to see which page or variant converts the best. AB testing can often double your conversion rates. In other words, you can essentially get twice as many leads for the same amount of traffic.

Tip of the iceberg

It stands to reason that we have only scratched the surface when it comes to digital advertising. This chapter could have easily turned into its own book on digital dental marketing (it almost did). We are fully aware that we did not dive into many topics or exhaust the topics we covered. This content is meant to awaken you to the options available and the concepts that are most important to your growth via online advertising. Most importantly, it is meant to arm you with the necessary knowledge to carefully select and vet your service providers. We hope this chapter has brought value to your practice.

Instagram and Growth

Did you really think I was going to finish this book without talking about Instagram?

Purpose

It is no secret that Instagram has been a great platform for me. I have been blessed with a large following that not only like and respect what I do but also provide important feedback and education. If you are thinking of starting a dental Instagram account, or you already have one and want to grow it, I would like to share my perspective.

The first thing you need to have is a purpose. What are you trying to do? Who is your target audience? If your answer is prospective patients, then you can skip everything that I am about to write. Patients do not like teeth, preps, gums, impressions, treatment, or anything dental related. If you think you can have a cool Instagram account with tips and facts for them, good luck with that. Who wants to follow their dentists? Exactly, nobody. Instagram is not a platform for organically finding patients. It can be done as part of paid ads like we have discussed but not as a daily organic content-producing account.

In my opinion, a dental Instagram account is for interacting with other dental professionals. If that is your goal, then let's dive into a few aspects of the platform that I have become familiar with.

Growth and the Instagram of our times

Four years ago, Instagram was an up-and-coming platform. At that point, and with hundreds of millions fewer users, we were all impressed by the quality and unique photography of many Instagram users. At that point, we were amazed by something we had never seen before. Posting a high-quality image would generate a high engagement rate because you were not competing with many other accounts. Likes and Comments were much easier to get. At that point, everything was new and different. Just as you were positively surprised by every unique post, your followers would have that same enthusiasm for your content. This tiny community grew fast. Small accounts exploded. For many of us, high-quality content was relatively easy to generate.

It is important to understand that Instagram is an ever-evolving and increasingly dynamic platform. As the algorithms get tighter, users get settled on the number and kind of accounts they follow. Instagram makes a decision for which accounts interact with each other. Breaking through is a bit harder. The growth rate is not as high as it used to be in the early days. Regardless, if you want to have an account and join us in this beautiful community, it is never too late. Just remember that content beats algorithm every time. Find your voice. Care about your followers and show us what you got!

Rules of engagement

Haters not allowed

At some point in time, there was a meeting that occurred in the development of the "dental Instagram niche" movement. I am happy to say that I was part of that meeting. The topic was how to deal with haters and bullies. Many of us were coming out of a Facebook dental community that is known for its negativity, with people being mean to other colleagues for no reason, leaving ugly comments, and engaging in bullying-type behavior. We wanted to change that. The consensus was strong and simple. Dental Instagram accounts are here to share, express, educate, and most importantly, to construct bridges among colleagues and generate healthy collaboration. We were not going to hate. We were going to protect each other and those who were subject to cyber bullying. I am happy to say that I believe it has worked. Today, it is an unspoken Instagram rule that if you do not like a case on a post, you just move on. If you do not like a story, just skip it.

In addition, I have come to rely on several rules of my own that I live by. I treat everyone with respect. If you message me, I will do my best to respond. If you need help, I will attempt to help you to the best of my abilities. Sometimes that means having about 500 to 800 conversations a day, all going at the same time. Having a large account generates that kind of engagement. I believe everyone deserves attention. I try.

Collaboration

One of the most beautiful aspects of my Instagram life has been the amount of professional collaboration that I have encountered. I have met colleagues with whom I have collaborated on many different projects. Several of them I now call my friends. I have traveled all over North America meeting thousands of dentists, listening to their stories, and sharing courses, dinners, and moments. Instagram has been the nexus between the rest of the profession and myself.

Education

At some point, there was an argument going around Instagram. The argument was whether real dental education could be achieved on the platform. I never engaged in the deliberations. To me the answer was always clear. Yes, Instagram is a great platform for learning. I learn every day. Most of the time I learn what not to do. I believe that learning what not to do is more important than its counterpart. Avoidance of hurting a patient by learning from someone else's hardships and failures is extremely valuable. I also learn about new techniques, materials, trends, tips, and tricks. Lastly, I—along with other colleagues—have generated several dental courses where learning takes place in person. All of this is a result of Instagram.

Inspiration

Not all accounts are created equally. Some of them are just special, and behind them exists a group of individuals that possess the most important qualities: humility, character, and talent. Here are my top recommendations:

@dr. randold.binns
Learn to plan, execute, and deliver complex cases at the hands of one of the most talented prosthodontists the earth has ever seen.

@_carlosdecarvalho
A true leader. Unrivaled knowledge. Gifted educator. I dare you to find someone who knows more about adhesive dentistry than him.

@sthepaniezeller
She is here to change the way you think about the future of dentistry, the digital landscape, the gender gap, everything. She is the future.

@midwestdentalarts
When a group of talented people get together with the goal to help dentists develop protocols for better patient care, this is what you get. One of the best labs in the country with one of the most interesting accounts on Instagram. Pure dental laboratory magic, every day.

@Griya.rr
Do you ever wonder what real day-to-day dentistry looks like in the hands of a gifted clinician? Then follow this account. You will not be disappointed.

@sfdentalnerd
Unmatched originality meets comedy meets good dentistry. This is likely one of the most plagiarized accounts in the dental arena. This is the original prophet for "content beats algorithm."

@Dr_bedrossian
The creator of the crazy idea that you could have one meaningful dental post a day—now 3 years and counting. As good a prosthodontist as the West Coast has delivered in decades.

@thedroolingtooth
Truly original content, as good as it gets. Once you start scrolling down through her posts you just cannot stop. Simply gifted.

@bestofprosth
Duhhh. Where you can find those treatments that really deserve a shout-out. And no, we do not get paid to post them there. You actually have to be good. You cannot buy us.

@webistry
A group of extremely talented dental consultants that can help you reach the next level of exposure and increase conversion rates. Numbers speak louder than words.

@ibizadentallab
The best dental laboratory in Spain meets the human aspect of perfection. Si estas en España, tiene que probar este laboratorio.

Instagram's Rules of Success

- Good content beats algorithm.
- Treat your colleagues with respect.
- Do not judge.
- Share the knowledge you were given.
- Do not be a hater.
- Ignore haters.
- Do not buy followers.
- Learn to critique your own work.
- Be yourself.
- Put the phone down and hug your kids. You only have them for 18 summers, if you are lucky.

Acknowledgments

LIT is the result of countless hours of work on the ground, in my practice, on planes, and in courses, traveling the globe in search of my fix—my colleagues' smiles. I love the dental profession and I love photography. Teaching both is my passion.

LIT has my name on the cover, but that is a misrepresentation of what it takes to deliver this kind of project. This book would have never been created without the unconditional support of friends, family, and mentors. It takes a crazy mind (from Argentina, no less) to envision writing a book while working full-time in a clinic, delivering 35 courses in 33 different cities, and being a father of 3 children under 7 years of age.

This crazy vision would never have come to light without my parents' persistent work ethic and solid values while raising my brother and me in difficult socioeconomic circumstances. My parents, Nestor and Mabel, made sure that no matter how hard times were, I had everything I needed to be where I am today.

It would also not be possible without my brother, Carlos, who blazes the trail of a true man and whose footsteps I try to follow in order to be a good friend, father, and husband. Thank you to his wife, Silvina, and their children—Abril, Nacho, and Leire—for making me El Tio Loco. Loco de Amor.

Thank you also:
To my friends, for keeping me real. Tien, Samira, Lauren, Camille, Edu, Randold, Ghaith, Ryan, Santiago, Mauro, Ashley, Nick, Kanika, Bharat, Paiyal, Sam, and Alan. . . . But not to Rags.

To my mentors, who have walked the path in front of me many times before and selflessly take the time to check in and make sure I am not falling off the road. To Dr Neda Shah-Hosseini, Dr Faheem Rasool, Dr Lee Jameson, and Dr Rand Harlow.

To the entire Quintessence team who worked on *LIT* as hard as I did, especially Bryn Grisham and Sue Zubek.

To Christie for making the book even better.

To my boys: Lucas, Marcos, and Tadeo. I truly hope that one day you can pick up this book from a shelf and know it was all for you. I want to show you that nothing can stop you. If you want to do something, go do it. Work hard. Nothing is too difficult; it just takes honest hard work. With any luck, I'm paving the way so that it is a bit easier for you. I hope so. You are my all. Papa loves you more than you can ever imagine.

To Colleen. My wife. My guide. My inspiration. Nothing happens without your unconditional support. With every project, with every crazy idea, you say, "No, it can't be done," but you back me anyway, and we make it happen together. I saved the last words for you because you are the most important person in my life. Thank you for your care and affection. You are my foundation; you ground me and remind me what is most important. You and our family together, I owe you so much. I hope I can repay you someday.

Gracias... Totales.